D0163584

COMMUNITY HEALTH ANALYSIS

A Holistic Approach

G.E. Alan Dever, Ph.D., M.T.

Aspen Systems Corporation
Germantown, Maryland
London, England

Library of Congress Cataloging in Publication Data

Dever, G.E. Alan
Community health analysis.

Includes index.

1. Health planning. 2. Community health services—Evaluation. 3. Epidemiology. 4. Holistic medicine. I. Title. [DNLM: 1. Community health services. WA546.1 D491c]
RA393.D49 362.1'04'25 79-26291
ISBN 0-89443-161-7

Library of Congress Catalog Card Number: 79-26291
ISBN: 0-89443-161-7

Printed in the United States of America

1 2 3 4 5

To Georgie,
Tammy, and Jamie

Table of Contents

Preface

Community health analysis—holistic epidemiology—is designed to bring to the health care sector a body of knowledge that encompasses the many dimensions of health. Throughout this work the theme of holistic analysis has been stressed. The first chapter, about our belief systems and health, provides the cornerstone for the remaining chapters. I am convinced that our health beliefs must be altered not only in our pursuit of health as individuals but also in our analysis of health as it relates to communities. This latter aspect becomes the topic of the remaining nine chapters. In particular, Chapter 2, Holistic Health—An Epidemiological Model for Policy Analysis; Chapter 3, Planning and Evaluation for Health; Chapter 7, Health-Status Indicators and Indexes; Chapter 9, Computer Graphics in Health Planning; and Chapter 10, Holistic Health—Process and Risk-Factor Analyses, approach the analysis of health problems holistically. The statistical methods and the epidemiological principles for dealing with these health problems are provided in Chapter 4, Basic Statistical Measures for Community Health Analysis and in Chapter 5, Basic Epidemiological Methods. Finally, the analysis of health problems would not be complete without some understanding of surveys and resource analysis, the subjects of Chapters 6 and 8 respectively.

This book was engendered a few years ago and grew as I grew within the public health sector. In particular, my relationship with James Alley, M.D., an innovative and enlightened individual, provided me with significant opportunities for personal and professional growth, and close friend Jules Terry, M.D., always supported my needs through understanding and sound direction. I want to thank both of these men. Additionally, the staff of the Health Services Research and Statistics Section, which I directed for several years, have had a direct impact on the fruition of this volume. I want to thank Charles Plunkett for providing input for several chapters and Judy Morris for providing the typing and editorial needs throughout the entire project. Also, I wish to thank Sherry Dorris, Scott Barton, Mike Lavoie, Ann Allen Lavoie, Sybil Mitchell, Sara Odum, and Jenny Hopkins. Many thanks to all the individuals, agencies, and publishers who allowed me to reproduce their material for inclusion in this book.

G. E. Alan Dever
December 1979

Chapter 1

Health and Our Belief Systems

Health care in the 1970s has evolved with some interesting ideas. For instance, the traditional concerns of legislation, cost containment, accessibility, availability, quality, continuity, and acceptability have gained increased emphasis in the pursuit of health. The more significant aspects of health care of the 1970s, however—surely to continue into the 1980s—are the concerns with holism, wellness, and self-responsibility. These facets of being healthy reflect personal awareness or self-actualization in physical activity, nutrition, stress management, and overall individual life styling. The result has been the development of holistic health centers, wellness resource centers, health spas and resorts, and a more aware population concerned about its physical and mental condition. Jogging, tennis, basketball, bicycling, vitamins, health foods, and coping skills are consequently becoming part of the community's needs. The emphasis is obviously not on illness but on wellness, extending even to a plateau of high-level wellness. This is what community health care is and what it will be in the decades ahead. Indeed, the task is to create the space where people in communities may be transformed so that wellness becomes a typical part of their lives.

The major barriers to this transformation are our belief systems or memory tapes. Our beliefs are entrenched so deeply in our philosophy that the physician and the medical care system will have to provide major supports to enable us to overcome our life-death crises and to make us well. The physician and the medical care system are already doing everything humanly possible in the areas of curative and treatment services. Wellness, however, is a function of prevention and maintenance, and this involves self-responsibility. Our expectations from the medical field practitioners must be reduced. We cannot continue to abuse our bodies and then expect a medical team to make repairs—time after time after time. The focus must be on prevention, and this becomes the individual's responsibility.

BELIEF SYSTEMS AND EPIDEMIOLOGY

Belief systems are the concepts we use to run our lives. They are created by knowledge or data without experience. The trouble with a belief is that we get stuck in it. Most of us persist in thinking and doing what we learned long ago rather than act from our experience in response to whatever is happening now. Beliefs need to be updated. An example will illustrate this point.

> A young bride regularly cut off the ends of the ham before putting it in the pan to bake. After watching her do this several times, her husband asked her why. She answered that her mother always did it that way. So the husband asked his mother-in-law why she cut off the ends of the ham, to which she replied, "Because my mother always did it that way." The old grandmother is still alive, and the husband visited her one day and asked the same question. "I cut off the ends of the ham," she explained, "because we were poor and had only one pan for all our baking. To get a large ham into the small pan, we had to cut off the ends."[1]

Most of us are cutting off the ends of something in our lives to fit into a pan no longer too small.

Epidemiology is appropriately linked to concepts of health and causality. It must be emphasized that the evolution of these concepts reflects shifts in our disease patterns. Epidemiology is the study of the determinants and distribution of diseases in human populations. It may be viewed as the study of patients in clinics in an orientation toward medical epidemiology, or it may focus on the study of populations in communities to reflect social epidemiology. This book concentrates on the latter aspect.

Over the past 100 years, three generalized causal models have directed epidemiological studies. The models are intrinsically related to the concepts of health, health measurement, and certainly to the shift in disease patterns (Table 1-1).

Single Cause/Single Effect Model

The first and simplest epidemiologic causal model is the single cause/single effect pattern (Figure 1-1). A single cause is sufficient to produce an observed effect. This model is quite logical but operates only rarely. Epidemiologists used this approach in the late 1800s and early 1900s when

Table 1-1 Epidemiology, Concepts of Health, and Health Measurement: Evolution and Relationships

Time	Epidemiologic Methods	Concepts of Health	Health Measurement
1900	Single-Cause Model (Infectious Diseases)	Ecology Model (Agent-Host-Environment)	Mortality from Infectious Diseases (Death Rates: Crude, Specific, Adjusted)
1920	Multiple-Cause Model (Infectious/Chronic Diseases, Transition Cycle)	Social Ecological Model (Host, Environment, Personal Factors)	Morbidity Measurement (Incidence, Prevalence) Disability Measurement (Work Loss, Disability Days)
1940		W.H.O. Model (Physical, Mental, Social)	
		Holistic Model (Life Style, Environment, Biology, Health Care System)	Holistic and Wellness Measurement (HHA, RADAR, Prospective Measures)
1970	Multiple Cause/ Multiple Effect Model (Chronic Disease Cycle)	High-Level Wellness Model (Physical Exercise, Stress Management, Nutrition, Self-Responsibility)	
1980		Content/Context Model (What's in Health/How to Hold on to Health)	Measurement of the Content and Context of Health (Mind/Body Relationships)

Figure 1-1 Single Cause/Single Effect Model

Cause ⟶ Effect

disease patterns were infectious and a single bacterium or virus was sufficient to produce disease.

Multiple Cause/Single Effect Model

A second, more complex model is the multiple cause/single effect pattern (Figure 1-2). An obvious extension of the single cause/single effect model, the multiple cause/single effect approach is valid where disease patterns are in a transitory state, that is, in communities or areas where infectious diseases are declining and chronic diseases are increasing. Thus, such chronic disease patterns as heart disease, cancer, stroke, and motor vehicle accidents may be analyzed using the multiple cause/single effect model. Some infectious diseases, such as ''Legionnaire's'' disease, may also be investigated using this model.

Multiple Cause/Multiple Effect Model

The third model of causality, multiple cause/multiple effect, is extremely complex, indicating that several causes produce many observed effects (Figure 1-3). This model closely embraces the health concepts of holism and wellness and is quite applicable to the disease patterns of the 1980s. For instance, air pollution, smoking, and specific forms of radiation (causes) may produce lung cancer, emphysema, and bronchitis (effects).

These epidemiological models of causality have a number of applications relating to models of association.[2] Association refers to the relationships that may exist between the occurrence of one thing (a risk factor) and the occurrence of another (a disease). There are three possible relationships which could exist between the risk factor and the disease:

Figure 1-2 Multiple Cause/Single Effect Model

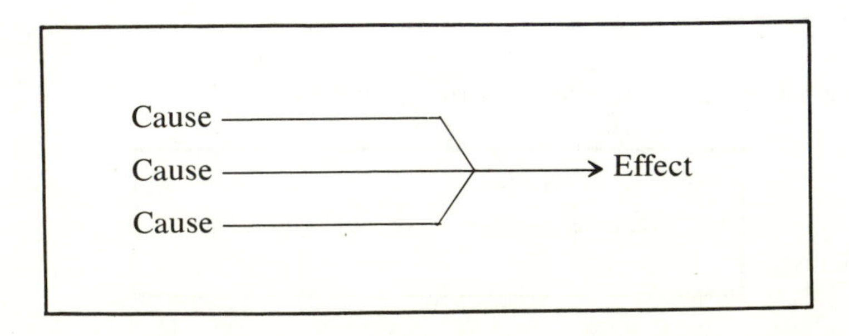

Figure 1-3 Multiple Cause/Multiple Effect Model

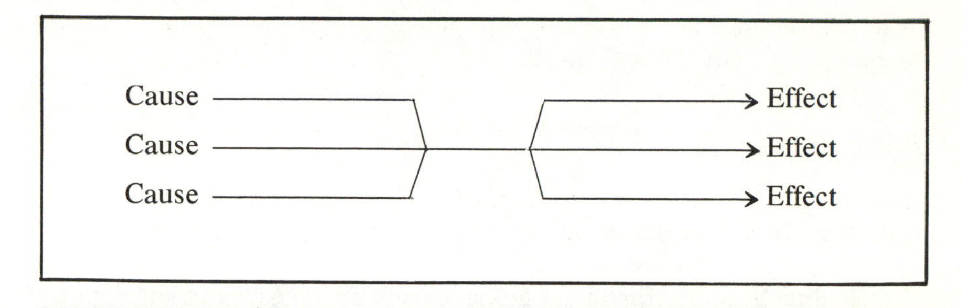

1. A positive association (they tend to occur together)
2. A negative association (they tend not to occur together)
3. No association (they occur independently)

Understanding the criteria of causality and association will aid in judging whether a relationship is causative or associative. These criteria are:

1. *Temporal relationship*. If A causes B, logically A should occur first.
2. *Specificity*. With high specificity, a cause leads to a single effect; with low specificity, a cause may be associated with multiple effects. In the latter case, for example, cigarette smoking can cause both lung cancer and bronchitis; low socioeconomic status can be associated with both illness and disability.
3. *Strength or intensity of association* or the degree of correlation between the cause and the effect. For infectious diseases the association of the pathogen with the disease process is usually high. For chronic diseases the association is a statistical or probabilistic association, allowing for a certain degree of uncertainty, as in the association of exercise and diet with lower rates of coronary heart disease. The three causal models are not quite logical in dealing with this problem, which requires statistical probability tests and broader concepts of health.
4. *Consistency*. When the same type of association consistently turns up in research studies of different designs, the chances are that it is real and likely to be causative.
5. *Coherence*. A supposed causal relationship should make sense in the light of existing biological facts. Contrary evidence suggests, however, that this point should not be heavily weighted, especially in the case of sugar consumption related to conditions like cancer and hypoglycemia.

These judgmental criteria are highly variable and operate quite effectively with the infectious disease cycle. The criteria do not, however, describe well the interactions within a holistic approach. For this we need to explore our concepts of health.

CONCEPTS OF HEALTH

A Shift in Disease Patterns

The turning points for infectious and chronic diseases in the United States occurred about 1925 (Figure 1-4). Collectively, deaths due to infectious diseases declined from about 650 deaths per 100,000 population in 1900 to about 20 deaths per 100,000 in 1970 (a decline of 96 percent). A major epidemic of influenza occurred in 1918, with the death rate mounting to 850 deaths per 100,000 population. Chronic diseases, on the other hand, collectively accounted for about 350 deaths per 100,000 population in 1900 and increased to about 690 deaths per 100,000 in 1970 (an increase of 97 percent). This disease transition—not unlike a demographic transition—represents a shift in our disease patterns. The reason is to be found in a societal shift from an agrarian to an industrialized type of society. Diseases which afflict a given segment of a culture vary with the social and physical conditions which characterize the society at the time. Thus, at the turn of the century, we emerged with our roots in a life style that was agricultural in nature; with the advent of industrialization, our societal roots changed, producing the shift in our disease patterns.

Our agrarian society generated a cycle of events that is portrayed in the infectious disease model (Figure 1-5). The agricultural era reflected high fertility; the needs were basic: food, shelter, and clothing. Thus, in 1900, 52 percent of our population was under 20 years of age, and 3 percent was over 65. (This type of population pyramid is typical of today's inner cities and developing countries where the infectious disease model is still applicable.) The results were devastating: with no specific treatment, parasitic diseases, infectious diseases, and malnutrition contributed to high infant and preschool mortality. In fact, 34 percent of all deaths occurred between birth and five years of age. In our agrarian culture, high fertility compensated for high mortality. Large families were also essential for harvesting food from the land.

Industrialization produced changes in our disease patterns. The cycle of diseases during the industrial period in our society is demonstrated by the chronic disease model (Figure 1-6). Because of its changing values, contemporary life can induce certain kinds of diseases; deleterious social,

Figure 1-4 Infectious and Chronic Disease Death Rates, United States, 1900–1970

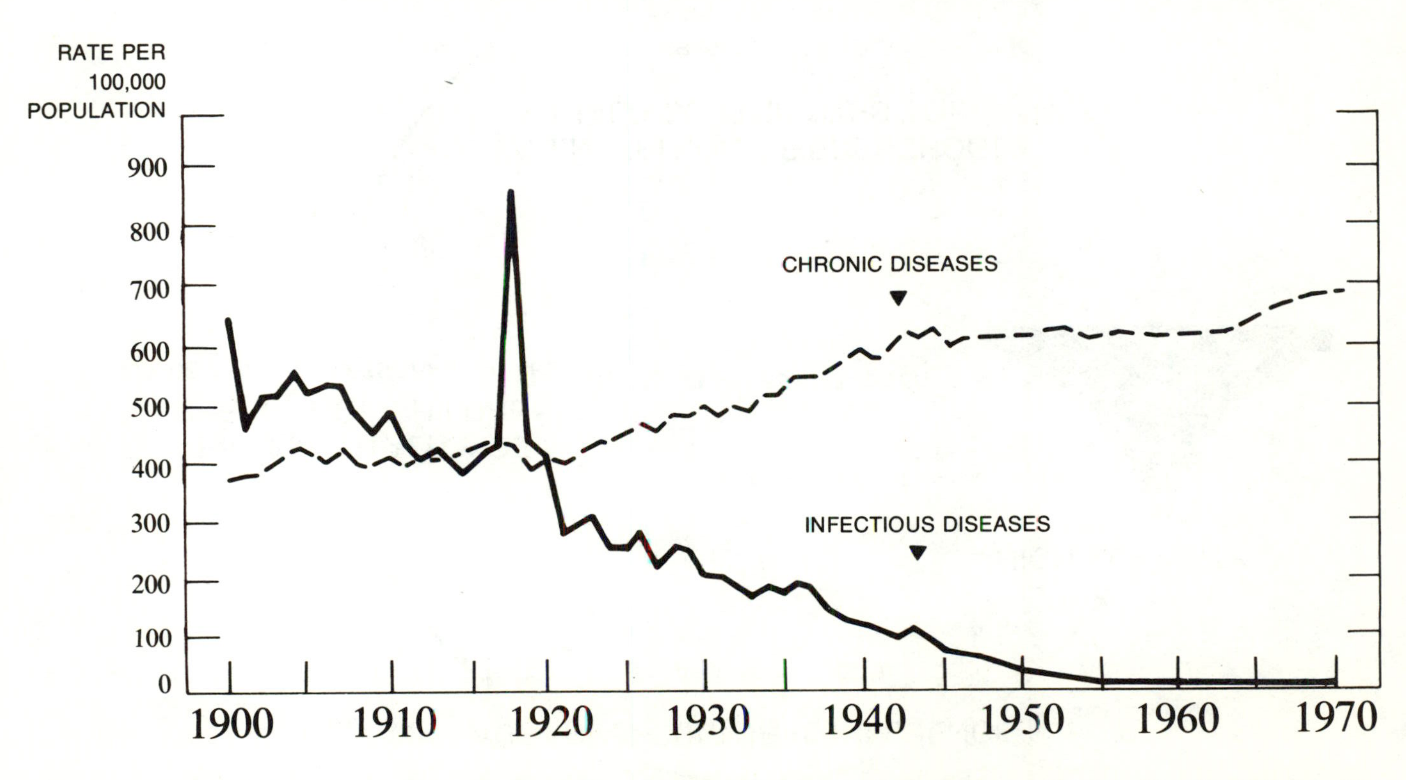

Source: C. L. Marshall and D. Pearson, *Dynamics of Health and Disease,* Appleton-Century Crofts, a division of Prentice-Hall, Inc., New York, New York, 1972, p. 131. Reprinted with permission.

Figure 1-5 Cycle of Disease Patterns, Infectious Disease Model

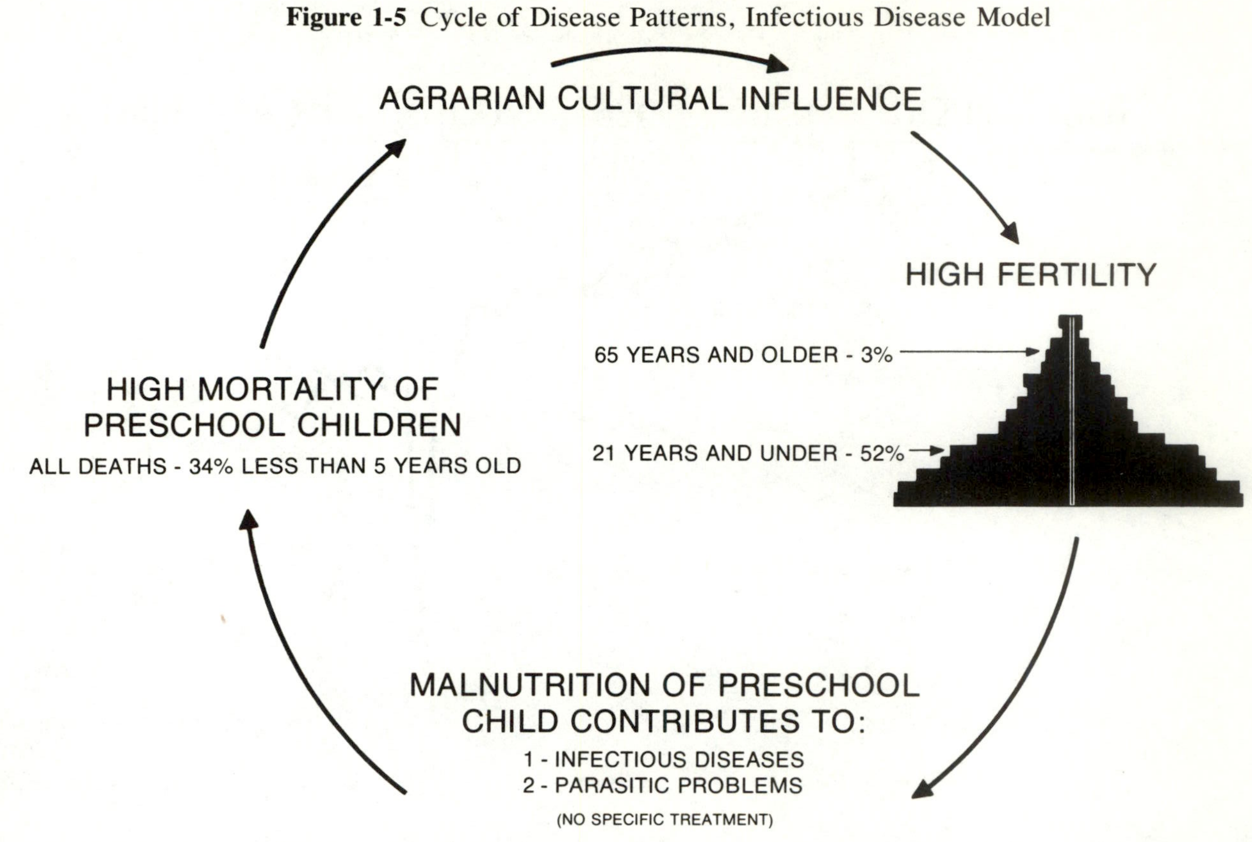

Source: G. E. Alan Dever, "The Pursuit of Health," *Social Indicators Research* 4, Figure 4, p. 485, 1977.

Figure 1-6 Cycle of Disease Patterns, Chronic Disease Model

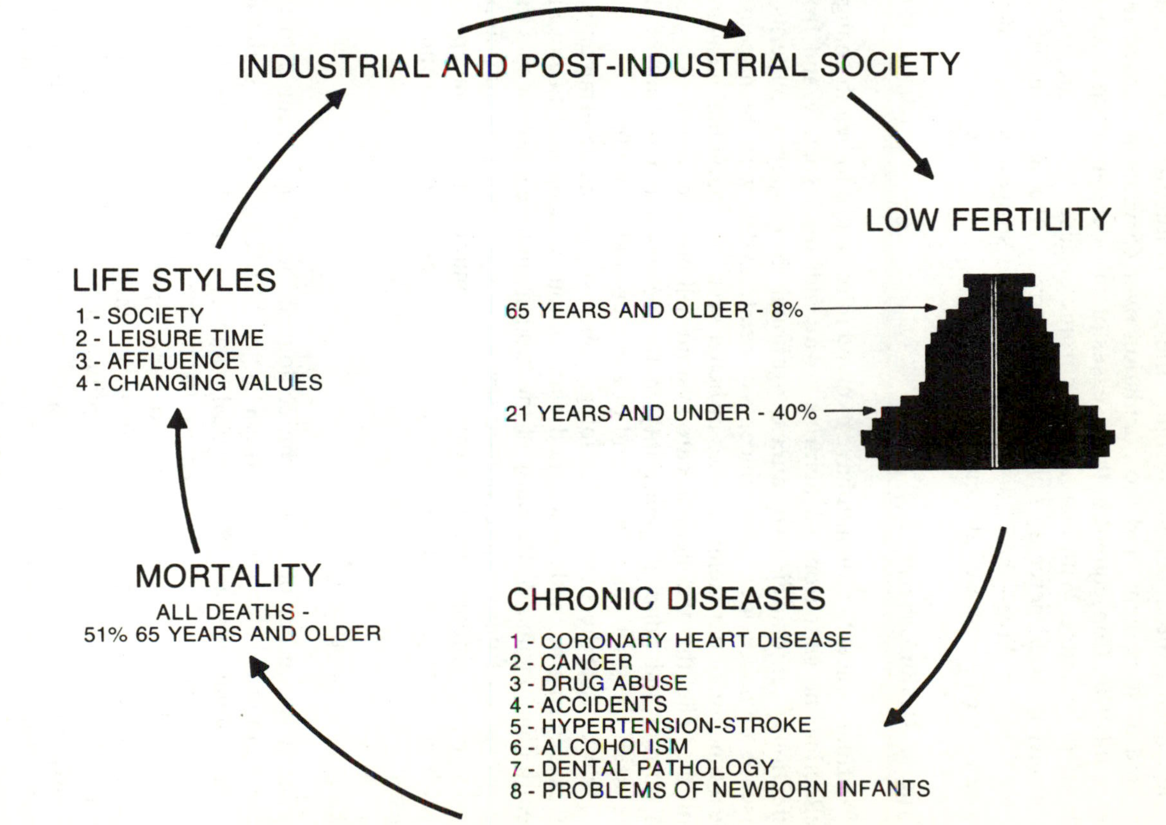

Source: G. E. Alan Dever, "The Pursuit of Health," *Social Indicators Research* 4, Figure 5, p. 486, 1977.

physical, emotional, and environmental ways of life have resulted from affluence, changing values, and increased leisure time. This overall societal change produced low fertility; the population under 20 years decreased to 40 percent, and the population over 65 years increased to 8 percent (1970). Consequently, the diseases of an older age group began to plague the country. With increases in chronic diseases and in the overall mortality level, 51 percent of all deaths occurred in the age group 65 and older. The big three—heart disease, cancer, and stroke—accounted for more than 60 percent of all deaths (1970).

Types of Health Concepts

Various concepts of health have evolved in response to health changes reflecting the shift from an agrarian to an industrial society and from infectious to chronic disease patterns. Although the changes in patterns of disease are now evident, our concepts of health to deal with them seem to be a function of our memory tapes or belief systems. Individual pleasures and the belief that the medical care system will provide the cures appear to outrank individual responsibility in the never-ending pursuit of decreased illness and disability—and of a better quality of life.

Health researchers and epidemiologists investigate the determinants of diseases using methods associated with various concepts of health and health components. While many of the fundamental health concepts that have evolved from the infectious disease cycle are not generally applicable to the chronic disease cycle, more comprehensive concepts of health provide a rational framework for the investigation of chronic diseases.

The Ecological Model

The first concept of health, the ecological model, is essential to the investigation of infectious diseases (Figure 1-7). This concept underlies the traditional approach of ecological balance. It involves a triad where the agent, the host, and the environment are in dynamic equilibrium. When the balance is upset, disease occurs. Upsets may happen when (1) the environment changes, (2) the agent's ability to infect man increases, and/or (3) the proportion of susceptibles increases in the population. Clearly, this concept has had successes in the control of infectious diseases. The concept allows drug therapy, sanitation, immunization, or surgery to tip the balance in favor of the host (man). This development was a natural consequence of the acceptance of the "germ theory" postulated by Koch.[3] It assumes a single causative agent (single cause/single effect model) based upon statistically absolute correlations. It is question-

Figure 1-7 The Ecological Model

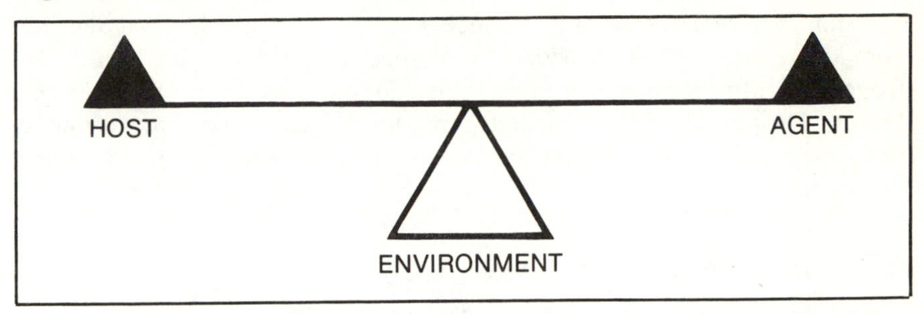

able whether this assumption is valid for the new disease patterns. Yet, despite its inherent limitations, the ecology model has been applied to a great many of our new illnesses, diseases, and hazards. Our belief system holds us to the ecology model (still cutting off the ends of something to make it fit into the pan), in the hope that it will aid in the curing of present-day illnesses and diseases. Because its methods of drug therapy, immunization, and surgery are borrowed from infectious disease epidemiology, however, the approach is outmoded for disease patterns of today.

The Social Ecological Model

A major improvement over the ecology model is the social ecological model provided by Morris[4] (Figure 1-8). Basically, this model replaces the agent (an infectious disease consideration) with personal behavior factors. The model suggests situations where there may be no specific etiologic

Figure 1-8 The Social Ecological Model

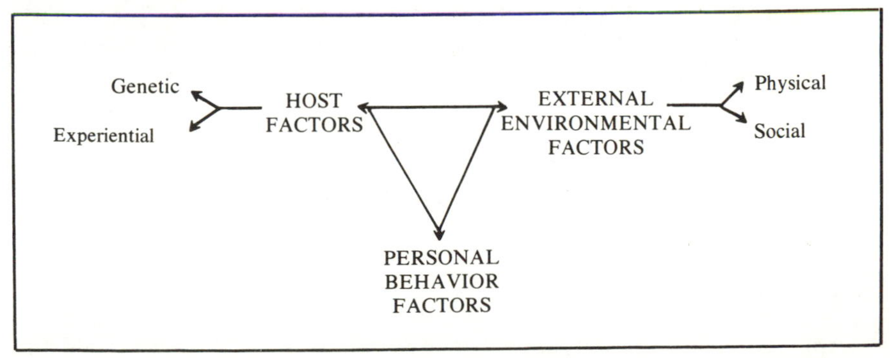

Source: Adapted from J. N. Morris, *Uses of Epidemiology*, 3rd ed. (Edinburgh: Churchhill Livingstone, 1975) p. 177.

agent (multiple cause/multiple effect or multiple cause/single effect). It recognizes that many factors influence a person's health. Thus, it does not consider medical care services as having an influence on health; iatrogenesis (illness caused by physicians), for example, is not considered a factor. The model illustrates that behavioral factors have more impact than the physical environment but that all aspects contribute to a dynamic balance.

World Health Organization Model

The concept of health held by the World Health Organization (WHO) is an expansion of the social ecological model. "Health is a state of complete physical, mental, and social well-being and not merely the absence of disease and infirmity." ("Constitution" of the World Health Organization, 1948. In *Basic Documents* 15th ed., WHO, Geneva, 1964.) This approach adds the dimension of mental well-being while retaining the social and physical characteristics. The basic difference between this concept and that of the previous model is that health is defined by WHO in terms of what should be, rather than in terms of the components or factors which constitute health. The WHO concept has been a major thrust toward changing our belief systems concerning the dimensions of health. Unrestricted by a specific definition of health, it has led to the development of multidimensional models that have broadened the framework of what constitutes health. These models can be described as holistic.

> Holistic means . . . viewing a person and his/her wellness from every possible perspective, taking into account every available concept and skill for the person's growth toward harmony and balance. It means treating the person, not the disease. The holistic approach promotes the interrelationship and unity of body, mind, and spirit. A holistic approach differs from simply following an "alternative" therapy. It is not an alternative to conventional medical practice. Rather, it includes judicious use of the best of modern Western medicine combined with the best health practices from East and West, old and new.[5]

Holistic Models

Apparently, health activities in many parts of the world (Sweden, the United States, and Canada) recognize the limitations of traditional concepts of health: ecology, social ecology, and WHO. The result is a new concept of health that is broad, comprehensive, and manageable from a policy point of view based upon new epidemiological needs. This, in turn, has fostered nontraditional approaches to health planning and policy making in an era of new disease patterns. The new holistic concepts of health as perceived by Blum, Lalonde, and Dever reach the same basic conclusion. Health, with its many dimensions, contains four fundamental attributes: environment, life style, human biology, and system of health care. Blum[6] calls it the "environment of health" (Figure 1-9), Lalonde[7] calls it

Figure 1-9 The Environment of Health Model

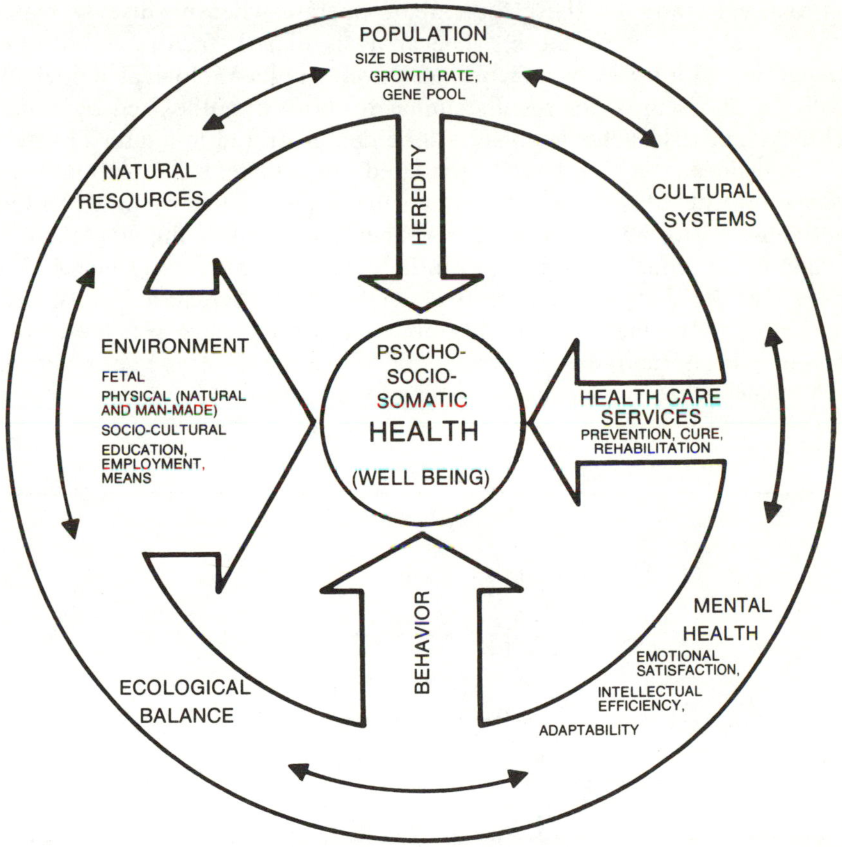

The width of the four large input-to-health arrows indicates assumptions about the relative importance of the inputs to health. The four inputs are shown as relating to and affecting one another by means of an encompassing matrix which could be called the "environment" of the health system.

Source: H. L. Blum, *Planning for Health—Developmental Application of Social Change Theory* (New York: Human Sciences Press, 1974) p. 3.

the "health field concept" (Figure 1-10), as Dever,[8] building on Lalonde's model, labels it "an epidemiological model for health policy analysis" (Figure 1-11). Blum suggests that the width of the four inputs contributing to health indicate assumptions about their relative importance. The four inputs relate to and affect one another by means of an encompassing wheel containing population, cultural systems, mental health, ecological balance, and natural resources. On the other hand, the assumptions of Lalonde and Dever are that the four inputs are weighted equally and must be in balance for health to occur. The important question to answer is, How do these four inputs operate when analyzed for specific diseases, or, alternatively, how do these four inputs operate when no disease exists (that is, a state of wellness)? The analysis of risk factors for disease categories within the framework of Dever's epidemiological model for policy analysis provides results similar to those hypothesized by Blum. This type of risk-factor analysis will be demonstrated in a later chapter.

These holistic models have engendered a new belief system about what constitutes health, but we still retain the belief that if we want to feel better we go to the physician. This belief is a result of the single cause/single effect model associated with the ecological concept of health. We have seen the changes in concepts of what constitutes health, but we have not let go of the medical care system as our only means to make us feel better. The alternative is the concept of wellness and the idea of giving up the medical care system as our means to survival.

Figure 1-10 The Health Field Concept

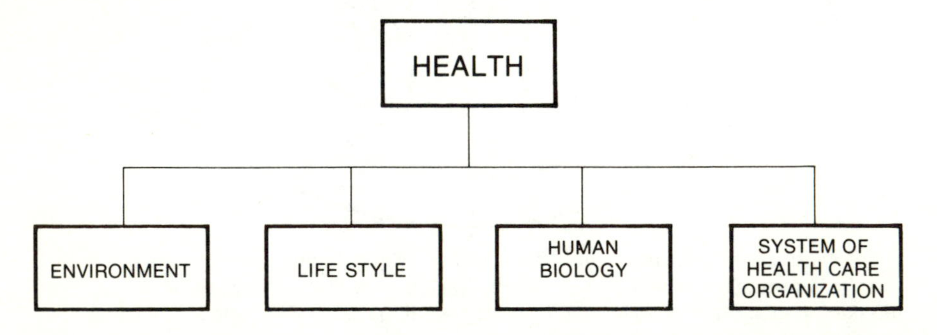

Source: M. Lalonde, *A New Perspective on the Health of Canadians* (Ottawa: Office of the Canadian Minister of National Health and Welfare, April 1974) p. 31.

Figure 1-11 An Epidemiological Model for Health Policy Analysis

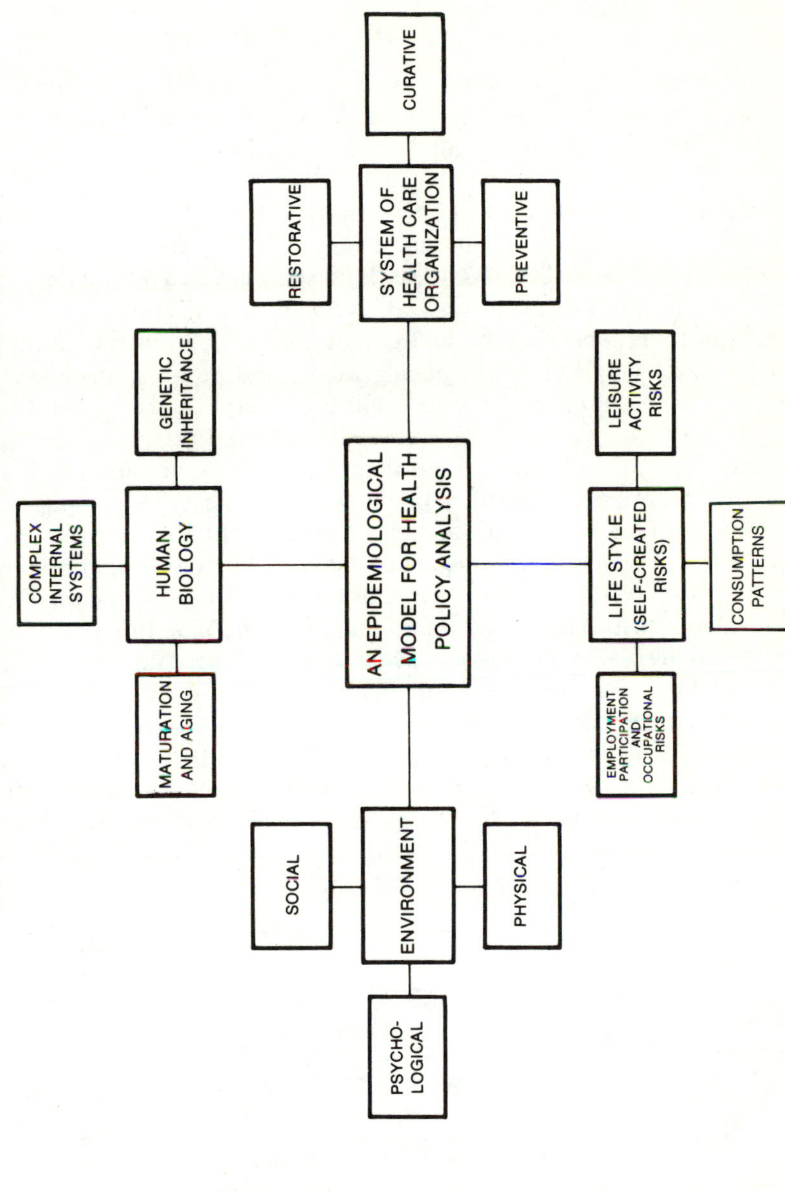

Source: G. E. Alan Dever, "An Epidemiological Model for Health Policy Analysis," *Social Indicators Research* 2, p. 455, 1976.

High-Level Wellness Model

The distinction between holism and wellness is made quite clear by Travis:

> The primary orientation of holistic health "is still towards healing conditions of illness. In contrast, the primary orientation of wellness is on increasing conditions of wellness."[9]

Specifically, the high-level wellness model focuses on four dimensions: (1) physical activity, (2) nutritional awareness, (3) stress management, and (4) self-responsibility. Wellness is a self-designed life style which allows one to *be* in order to *do* and to *have*. For instance, the *be* is a oneness of mind, spirit, body, and emotion by which nutritional awareness, physical activity, stress management, and self-responsibility become the *dos*, resulting in *having* a healthful life style and a high potential for well-being.

Travis illustrates wellness as an illness-wellness continuum[10] (Figure 1-12). The neutral point indicates no illness or wellness. Movement to the left shows poorer conditions of illness; movement to the right shows better levels of wellness. For instance, it is possible to be not quite physically ill, yet to experience depression, anxiety, frustration, and an overall dissatisfaction with life. While traditional medicine may bring one to the point of having no discernible physical illness, wellness goes beyond and deals with life experiences resulting in aliveness and enlightenment. This innovative concept of health is growing in popularity and is fast becoming a major portion of the health plans produced by Health Systems Agencies (HSAs) and public health departments. The only potential drawback to this approach (at least in the Wellness Resource Center, Mill Valley,

Figure 1-12 The Illness-Wellness Continuum

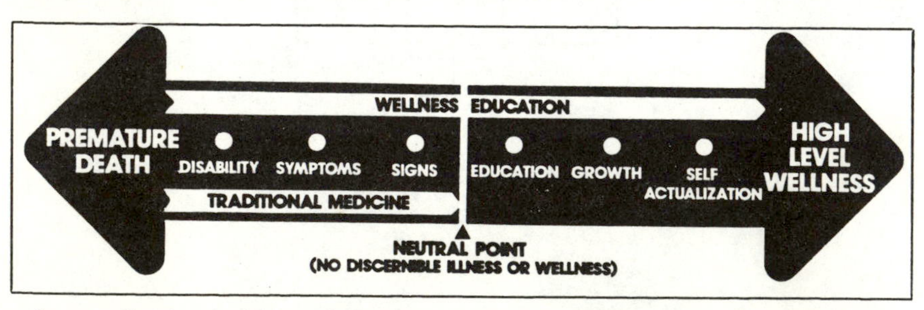

Source: Reprinted with permission from the *Wellness Workbook for Health Professionals*, copyright 1977, John W. Travis, M.D., published by the Wellness Resource Center, 42 Miller Ave., Mill Valley, CA 94941, p. 122.

California) is the lack of any physical assessment. A wellness center approach should meld a Travis model with an aerobics model like that of Dr. Kenneth Cooper in Dallas, Texas. Such a combination would encourage greater community participation, thereby resulting in higher levels of wellness for individuals in their communities.

THE CONTENT AND CONTEXT OF WELLNESS—THE WAY WE THINK ABOUT HEALTH

We really must ask ourselves, Do we think about health in the proper perspective? Or more precisely, How does wellness fit into the big picture? To answer the first question, consider the following scenario.

> It was 6:30 p.m. and time for Jack, age 23, to leave to pick up his date. Meeting her at 7:00 p.m., Jack drove his date to a dance, where they enjoyed dancing, food, and drink. After the dance, Jack took his date home.
>
> One hour later, a piercing ring suddenly awakened the household of Jack's family. The message was clear. Jack had been killed in an automobile accident while enroute from his girlfriend's house to his home.
>
> The death certificate recorded immediate cause of death: "Substantial head and chest injuries due to a motor vehicle accident" [Exhibit 1-1]. In addition, the car speed was estimated at 70 m.p.h., resulting in Jack's loss of control of the car, thereby hitting a bridge abutment.
>
> Reviewing Jack's behavior, we are able to determine the exact cause of his death. In actuality, Jack had been under extreme pressure from his parents to find a job. The party that night was to be a release from their subtle haranguing. At the party, he had fallen prey to the admonishments of his friends to "chug-a-lug just one more." After leaving his girlfriend, he became a victim of the lack of responsibility and inhibition which the excessive consumption of alcohol produced. He was also subject to the Mario Andretti syndrome—a sense of great power over an inanimate machine—hence the high speed and lack of caution.
>
> In essence, the death certificate recording should have been: (1) excessive alcohol intake; (2) failure to use seat belt; (3) excessive speed; and (4) societal pressure. In other cases, physical environmental factors may be the cause: (1) road under construction; (2) inclement weather; and (3) poor lighting [Exhibit 1-2].[11]

Exhibit 1-1 Certificate of Death—Coded by Disease Category (Motor Vehicle Accident)

REGISTRAR: CHECK CERTIFICATE CAREFULLY
Revised December 1, 1956

CERTIFICATE OF DEATH

State File No. 35142

BIRTH NO. | Militia Dist. No. | Custodian's No.

1. NAME OF DECEASED (Type or Print) a. (First) (b. (Middle) c. (Last)
2. DATE OF DEATH (Month) (Day) (Year)

3. Place of Death
County Baldwin
City or Town Milledgeville — In City Limits Yes ☐ No ☒ — LENGTH OF STAY (in this place)
Name of Hosp. or Institution Baldwin Co. Hospital — LENGTH OF STAY D.O.A.

4. Usual Residence (Where deceased lived. If institution: residence before admission)
State Georgia County Hancock
City or Town — In City Limits ☐ Yes No ☒ — LENGTH OF STAY (in this place) 22 yrs.
Street Address or R. F. D. and Box No.

5. SEX M | 6. RACE W | 7. BIRTHPLACE (State or foreign country) Alabama | CITIZEN OF WHAT COUNTRY? USA
15. Is residence on a farm? Yes ☒ No ☐
16. BURIAL ☒ REMOVAL ☐ CREMATION ☐ — DATE 6/4/74

8. DATE OF BIRTH 4/20/51 | 9. AGE (In years last birthday) 23 | IF UNDER 1 YEAR Months Days | IF UNDER 24 HRS. Hours Min.
NAME OF CEMETERY | LOCATION (City or Town) (County) (State)

10. MARRIED ☐ NEVER MARRIED ☒ WIDOWED ☐ DIVORCED ☐ SEPARATED ☐ | If Married or Widowed Give Name of Spouse
17. EMBALMER'S SIGNATURE | LICENSE NO.

11. USUAL OCCUPATION (Give kind of work done during most of working life, even if retired) loom cleaner | KIND OF BUSINESS OR INDUSTRY textiles
18. MORTICIAN

12. WAS DECEASED EVER IN U. S. ARMED FORCES? (Yes, no, or unknown) no | (If yes, give war or dates of service) | SOCIAL SECURITY NO.
19. MORTICIAN'S ADDRESS

13. FATHER'S NAME
20. INFORMANT | Relationship

14. MOTHER'S MAIDEN NAME
21. INFORMANT'S ADDRESS

MEDICAL CERTIFICATION

22. CAUSE OF DEATH [Enter only one cause per line for (a), (b), and (c).]
PART I. DEATH WAS CAUSED BY:
IMMEDIATE CAUSE (a) HEAD AND CHEST INJURIES — INTERVAL BETWEEN ONSET AND DEATH: MINUTES
Conditions, if any, which gave rise to above cause (a), stating the underlying cause last.
DUE TO (b) MOTOR VEHICLE ACCIDENT
DUE TO (c)
DO NOT WRITE IN THIS SPACE 1. 2. 3. 4. 5. 6.

PART II. Other significant conditions contributing to death but not related to the terminal disease condition given in Part I (a)
23. AUTOPSY? Yes ☒ No ☐

24. ACCIDENT ☒ SUICIDE ☐ HOMICIDE ☐ | PLACE OF INJURY (e.g., in or about home, farm, factory, street, office bldg., etc.) | INJURY OCCURRED While at Work ☐ Not While at Work ☐
(CITY OR TOWN) (COUNTY) (STATE) Milledgeville, Baldwin, Ga. | TIME OF INJURY (Month) (Day) (Year) (Hour) 6/1/74/7:25p.m.
HOW DID INJURY OCCUR? Est. speed 70MPH, lost control of pick up truck hit bridge abutment

27. I hereby certify that I attended the deceased from ______ 19___ to ______ 19___, that I last saw the deceased alive on D.O.A. ______ 19___, and that death occurred at 7:30 p.m., from the causes and on the date stated above.
28. SIGNATURE | Degree or Title Medical Exam.

25. DATE REC'D BY LOCAL REG. 6/3/74 | 26. REGISTRAR'S SIGNATURE | ADDRESS | DATE SIGNED 6/2/74

Georgia Department of Public Health, Division of Vital Records, Atlanta 3, Georgia | ADM-5.3 | Department of Health, Education, and Welfare, U. S. Public Health Service

Source: Modified from G. E. Alan Dever "The Pursuit of Health," *Social Indicators Research* 4, p. 491, 1977.

Exhibit 1-2 Certificate of Death—Coded by Causes (Speed, Excessive Alcohol, Failure to Use Seat Belt)

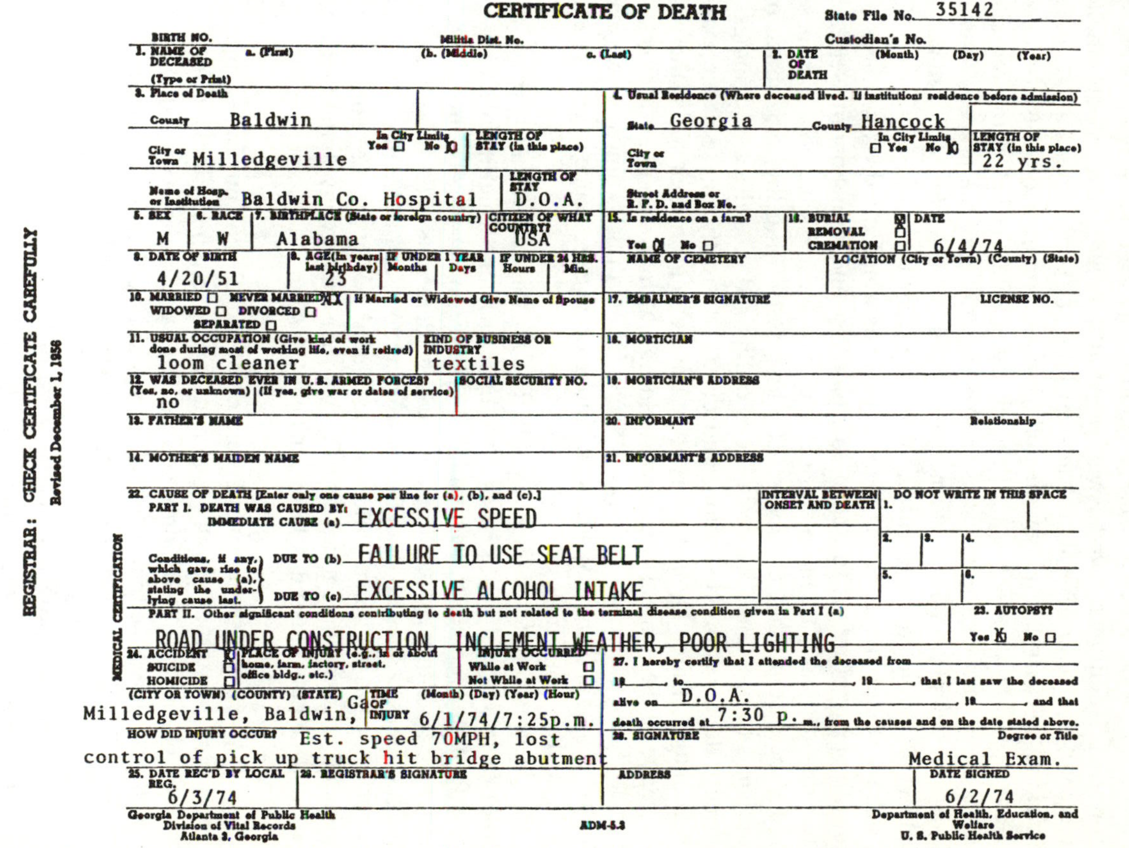
REGISTRAR: CHECK CERTIFICATE CAREFULLY
Revised December 1, 1956

CERTIFICATE OF DEATH
State File No. 35142
BIRTH NO. Militia Dist. No. Custodian's No.
1. NAME OF DECEASED (Type or Print) a. (First) (b. (Middle) c. (Last)
2. DATE OF DEATH (Month) (Day) (Year)
3. Place of Death
County Baldwin
City or Town Milledgeville In City Limits Yes ☐ No ☒ LENGTH OF STAY (in this place)
Name of Hosp. or Institution Baldwin Co. Hospital LENGTH OF STAY D.O.A.
4. Usual Residence (Where deceased lived. If institution: residence before admission)
State Georgia County Hancock
City or Town In City Limits ☐ Yes No ☒ LENGTH OF STAY (in this place) 22 yrs.
Street Address or R. F. D. and Box No.
5. SEX M 6. RACE W 7. BIRTHPLACE (State or foreign country) Alabama CITIZEN OF WHAT COUNTRY? USA
15. Is residence on a farm? Yes ☒ No ☐
16. BURIAL ☒ REMOVAL ☐ CREMATION ☐ DATE 6/4/74
8. DATE OF BIRTH 4/20/51 9. AGE (In years last birthday) 23 IF UNDER 1 YEAR Months Days IF UNDER 24 HRS. Hours Min.
NAME OF CEMETERY LOCATION (City or Town) (County) (State)
10. MARRIED ☐ NEVER MARRIED XX WIDOWED ☐ DIVORCED ☐ SEPARATED ☐ If Married or Widowed Give Name of Spouse
17. EMBALMER'S SIGNATURE LICENSE NO.
11. USUAL OCCUPATION (Give kind of work done during most of working life, even if retired) loom cleaner KIND OF BUSINESS OR INDUSTRY textiles
18. MORTICIAN
12. WAS DECEASED EVER IN U. S. ARMED FORCES? (Yes, no, or unknown) no (If yes, give war or dates of service) SOCIAL SECURITY NO.
19. MORTICIAN'S ADDRESS
13. FATHER'S NAME
20. INFORMANT Relationship
14. MOTHER'S MAIDEN NAME
21. INFORMANT'S ADDRESS

MEDICAL CERTIFICATION
22. CAUSE OF DEATH [Enter only one cause per line for (a), (b), and (c).]
PART I. DEATH WAS CAUSED BY:
IMMEDIATE CAUSE (a) EXCESSIVE SPEED
Conditions, if any, which gave rise to above cause (a), stating the underlying cause last.
DUE TO (b) FAILURE TO USE SEAT BELT
DUE TO (c) EXCESSIVE ALCOHOL INTAKE
INTERVAL BETWEEN ONSET AND DEATH
DO NOT WRITE IN THIS SPACE 1. 2. 3. 4. 5. 6.
PART II. Other significant conditions contributing to death but not related to the terminal disease condition given in Part I (a)
ROAD UNDER CONSTRUCTION, INCLEMENT WEATHER, POOR LIGHTING
23. AUTOPSY? Yes ☒ No ☐
24. ACCIDENT ☒ SUICIDE ☐ HOMICIDE ☐ PLACE OF INJURY (e.g., in or about home, farm, factory, street, office bldg., etc.) INJURY OCCURRED While at Work ☐ Not While at Work ☐
(CITY OR TOWN) (COUNTY) (STATE) Milledgeville, Baldwin, Ga TIME OF INJURY (Month) (Day) (Year) (Hour) 6/1/74/7:25p.m.
HOW DID INJURY OCCUR? Est. speed 70MPH, lost control of pick up truck hit bridge abutment
27. I hereby certify that I attended the deceased from 19 to 19 that I last saw the deceased alive on D.O.A. 19 and that death occurred at 7:30 p.m., from the causes and on the date stated above.
28. SIGNATURE Degree or Title Medical Exam.
ADDRESS DATE SIGNED 6/2/74
25. DATE REC'D BY LOCAL REG. 6/3/74 26. REGISTRAR'S SIGNATURE
Georgia Department of Public Health Division of Vital Records Atlanta 3, Georgia
ADM-5.3
Department of Health, Education, and Welfare U. S. Public Health Service

Source: Modified from G. E. Alan Dever "The Pursuit of Health," *Social Indicators Research* 4, p. 492, 1977.

It is quite clear—and it is important to be clear on this—that we are not thinking about health in the proper perspective. Death certificates code diseases; they do not code causes. Traditionally we ask, What is the cause of death? Traditionally we answer, heart attack, lung cancer, automobile accident, and so on. We should answer lack of exercise, inadequate diet, smoking, excessive drinking, air pollution, and depression. Disease classifications should incorporate these changes, and the list of top ten diseases should be the top ten causes. We are attacking the process after it has been completed. Thus, we never expand our knowledge. More accurately, we do not think about health in the right way.

The first step in answering the second question, How does wellness fit into the big picture? is to find a "big picture" and somehow fit wellness into that picture. The big picture is life, and wellness is about aliveness and experiencing that aliveness. The task is to bring the experience of aliveness to life. The picture of life is composed of wellness, happiness, money, depression, frustration, and death. Basically, these aspects are the content of life. Though everybody has content in their lives, the significance of the content is how we hold onto it in the context of life. We can do this in either of two ways. We can let life drag us down, or we can realize that that is the way life is and move on to experience aliveness and to make life work for us.

Wellness is about making life work. The reason life doesn't work or we don't experience aliveness is that we have barriers which prevent aliveness from happening. For example, the failure to participate and to share and the lack of money and time are the considerations in life which lead to holistic illness. These barriers exist as functions of our memory tapes or belief systems. As noted earlier in the "ham" story, we are still cutting the ends off something to make it fit. Another analogy involving men and rats and tunnels illustrates how our belief systems work.

> If you put a rat in front of a bunch of tunnels and put cheese in one of them, the rat will go up and down the tunnels looking for the cheese. If, every time you do the experiment, you put the cheese down the fourth tunnel, eventually you'll get a successful rat. This rat knows the right tunnel and goes directly to it every time.
>
> If you now move the cheese out of the fourth tunnel and put it at the end of another tunnel, the rat still goes down the fourth tunnel. And, of course, gets no cheese. He then comes out of the tunnel, looks the tunnel over, and goes right back down the cheeseless fourth tunnel. Unrewarded, he comes out of the tunnel, looks the tunnel over again, goes back down the fourth

> tunnel again, and again finds no cheese. (REMEMBER—TIME AFTER TIME AFTER TIME, WE CANNOT EXPECT THE MEDICAL CARE SYSTEM TO MAKE REPAIRS.)
>
> Now the difference between a rat and a human being is that eventually the rat will stop going down the fourth tunnel and will look down the other tunnels, and a human being will go down the tunnel with no cheese forever. Rats, you see, are only interested in cheese. But human beings care more about going down the right tunnel.
>
> It is belief which allows human beings to go down the fourth tunnel ad nauseam. They go on doing what they do without any real satisfaction, without any nurturing, because they come to believe what they are doing is right. And they will do this forever, even if there is no cheese in the tunnel, as long as they believe in it and can prove that they are in the right tunnel.[12]

PEOPLE WHO ARE EXPERIENCING ALIVENESS IN LIFE DON'T HAVE TO PROVE THEY ARE IN THE RIGHT TUNNEL.

By applying this notion of belief systems to health care, we can expand our knowledge and create the space in which we have the potential to transform holistic illness into holistic wellness.

Travis has identified an illness/wellness and atomistic/holistic continuum which focuses on line functions (see Figure 1-12). A modification of this would be to concentrate on the areas and the functions within the areas (Figure 1-13). Thus, we arrive at atomistic illness, atomistic wellness, holistic illness, and holistic wellness. To show how our belief systems are major reinforcements to our seeking medical care from the physician or, alternatively, to show how our belief systems are major barriers to the acceptance of holism and wellness and to less dependence on the medical care system and the physician, it is necessary to focus on the specific areas noted in Figure 1-13.

Our belief systems have produced habits resulting in patterns which at one time provided solutions but now provide problems. Atomistic illness (the smallest recognizable component) is a result of the infectious disease cycle where a single cause produced a single effect. Examples include polio, diphtheria, measles, and whooping cough. Our belief system at the time set up a habit which impelled us to go to the physician or clinic to get the solution to our infectious disease problem. We did this frequently enough to establish a pattern—to feel better, go to the physician to get a shot for the illness. At that point, the solution was a single interaction—usually, immunization. The result of this pattern was atomistic wellness (at least no discernible illness). Thus, if we wanted to keep well from

Figure 1-13 Modification of the Illness-Wellness Continuum

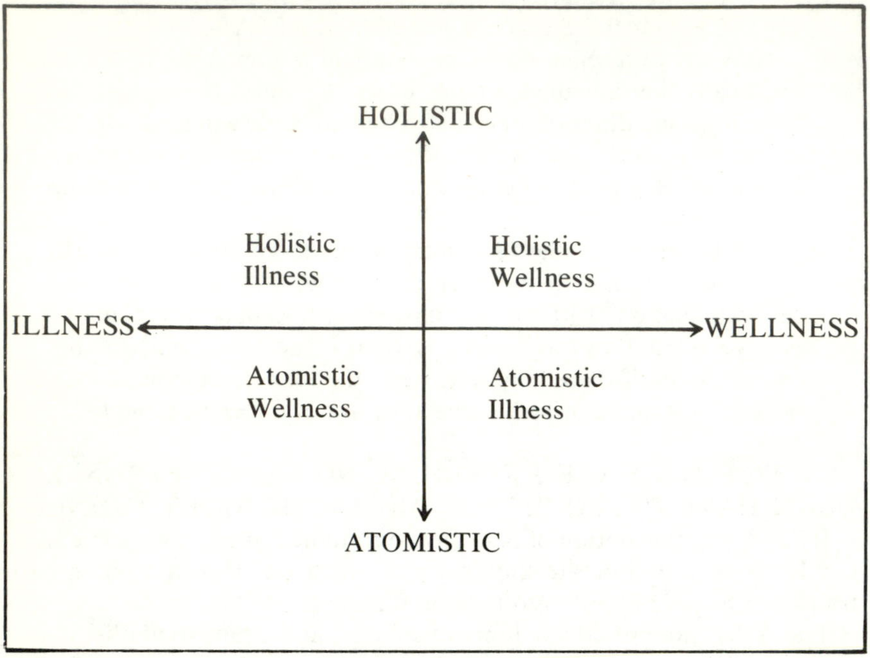

HOLISTIC

Holistic Illness

Holistic Wellness

ILLNESS ← → WELLNESS

Atomistic Wellness

Atomistic Illness

ATOMISTIC

Source: Adapted and reprinted with permission from the *Wellness Workbook for Health Professionals,* copyright 1977, John W. Travis, M.D., published by the Wellness Resource Center, 42 Miller Ave., Mill Valley, CA 94941, p. 123.

---

infectious diseases, we would go and get shots. We played this memory tape or belief system over and over again because—you know what?—it worked! Our disease patterns changed, however, and now we are faced with the major chronic diseases. The result: holistic illness.

Holistic illness results from the multiple cause/multiple effect model. The multiple causes are smoking, diet, drinking, lack of exercise, poor sleeping habits, stress, and depression. The multiple effects are heart disease, cancer, stroke, suicide, homicide, motor vehicle accidents, and so on. Because of our old memory tapes or belief systems (going down the same tunnel), we go to the physician and expect the holistic illness to be taken care of. The interventions for holistic illnesses are multiple—stress management, nutritional awareness, physical activity, and an overall life style to bring about enlightenment and the capability to make our life work. If we want to experience holistic wellness and aliveness, the majority of the responsibility is our own. Our previous pattern of going to the physician for wellness now becomes the problem instead of the solution, because after we develop the illness the physician can do very little to make it better. Thus, holistic wellness becomes a function of the individual and not the physician. But as long as we continue to play our old memory tapes (go down the same tunnel), it will be extremely difficult to achieve holistic wellness. It is apparent that these memory tapes are the barriers to wellness. As long as we feel the physician can take care of our illness, we do not have to be personally responsible for our own health—a situation that was true for the infectious diseases but not for the chronic diseases.

To make change, we must discard our memory tapes, that is, go down a new tunnel, and begin to remove the barriers which keep us stuck in the same tunnel. That means we must participate, share, and communicate and find the time and the money. In other words, we must change the context of life or how we hold onto life. We must transform and overcome the barriers and experience aliveness and make life work and be well. It's time to change tunnels and find the cheese.

SUMMARY

Health in the 1980s will be primarily a function of self-responsibility and authority—the main components of good management. Our dependence on the medical care system and the physician will decrease and be replaced by holistic and wellness approaches to health.

The epidemiological causal models and concepts of health are related to the shift in disease patterns. Our belief systems impact immensely on the way we think about health care and on how we seek positive health. It is essential that we change our belief systems if we want to experience wellness.

The relevance and appropriateness of the concepts discussed in this chapter will be assessed in the analysis of community health problems.

NOTES

1. Adelaide Bry, *Est* (New York: Avon Books, August 1976).

2. I have not discussed the concept of "association" as it relates to causation; however, the reader may find a brief but excellent comparison of causation and association in Donald F. Austin and S. Benson Werner, *Epidemiology for the Health Sciences* (Springfield, Ill.: Charles C Thomas, 1974). For a more sophisticated interpretation of causality in epidemiology, see: P. O. Woolley et al., *Syncrisis: The Dynamics of Health* (Washington, D.C.: U.S.

Government Printing Office, June 1972); and M. Susser, *Causal Thinking in the Health Sciences*, (New York: Oxford University Press, 1973).

3. Austin and Werner, *Epidemiology for the Health Sciences*, p. 42.

4. J. N. Morris, *Uses of Epidemiology*, 3rd ed. (Edinburgh: Churchill Livingstone, 1975), p. 173–180.

5. D. B. Ardell, *High Level Wellness, An Alternative to Doctors, Drugs, and Disease* (Emmons, Pa.: Rodale Press, 1977), p. 5.

6. H. L. Blum, *Planning for Health—Development and Application of Social Change Theory* (New York: Human Sciences Press, 1974), pp. 2–4.

7. M. Lalonde, *A New Perspective on the Health of Canadians* (Ottawa: Office of the Canadian Minister of National Health and Welfare, April 1974), pp. 31–34.

8. G. E. A. Dever, "An Epidemiological Model for Health Policy Analysis," *Social Indicators Research* 2 (1976): 453–466.

9. J. W. Travis, *Wellness Workbook for Health Professionals* (Mill Valley, Calif.: Wellness Resource Center, 1977), p. 4.

10. Ibid., p. 6.

11. G. E. A. Dever, "The Pursuit of Health," *Social Indicators Research* 4 (1977): 475–497.

12. Bry, *Est*, pp. 15–16.

Chapter 2

Holistic Health—An Epidemiological Model for Policy Analysis

The purpose of this chapter is to develop an innovative epidemiological model which may be used in policy analysis for community health programs.[1 2 3] This model would be applicable in such community settings as HSAs, public health departments, health maintenance organizations, and medical care foundations. Community health programs that need health and related data have been largely unsuccessful because they have lacked a rational framework for analysis. In the previous chapter, a cursory analysis of present disease patterns revealed chronic conditions for which the present system of organized medical care has no immediate cures or solutions. Moreover, our individual belief systems were shown to be stuck in the solutions of the disease patterns of the 1900s. Though the infectious disease cycle of the 1900s has been all but eliminated by vaccines and antibiotics, we will be unable either to prevent or to arrest the current disease pattern until we change our belief systems and adopt a new concept of health. This will allow us to reorganize the health field into more manageable elements in order to develop creative areas for epidemiological models.

It is essentially irrelevant how we use health data if we fail to recognize what is needed to develop solutions to our disease patterns. Typically, we have correlated, rigorously factored, and canonized data in an effort to squeeze out all meaningful relationships. The results, for the most part, have had questionable utility. We have also displayed data in graphs, tables, and maps to demonstrate trends, distributions, and patterns. These efforts have increased awareness relative to the magnitude of the problems, but they have not been significantly instrumental in changing disease patterns. We have planned, implemented, and evaluated many health programs with little or no reduction of morbidity or mortality. Pure research and clinical investigations certainly have merit, but these approaches, when viewed in the overall scheme of current disease patterns, have had a negligible effect in bringing about major disease reduction. The net result of these approaches to disease investigation, prevention, and cure has been the alarming increase of health dollar expenditures with a parallel increase in health problems. For these reasons, we need a conceptual framework that allows the health field to be divided into more manageable elements.

We do not need better data analysis, data presentation, programmatic involvement, or privately dominated research. Rather we need a new epidemiological approach which employs the above concerns in a more meaningful way and which considers the health field from a different point of view (finds a new tunnel). Such an epidemiological model, combined with a change in our belief systems, will enable us to provide a policy analysis to deal more realistically with the current health needs of our population.

AN EPIDEMIOLOGICAL MODEL FOR HEALTH POLICY ANALYSIS

Only recently have we changed our views about epidemiology and what it involves. The change still falls well below our expectations, however, in terms of how we prevent or arrest a disease process.

In 1900, disease was primarily infectious in nature, and major barriers were overcome. Presently disease is noninfectious, and major barriers still exist because we continue to apply 1900 solutions. The 1900 model is antiquated because infectious diseases in the United States are all but eradicated.

For these reasons, an epidemiological model for health policy analysis that addresses the problems concerned with changing disease patterns is required. The need to break the problem of health policy into more manageable segments has been expressed elsewhere.[4] [5] [6] Indeed, recent Canadian publications have developed this theme into a health field concept.[7] [8]

Components of the Model

An epidemiological model that supports health policy analysis and decisiveness must be broad and comprehensive, including all matters affecting health. Four primary divisions have been identified: (1) system of medical care organization, (2) life style (self-created risks), (3) environment, and (4) human biology (See Figure 1-11). This epidemiological model is said to provide a more balanced approach to the development of health policy when compared with the limiting, traditional divisions of prevention, diagnosis, therapy, and rehabilitation, or with public health, mental health, and clinical medicine.[9] Figure 1-11 shows the pertinent subdivisions that allow a more intense investigation of disease.

System of Medical Care Organization

A system of medical care organization may be divided into three elements: curative, restorative, and preventive. The system itself consists of the availability, quality, and quantity of resources to provide health care. Its restorative elements include hospital, nursing home, and ambulance services. Its curative elements include medical drugs, dental treatments, and medical professionals. The system has a very limited input of preventive elements. Efforts and expenditures to improve health in the United States have been directed almost totally toward the system of medical care organization. Yet, the morbidity and mortality disease patterns of today are deeply entrenched in the other three divisions of our epidemiological model. The huge sums of money spent for restoring and curing should be earmarked for prevention of disease in the population. Rather than concentrate on the failures of the system of medical care organization, we would find it more advantageous to promote the positive points of the other three divisions: life style, environment, and human biology.

Life Style

Life styles or, more accurately, self-created risks may be divided into three elements: leisure activity risks, consumption patterns, and employment participation and occupational risks. This division of the epidemiological model consists of the aggregation of decisions by individuals which affect their health and over which they have more or less control.[10] Bad or incorrect decisions result in destructive modes of health that contribute to an increased level of illness or premature death.

Leisure activity risks. Some self-imposed destructive modes are the result of leisure activity risks. For instance, lack of recreation is strongly associated with hypertension and coronary heart disease. Similarly, lack of exercise aggravates coronary heart disease, leads to obesity, and results in a total lack of physical fitness. These examples (and there are many more) point up the need to focus more specifically on the other divisions of the epidemiological model. Indeed, such a shift in focus is imperative if we wish to reduce disability and promote a better quality of life.

Consumption patterns. Another kind of self-imposed risk is in the area of "consumption patterns." These include (1) overeating, leading to obesity and subsequent consequences; (2) cholesterol intake, contributing to heart disease; (3) alcohol addiction, leading to cirrhosis of the liver; (4) alcohol consumption, leading to motor vehicle accidents; (5) cigarette smoking, causing chronic obstructive pulmonary disease (chronic bronchitis, emphysema) and lung cancer and aggravating heart disease; (6) drug dependency and social drug use, leading to suicide, homicide, malnutrition, accidents, social withdrawal, and acute anxiety attacks; and (7) abundant glucose (sugar) intake, contributing to dental caries, obesity, and hyperglycemia with its concomitant problems.

Employment/occupational risks. Destructive life styles resulting from employment participation and occupational risks are equally significant but far more difficult to identify. Work pressures lead to stresses, anxieties, and tensions which, in turn, may cause peptic ulcers and hypertension. Other habits (admittedly difficult to categorize) such as careless driving lead to accidents, while sexual promiscuity often results in syphilis or gonorrhea.[11]

The life-style component of the epidemiological model is a major contributing factor to our present disease patterns. It is, however, a component which is viewed with considerable pessimism. The main reason for this "Achilles' heel" is self-pleasure. A change in hedonistic behavior occurs only after a life-death event, and even this change wanes considerably as the length of time increases from the onset of the initial event. The consequence of this pleasure principle is that we have at best little change and at worst no change in the major disease patterns that affect our population.[12] We must thus alter our belief systems and realize that the solutions to our disease patterns are in "new tunnels" in order to achieve a wellness and a life that works.

Environment

The environment in the epidemiological model is defined as events external to the body over which the individual has little or no control. This element may be subdivided into physical, social, and psychological dimensions.[13]

The physical dimension. In a physical environment certain hazards show a close relationship to the use of energy (oil) by an expanding population. Per capita energy consumption is increasing concomitantly with the population and the standard of living. Thus, health hazards stemming from air, noise, and water pollution will almost assuredly also increase steadily. The resulting diseases and problems include hearing loss, infectious diseases, gastroenteritis, cancer, emphysema, and bronchitis. In limiting cases, ionizing and ultraviolet radiation have health implications in terms of skin cancer and genetic mutation.[14]

The social and psychological dimensions. The social and psychological divisions of environmental health encompass major factors involving behavior modification, perceptional problems, and interpersonal relationships. For example, crowding, isolation, rapid and accelerated rates of change, and social interchange may contribute to homicide, suicide, decisional stress, and environmental overstimulation.[15] [16]

The environmental conditions we have described create risks which are a far greater threat to health than any present inadequacy of the system of medical care organization. The resulting health problems will be resolved only by imposing standards and controls on the responsible agencies and industries.

Human Biology

The final division of the epidemiological model is human biology. This element, focusing on the human body, is concerned with man's basic biologic and organic makeup as an individual. Thus, the genetic inheritance of the individual creates genetic disorders, congenital malformations, and mental retardation. The maturation and aging process is a contributing factor in arthritis, diabetes, atherosclerosis, and cancer. Obvious disorders of the skeletal, muscular, cardiovascular, endocrine, and digestive systems can be included in a subcomponent of complex internal systems. Disease categories relative to human biology must be weighted in accordance with the other divisions of the epidemiological model. Genetic counseling of parents with possible Tay-Sachs disease is a step in the right direction. If we can overcome the problems resulting from the human biology of man, we would be able to save many lives, decrease misery, and reduce the cost of treatment services. This is an obligation to humanity.

Advantages of the Model

The combination of the four divisions—system of medical care organization, life style, environment, and human biology—into an epidemiological model for health policy analysis has many advantages. Lalonde cites these:

1. "This model raises Life Style, Environment, and Human Biology to a level of categorical importance equal to that of the System of Medical Care Organization.

2. "The model is comprehensive. Any health problem can be traced to one or a combination of the four divisions.
3. "The model allows a system of analysis by which a disease or pattern may be examined under the four divisions in order to assess relative significance and interaction (i.e., what percentage or proportion of Life Style, Environment, Human Biology, and System of Medical Care Organization contributes to suicide?).
4. "This model permits further subdivision of the four major factors; for example, Environment is subdivided into physical, social, and psychological.
5. "This model provides a new perspective (a new tunnel) on health that creates a recognition and exploration of previously neglected fields."[17]

APPLICATIONS OF THE EPIDEMIOLOGICAL MODEL

The application of this model involves four steps: (1) the selection of diseases that are of high risk and that contribute substantially to overall mortality and morbidity, (2) the proportionate allocation of the contributing factors of the disease to the four elements of the epidemiological model, (3) the proportionate allocation of total health expenditures to the four elements of the epidemiological model, and (4) the determination of the difference in proportions between (2) and (3) above. In a later chapter, we will see the application of this approach to a risk-factor analysis model which analyzes each disease specifically in support of program management decisions.

Application to Disease Patterns in Georgia

For purposes of illustration, the top 13 diseases in Georgia were selected for analysis (Step one). Table 2-1 shows the percentage distribution of deaths by age group and disease. Cancer, heart disease, and stroke ranked first, second, and third, respectively, with high-risk groups concentrated in ages over 55. Deaths due to automobile accidents and other accidents were concentrated in the 15–34 age group. Two other diseases, homicide and suicide, showed concentrations of high risk in the 15–34 and the 35–54 age groups, respectively. Thus, the major cripplers and killers of Georgians were represented in multiple age groups in terms of high risk and in multiple etiologies in terms of determining preventive measures.

Using the 13 selected diseases, the analysts next allocated proportionately the contributing factors of each disease to the four components

Table 2-1 Percentage Distribution of Deaths by Age Group for Selected Important Causes of Mortality in Georgia, 1973

Cause of Mortality	Total, All Causes	% of Deaths per Disease	% of Total Deaths	Percentage Distribution by Age Group									
				Under One	1-4	5-14	15-24	25-34	35-44	45-54	55-64	65-74	75 +
TOTAL, ALL AGES	43,910	100.0	100.0	3.7	0.8	1.1	3.2	3.4	5.1	10.6	18.4	22.2	30.5
Diseases of the heart	14,922	100.0	34.0	0.1	0.1	0.1	0.2	0.7	2.8	9.6	20.3	28.2	37.8
Cancer	6,532	100.0	14.9	0.1	0.4	0.8	1.0	1.6	4.6	14.5	26.8	28.1	22.2
Cerebrovascular	5,897	100.0	13.4	0.0	0.1	0.1	0.4	0.8	2.3	6.2	14.1	25.9	50.1
Motor vehicle accidents	1,847	100.0	4.2	0.9	3.4	8.0	28.2	17.5	11.9	10.4	9.4	6.7	3.7
All other accidents	1,657	100.0	3.8	4.6	5.3	7.5	14.5	12.6	10.6	12.3	11.5	8.6	12.6
Influenza and pneumonia	1,648	100.0	3.8	11.6	2.2	0.8	1.6	2.1	4.7	8.4	11.4	18.9	38.2
Diseases of the respiratory system	1,179	100.0	2.7	2.4	0.9	0.6	0.8	2.0	2.6	9.4	22.6	30.4	28.2
Diseases of the arteries, veins, and capillaries	1,120	100.0	2.6	0.2	0	0.1	0.1	0.2	2.1	4.3	12.2	23.7	57.1
Homicides	985	100.0	2.2	0.5	0.7	1.3	22.8	26.9	21.2	13.0	9.2	2.9	1.3
Birth injuries and other diseases of early infancy	834	100.0	1.9	99.8	0.2	0	0	0	0	0	0	0	0
Diabetes mellitus	772	100.0	1.8	0	0	0.1	0.5	1.9	3.5	11.0	22.0	34.5	26.4
Suicides	630	100.0	1.4	. . .	. . .	0.8	15.6	17.0	19.0	22.1	14.4	7.8	3.3
Congenital anomalies	351	100.0	0.8	66.4	10.0	6.3	4.0	3.1	3.4	1.4	2.3	2.3	0.9

Source: G. E. Alan Dever in *Social Indicators Research* 2, pp. 460–461, 1976.

of the epidemiological model (Step two). Table 2-2 clearly shows that the major contributing factors to the selected diseases are deeply rooted in life style, environment, and human biology. It also indicates that the system of medical care organization has limited impact with respect to disease prevention.

In Table 2-2 the allocation of diseases to the four categories was achieved by polling 40 professionals and paraprofessionals to determine

Table 2-2 An Epidemiological Model for Health Policy Analysis—Disease Evaluation

Percent Distribution of Total Deaths*	Cause of Mortality	Percentage Allocation of Mortality to the Epidemiological Model**			
		System of Medical Care Organization	Life Style	Environment	Human Biology
34.0	Diseases of the heart	12	54	9	28
14.9	Cancer	10	37	24	29
13.4	Cerebrovascular	7	50	22	21
4.2	Motor vehicle accidents	12	69	18	1
3.8	All other accidents	14	51	31	4
3.8	Influenza and pneumonia	18	23	20	39
2.7	Diseases of the respiratory system	13	40	24	24
2.6	Diseases of the arteries, veins, and capillaries	18	49	8	26
2.2	Homicides	0	66	30	5
1.9	Birth injuries and other diseases of early infancy	27	30	15	28
1.8	Diabetes mellitus	6	26	0	68
1.4	Suicides	3	60	35	2
0.8	Congenital anomalies	6	9	6	79
	Percent Allocation—Average	11	43	19	27

*1973.
**Due to rounding, the percent allocation may not add to 100%.
Source: G. E. Alan Dever, *Social Indicators Research* 2, p. 462, 1976.

what factors of life style, environment, human biology, and system of health care organization contributed to each cause of mortality listed. The 40 responses were then summed and averaged to determine the potential impact of the four factors on each disease. It is recommended that, if an agency uses this model, it form a similar group of professionals to do this task. Though the analysis in Table 2-2 is subjective and, in most instances, judgmental, it does agree with the majority of medical literature.[18] [19] [20]

Step two, then, allows programmatic areas dealing with specific diseases to set priorities and to decide upon health policy. This type of health policy analysis may reveal gaps in the delivery of our health services. A reduction of mortality will undoubtedly occur only if the health program is proportionately directed toward each element of the epidemiological model.

A total of $29.2 billion was spent for health by the federal government in 1974. This amount was estimated to increase to $35.0 and $37.7 billion for 1975 and 1976, respectively.[21] Table 2-3 shows the distribution of federal outlays for health activities by category. In its present form, the table

Table 2-3 Federal Outlays for Medical and Health-Related Activities by Category (in millions of dollars)

	Outlays		
Health Programs	**1974 Actual**	**1975 Estimate**	**1976 Estimate**
Development of health resources, total	4,383	5,242	5,362
Health research	2,085	2,424	2,512
Training and education	1,146	1,324	1,145
Construction	761	967	1,108
Improving organization and delivery	392	527	596
Provision of hospital and medical services, total	23,918	28,783	31,348
Direct federal services	4,797	5,390	5,828
Indirect services	19,120	23,393	25,520
Prevention and control of health problems, total	888	1,019	989
Disease prevention and control	419	458	405
Environmental control	90	129	137
Consumer protection	378	432	446
Total, Health Programs	29,189	35,044	37,699

Note: Fiscal data are not available for Georgia, therefore, the U.S. fiscal data are used.
Source: Adapted from Federal Health Programs, Office of Management and Budget, Special Analysis K, Budget of the U.S. Government, 1976, p. 169.

provides very little information in terms of the proposed epidemiological model for health policy analysis. For this reason, Table 2-4 was prepared to correspond to the four elements of the epidemiological model (Step three). Over the three years, the majority of expenditures by the federal government, an average of 90.6 percent, was allocated to the system of medical care organization (Table 2-5). The elements of human biology, environment, and life style accounted for an average of 6.9 percent, 1.2 percent, and 1.5 percent, respectively.

Finally (Step four), a comparison of Tables 2-2 and 2-4 shows a disproportionate amount of money allocated for the system of medical care organization, despite the fact that the means for reducing mortality and morbidity are deeply rooted in Life Style, Environment, and Human Biology elements and that only minimal reductions in mortality and morbidity can be expected from the system of medical care organization (Table 2-5). The conclusion is obvious. Unless we dramatically shift our health policy from current procedures for reducing mortality and morbidity, we will see little or no change in our present disease patterns. In fact, with our aging population we might very well see dramatic increases in mortality and morbidity.

It is clear that present policies do not support methods most likely to improve health status. If, however, we apply the foregoing epidemiological model to health status (disease specific), we will have a basic framework for specifying goals and objectives. This will lead to recommendations for programming actions at the state and area levels to improve health status. The goals developed would relate to both health status and health system, the latter type describing the desired system and giving considerable attention to services for promoting health and preventing disease.

In any case, a major effort should be unleashed to engineer holistic and wellness policy statements. Without such an approach, we will continue our present tunnel-vision analysis, leading to greater dependence on the system of medical care organization, which includes the concepts of a growing medical technology and a concomitant increase in specialized manpower. This is a very mechanistic and reductionistic[22] avenue to medical care at a time when there is an essential need for a return to the "community."

The question that remains is, How do we change our short range, hedonistic model so that diseases resulting from life styles may be significantly altered or reduced? Two possibilities are social health marketing and social engineering.[23] [24] The major need, however, is to erase from our memory tapes the single cause/effect model and dependence on the physician to make us better. A new belief system is required which reflects

Table 2-4 Allocation of Federal Health Expenditures in Accordance with the Epidemiological Model for Health Policy Analysis; 1974, 1975 and 1976

Elements of the Epidemiological Model for Health Policy Analysis	Federal Outlay (in millions)		
	1974 Actual	1975 Estimate	1976 Estimate
Total federal health expenditures	29,189	35,044	37,699
Systems of medical care organization	26,216	31,601	34,197
Training and education	1,146	1,324	1,145
Construction of health care facilities	761	967	1,108
Improving organization and delivery	392	527	596
Provision of hospital and medical services	23,918	28,783	31,348
Direct federal services	4,797	5,390	5,828
Indirect services	19,120	23,393	25,520
Percent of total federal health expenditures	89.8%	90.1%	90.7%
Life style	420	458	405
Disease prevention and control	420	458	405
Percent of total federal health expenditures	1.4%	1.3%	1.1%
Environment	468	561	583
Environmental control	90	129	137
Consumer safety	378	432	446
Percent of total federal health expenditures	1.6%	1.6%	1.5%
Human biology	2,085	2,424	2,512
Health research	2,085	2,424	2,512
Percent of total federal health expenditures	7.1%	6.9%	6.7%

Source: G. E. Alan Dever, *Social Indicators Research* 2, p. 464, 1976.

holism and wellness and leads to less dependence on the physician and more dependence on the self to make us alive and well. The combination of a new health concept and a new belief system will result in a life which works with aliveness.

Application to U.S. Mortality, 1975

A refreshing and creative use of the epidemiological model for health policy analysis has been outlined by the Center for Disease Control.[25] Building on the initial model design by Dever, the Center analyzed the top

Table 2-5 Comparison of Federal Health Expenditures to the Allocation of Mortality in Accordance with the Epidemiological Model for Health Policy Analysis

Epidemiological Model for Health Policy Analysis	Federal Health Expenditures 1974-76 (percentage)	Allocation of Mortality to the Epidemiological Model (percentage)
System of medical care organization	90.6	11
Life style	1.2	43
Environment	1.5	19
Human biology	6.9	27
Total	100.2*	100

*Percentages do not add to 100.0 due to rounding.
Source: G. E. Alan Dever, *Social Indicators Research* 2, p. 465, 1976.

ten diseases by race and sex in terms of years of potential life lost (before age 75 and before age 65) and of total mortality of one-plus years of age. The data in Table 2-2 were used by the Center as the basis for the proportional allocation of the contributing factors of premature mortality to the four elements of the epidemiological model. The results for the ten leading causes of death among the total population of one-plus years of age, ranked by number of years of life lost before age 65 (United States, 1975), are given in Table 2-6. Figure 2-1 presents the data in Table 2-6 and graphically, showing differences when total mortality (one-plus years of age) and years of life lost (before age 75) are used as different points of departure. For the years of life lost before age 65, it is evident that life style and environment (53.1 percent and 21.7 percent, respectively) are significant factors contributing to premature mortality for the total U.S. population (Table 2-6). In contrast, the contributions from human biology and the medical care system are substantially lower.

Again, the conclusion is obvious. To reduce morbidity, mortality, and disability in this country, we must shift our resources. More importantly, we must change our belief systems.

SUMMARY

This chapter has proposed a new holistic epidemiological model to deal with present disease patterns. The elements of life style, human biology,

Table 2-6 Proportional Allocation of the Contributing Factors of Premature Mortality to the Four Elements of the Epidemiological Model. Ten Leading Causes of Death among the Total Population 1+ Years of Age Ranked by Number of Years of Life Lost before Age 65, U.S.A., 1975

Ten Leading Causes of Death	Years of Life < 65 Lost	%	Health System*	Life Style*	Environment*	Human Biology*
Cancer	1,802,820	17.5	10	37	24	29
Heart disease	1,769,180	17.2	12	54	9	28
Motor vehicle accidents	1,424,823	13.8	12	69	18	1
All other accidents	1,166,793	11.3	14	51	31	4
Homicide	621,846	6.0	0	66	30	5
Suicide	583,751	5.7	3	60	35	2
Cerebrovascular disease	352,524	3.4	7	50	22	21
Cirrhosis of the liver	320,457	3.1	3	70	9	18
Influenza and pneumonia	206,673	2.0	18	23	20	39
Diabetes	118,119	1.1	6	26	0	68
Percent Allocation—Average			9.8	53.1	21.7	16.8

Note: In the CDC report, the years of potential life lost were determined by computing the mean age of death for each cause, subtracting that number from either 65 or 75, and multiplying the difference by total number of cause-specific deaths. This was calculated for deaths of one-plus years.

*Percentages are based on Table 2-2.

Source: U.S. Department of HEW, PHS, Center for Disease Control. "Ten Leading Causes of Death in the United States, 1975." Atlanta, Georgia Bureau of State Services, Health Analysis and Planning for Preventive Services, p. 46, 1978.

environment, and system of medical care organization have been applied to the disease patterns of Georgia and the United States. The results clearly indicate that our present policies of allocating resources are not solving the existing problems.

We recommend that health policy analysts reconstruct this model and apply it with their own health agencies. A shift in our health policy is essential if we want to reduce morbidity, disability, and mortality. Such a shift, however, must be accompanied by a change in our belief systems. We are presently applying old solutions to new problems. What we need are new solutions (a new tunnel). Our memory tapes get stuck, and we

Figure 2-1 Proportional Allocation of the Contributing Factors of Mortality to the Four Elements of the Health Field Based on the Ten Leading Causes of Death Among the Total Population 1 + Years of Age, U.S.A., 1975

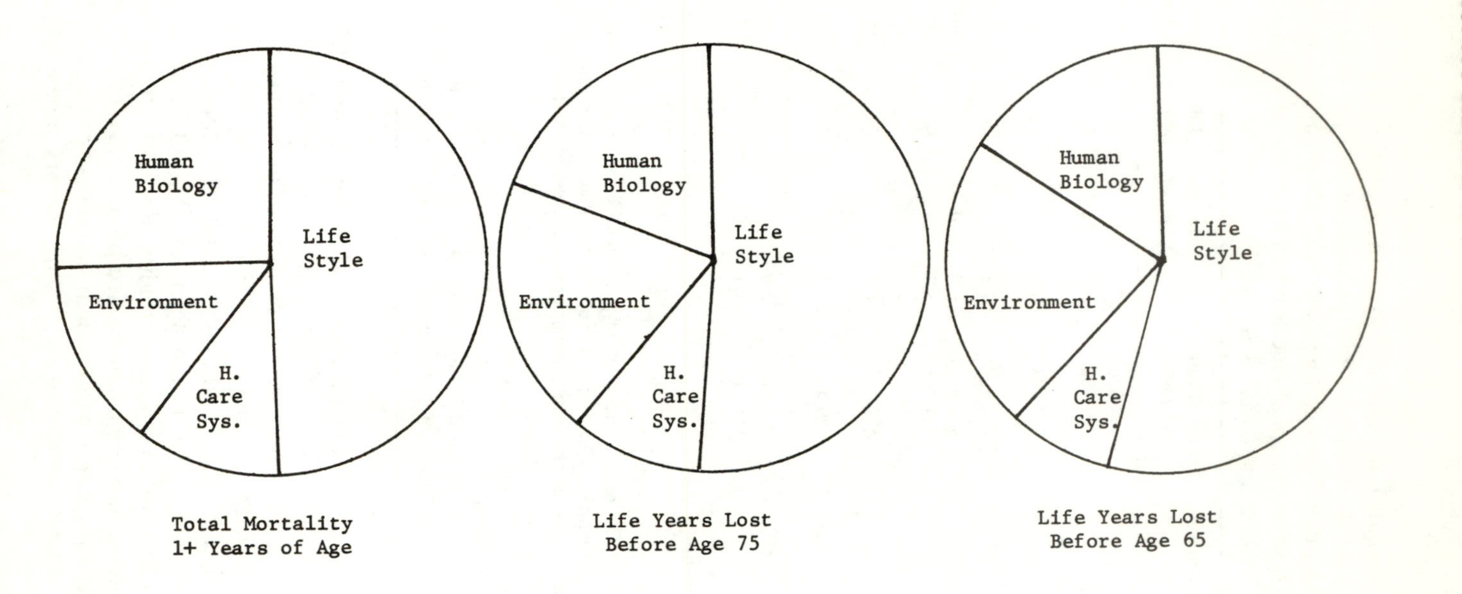

Source: U.S. Department of HEW, PHS, Center for Disease Control. "Ten Leading Causes of Death in the U.S., 1975." Atlanta, Georgia Bureau of State Services, Health Analysis and Planning for Preventive Services, p. 35, 1978.

continue to cut the ends off of something to make it fit. Our memory tapes prevent us from being alive, and our barriers keep us stuck in the tunnel. Two new approaches are critical to the development of a well population who are able to experience aliveness: New belief systems must be developed and our health policies must be changed to create a new context of health in the 1980s.

NOTES

1. Most of this chapter is based on an earlier article by the author (Dever, "An Epidemiological Model for Health Policy Analysis," *Social Indicators Research* 2 (1976): 453–466). Parts are taken from consultations with personnel of HSAs and public health departments.
2. M. R. Burt, *Policy Analysis—Introduction and Application to Health Programs* (Washington, D.C.: Information Resources Press, 1974), p. 136.
3. N. K. Newell, "Public Health Research: Possibilities and Opportunities," *WHO Chronicle* 29: 3–5.
4. Blum, *Planning for Health,* p. 622.
5. Burt, *Policy Analysis,* p. 136.
6. H. L. LaFramboise, "Health Policy: Breaking the Problem Down into More Manageable Segments," *Journal of the Canadian Medical Association* 108: 388–393.
7. Lalonde, *A New Perspective,* April 1974, p. 76.
8. Minister of Industry, Trade, and Commerce, *Perspective Canada: A Compendium of Social Statistics* (Ottawa: Information Canada, Office of the Senior Advisor on Interpretation, Statistics Canada, 1974), p. 321.
9. LaFramboise, "Health Policy," pp. 388–393.
10. Lalonde, *A New Perspective,* April 1974, p. 76.
11. Minister of Industry, Trade, and Commerce, "Perspective Canada," p. 321.
12. Dever, "The Future of Health Services in Georgia" (Paper presented at a Workshop on Change, Armstrong State College, Savannah, Ga., 1974), p. 15.
13. Dever, "Dimensions of Environmental Health" (Paper presented at the Georgia Public Health Association annual convention, Macon, Ga., 1974), p. 11.
14. U.S. Department of Health, Education, and Welfare, "Man's Health and the Environment—Some Research Needs," in *Report of the Task Force on Research Planning in Environmental Health Sciences* (Washington, D.C.: U.S. Government Printing Office, March 10, 1970), p. 258.
15. J. B. Cullingworth, ed., *Problems of an Urban Society,* vol. 3, *Planning for Change* (Toronto, Canada: University of Toronto Press, 1973), p. 195.
16. Alvin Toffler, *Future Shock* (New York: Random House, Bantam Books, 1970), p. 562.
17. Lalonde, *A New Perspective,* p. 76.
18. C. L. Erhardt and Joyce E. Berlin, eds., *Mortality and Morbidity in the U.S.,* Vital and Health Statistics Monographs, American Public Health Association (Cambridge, Mass.: Harvard University Press, 1974), p. 289.
19. J. M. Hunter, ed., *The Geography of Health and Disease,* Papers of the First Carolina Geographical Symposium (Chapel Hill, N.C.: University of North Carolina, 1974), p. 193.

20. A. M. Lillefeld and A. J. Gifford, eds., *Chronic Diseases and Public Health* (Baltimore: Johns Hopkins Press, 1966), p. 846.

21. Office of Management and Budget, *Special Analyses, Budget of the United States Government, 1976, Federal Health Programs, Special Analysis K, Feb. 1976*, pp. 169–196.

22. Reductionistic is defined here as an attempt by the medical establishment to reduce the physical, social, and mental well-being of individuals into very specific entities. It is also an attempt to explain away causes of diseases by simple means when, in fact, the causes are quite complex.

23. P. Kitler and G. Zaltman, "Social Marketing: An Approach to Planned Social Change," *J. Marketing* 35 (1971): 3–12.

24. G. Zaltman and I. Vertinsky, "Health Service Marketing: a Suggested Model," *J. Marketing* 35 (1971): 19–27.

25. U.S. Dept. of HEW, Public Health Service, Center for Disease Control, *Ten Leading Causes of Death in the United States, 1975* (Atlanta, Ga.: Bureau of State Services, Health Analysis and Planning for Preventive Services, 1978), p. 70.

Chapter 3

Planning and Evaluation for Health

Just as holism and wellness evolved from concern with the entire well-being of the individual, so must planning concern itself with the entire fabric of society and its institutions. Planning for one institution or for one dimension of health without full consideration of the interdependencies with other parts of society ignores the fact that the institution is part of a larger system. Community health must be planned with this concept of a system.

Van Gigch defines a system as "an assembly or set of related elements."[1] He explains that a system's elements can be concepts (as in language), objects (like a typewriter), subjects (as in a football team), or a combination of concepts, objects, and subjects (as in a man-machine system). A hospital is an example of the latter system, with the concepts of medical care, the objects of medical equipment, and the subjects composed of health workers, patients, and administrators. The system can be further divided into subsystems which, in turn, may become subsystems of some other larger system.

Ackoff defines the systems approach as focusing on "systems taken as a whole, not on their parts taken separately."[2] Such an approach concerns total-system performance where properties of the system can only be analyzed correctly from a holistic point of view. Even though every part of a system performs perfectly, if the total system is imperfectly organized it will not be able to attain its objectives because of the relationships between the parts.

Health, then, can be considered an element of a system called life. Indeed, as WHO recognizes, the holistic approach to health and health planning "conceives of health as the essence of productive life."[3] The medical care system is one element, or subsystem, within society which seeks to ensure the health of society's members. This subsystem interacts with other subsystems in carrying out society's goals. In planning for the health system, we must concern ourselves with the interactions both within the system (medical care) and with other systems (life style, environment, and biology).

In this chapter, rather than develop a step-by-step approach, we present a framework for the systems approach to holistic health planning. The community health planner is referred to the many excellent sources on planning for detailed steps in the planning process.[4 5 6 7 8]

PLANNING—A SYSTEMS APPROACH TO CHANGE

Several authors have offered excellent guidelines for a systems approach to health planning.[9 10 11 12] In this section, the systems approach is presented in terms of what Jantsch calls the "new" planning.[13] The three essential features of this approach are:

1. "The general introduction of *normative thinking* and *valuation* into planning, making it nondeterministic and futures-creative, and placing emphasis on invention through forecasting.
2. "The recognition of *system design* as the central subject of planning, making it nonlinear (i.e., acting upon structures rather than variables of systems) and simultaneous in its general approach; and, following from the two preceding points:
3. "The conception of three levels—normative or policy planning (the 'ought'), strategic planning (the 'can'), and tactical or operational planning (the 'will')—in whose interaction the 'new', futures-creative planning unfolds."[14]

If we consider these three features as forming a framework, we can develop a holistic approach to health planning:

1. Health planning should attempt to define what should be, rather than simply identify problems.
2. Health planners should free themselves from an incremental, systems improvement attitude and move to a creative, systems design approach. As Van Gigch indicates, systems improvement implies that the system is designed and that norms or standards (that is, memory tapes or belief systems) have been set and accepted, whereas systems design is a creative process that questions the assumptions upon which old forms have been built.[15] This means a rejection of an incremental approach and the acceptance of a holistic approach to health care, in which we become concerned with the design of a new system emphasizing prevention, productive living,

and the well-being of the whole person in relation to his or her environment.

3. Health planners must recognize the level of planning appropriate to a given situation. The situation is defined by the particular subject being planned for, by the organizations involved (both in planning and in carrying out the plans), and by the requirements to achieve successful change.

Three Levels of Planning

Policy Planning

The policy level of planning is the most conceptual, and the most important, in establishing the system design. It deals with society's value structure or what society considers to be important. Planning at this level is normative, idealistic, or futures-creative, dealing with what ought to be. It is defined by Hyman as goal-oriented planning or new system creating.[16] Emphasis is placed both on desired ends and on the means to these ends. Bailey defines a policy analysis model as involving ". . . a careful, logical analysis of a complex of different problems at the policy level . . . for the purpose of making all assumptions more explicit, recognizing constraints more clearly, drawing conclusions from the assumptions in a more reliable manner, and so on."[17]

Several models may be used, including the following:

1. Technical models, aimed at providing scientific understanding of behavior, for example, the population dynamics of diseases, and at forecasting possible outcomes of intervention with goals of optimum health. Demographic and manpower models fall in this category.
2. Systems models, dealing with interactions among technical models.
3. Information system models, dealing with the flow of information for decision making.[18]

At this level, epidemiological principles are most important to the planning process. Such principles aid in describing the distribution and size of disease and disability; in providing data for planning, implementation, and evaluation; and in identifying etiological factors.[19]

Kostrzewski notes the following:

> The health needs and demands of a population should be taken into account, and consideration should be given to health promotion and protection in all its aspects: prevention, restoration of impaired health, rehabilitation, and social welfare. Adequate in-

formation about the health services required should be collected and evaluated; this would include manpower, investment, equipment, financing, and management.[20]

At this level, the community establishes its values, goals, and objectives. At this level, too, a particular holistic model of health is adopted. Such a model will indicate the interactions of man with his social, psychosocial, and physical environment within a total system.[21 22 23 24]

Community involvement in policy planning is essential to establish the values and norms of the system. The health planning agency should seek the involvement of all relevant sectors of the community, including business and civic leaders, residents, and "victims."[25] In an early study of community health planning, several factors were found to be important in establishing an effective process. The major factors were the involvement and the influencing of economic, political, and professional sectors of the community and the recognition that health is only a part of the total community system.[26] Total community commitment to health values is attained in this phase. If not attained, consensus at a later time is often impossible to achieve.

Sigmond offers the following suggestions as steps toward more effective health planning:

1. Achieve a consensus.
2. Identify and fill in gaps in knowledge.
3. Assist health agencies.
4. Provide incentives.[27]

Each suggestion should relate to health goals as they provide for optimum health services.

Finally, at the policy level of planning, forecasting becomes essential to developing the succeeding levels. Forecasting is the process of modeling the likely future or anticipating what will happen or be in existence in a future period. Some indication of what the future will contain is a basic need in planning for the future. Although specific techniques of forecasting are not within the realm of this chapter, three broad approaches are possible:

1. Extrapolation of base data to the future. This can vary from simple straight-line extrapolation based on past history to complex multivariate predictive models involving causal assumptions, past trends, and indicators.

2. Delphi or the "expert opinion" forecast. The essential components of this approach consist of soliciting the opinions of many experts on a subject concerning future events, averaging the expectations, presenting the results, and reiterating the process to refine the forecast. Anonymity of responses is essential to the process. The result is an expert consensus of the future.
3. Brainstorming or an open discussion of forecasting. Members of a group present their opinions on future events and hold discussions to alter or accept specific opinions. As in the Delphi technique, consensus is sought, but individual responses are public, leading to possible domination of the forecast by a person with a strong personality or position of authority.

Each of these methods has strengths and weaknesses based on the desired results and the nature of the forecast. Brainstorming or Delphi techniques offer strength in areas where relatively little data are available to indicate trends or where causal relationships are unclear, whereas extrapolation techniques require good baseline data. Predictive models generally require an understanding of causal relationships and more extensive baseline data. The larger data base makes it possible to model future events more precisely and to alter certain variables more selectively so that the sensitivity of the model to changes in the predictive variable can be measured.

At the policy level, the emphasis is on design. Efforts are made to deal with what should be, rather than what is. This level deals with the "invention of anticipations, the design of social systems with preferred dynamic characteristics, the definition of roles for and the creation of institutions, and the feedback interactions between them."[28] Jantsch identifies institutions like education, the family, government, or religion as concepts; he defines schools, universities, marriage, forms of government, or churches as "instrumentalities," which become the means of implementing institutions.

Jantsch indicates how the policy level of planning is combined with the other two levels of strategies and tactics or operations (see Figure 3-1). Movement through the planning process proceeds from left to right and from top to bottom. Thus, at the policy level, society's values establish norms leading to anticipations, to understanding of the interdependencies of the total system, to systems designed to effect behavior, and to the creation of institutions. At this level, forecasting consists of the creation of anticipated futures, and planning deals with establishment of the total system and its dynamics. Decision making is the process of determining that a system causes behavior to change and of creating institutions to effect the change.

Figure 3-1 A Paradigm for Planning

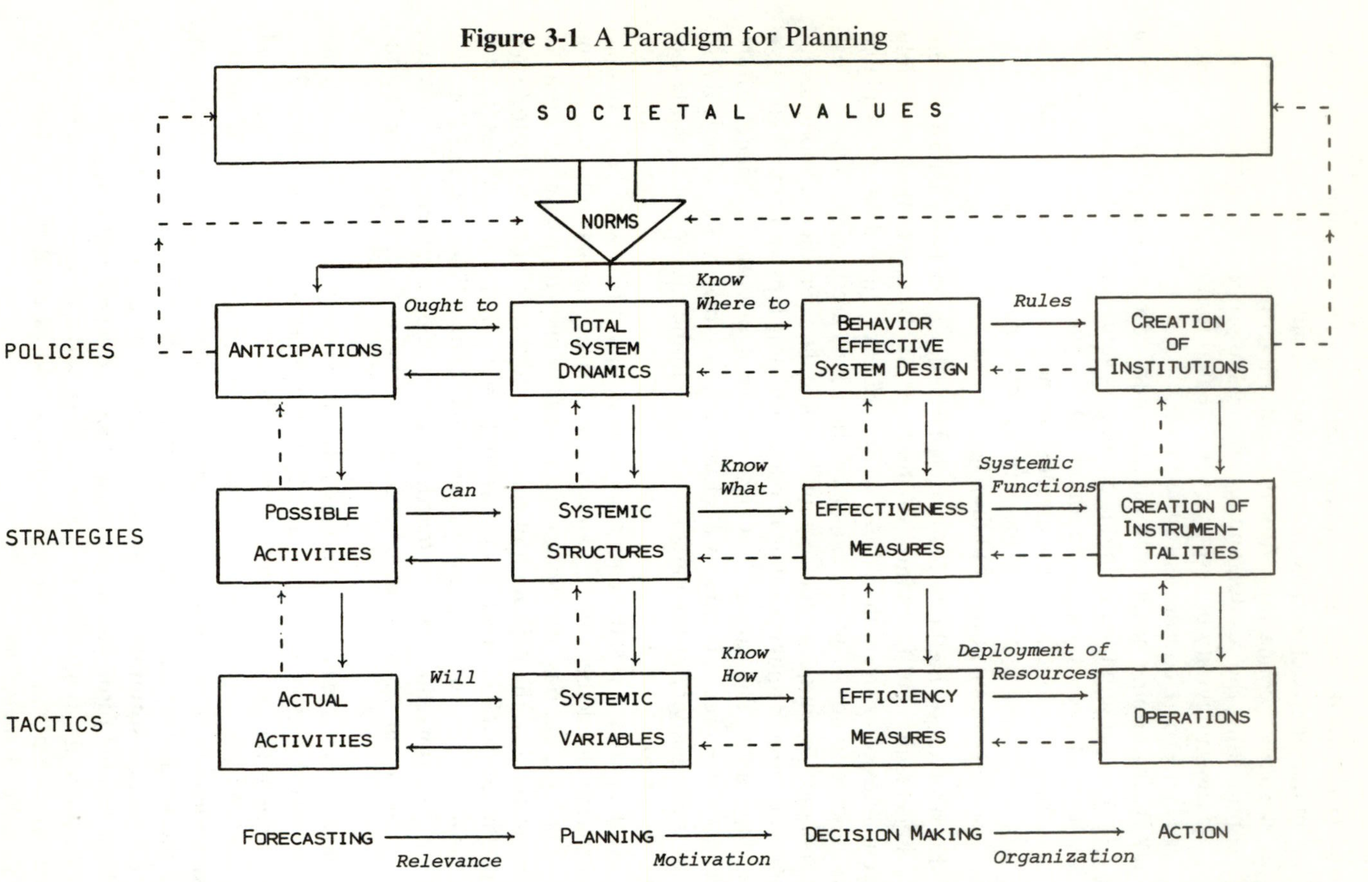

Source: Modified from Erich Jantsch, *Technological Planning and Social Futures* (London: Associated Business Programmes, 1972), p. 16.

Strategic Planning

Strategic planning is the "can" level of planning. Here we are dealing with "the conception of possible activities, their implications for system structures and system effectiveness, and the creation of instrumentalities. . . . Emphasis is on analysis: system analysis, policy analysis, need analysis, institutional analysis, market analysis."[29] At this point, "the community health planning body converts the general goals of the health aims of the community into specific objectives and criteria for health and health services which the community's operating or delivery systems will be asked to meet."[30] This would be equivalent to Sigmond's second element of planning: "advance thinking as a basis for doing"[31] or thinking about how to carry out plans.

At the strategic level, long-range goals are established and the possible means of achieving these goals are considered. As seen in Figure 3-1, strategic forecasting deals with the examination of possible activities to carry out the anticipations of society. From that point, specific system structures are established, effective outcome indicators are defined, and instrumentalities or means to operationalize institutions are created.

Operational Planning

The final level of planning consists of developing the detailed plans for carrying out the strategies developed at the second level. Blum indicates that, at this phase of planning, people and resources are organized to carry out the community's objectives.[32] Sigmond warns that "planning can be transmitted into action only by those with operational responsibility for the action."[33] Thus, at this level we are concerned with specific implementation of a plan or with what will be done. The final outcome is the operation of the system. The important point is that the operational plan must be implemented. To be capable of being implemented, it must fit within the operational framework of the organization.

Planning for Holistic Health

Each of the three levels of planning deals with specific requirements to bring about change in society. In the context of health, each level fits into a holistic health system plan (Figure 3-2).

At present, only the medical care system, the traditional boundary of health care planning, is involved in operational planning (the "will" aspect). Life style, environment, and biology are still evolving from the strategic level (the "can" aspect) and the policy level (the "ought to" concept). In other words, while our memory tapes or belief systems

Figure 3-2 The Traditional Relationship of Planning Levels to Holistic Health Components

LEVELS OF PLANNING

HOLISTIC HEALTH COMPONENTS

MEDICAL CARE SYSTEM

BIOLOGY, LIFE STYLE, ENVIRONMENT

OPERATIONAL

Manpower + *Technology, Transportation, Communication* + *Facilities* + *Financing*

CARE

SERVICES

DELIVERY

ORGANIZATION

+ CONSUMERS = MEDICAL CARE ORGANIZATION

HUMAN BIOLOGY

HEALTH

ENVIRONMENT

LIFE STYLE

Boundary of Medical Care System Planning

STRATEGIC

Surveillance and Control by Public Agencies (State Health Department City and County Health Departments Social Agencies)

Evaluation and Planning by Public Agencies (HSA, SHPDA)

POLICY

Public Policy Setting (SHCC, Boards, Legislative Bodies)

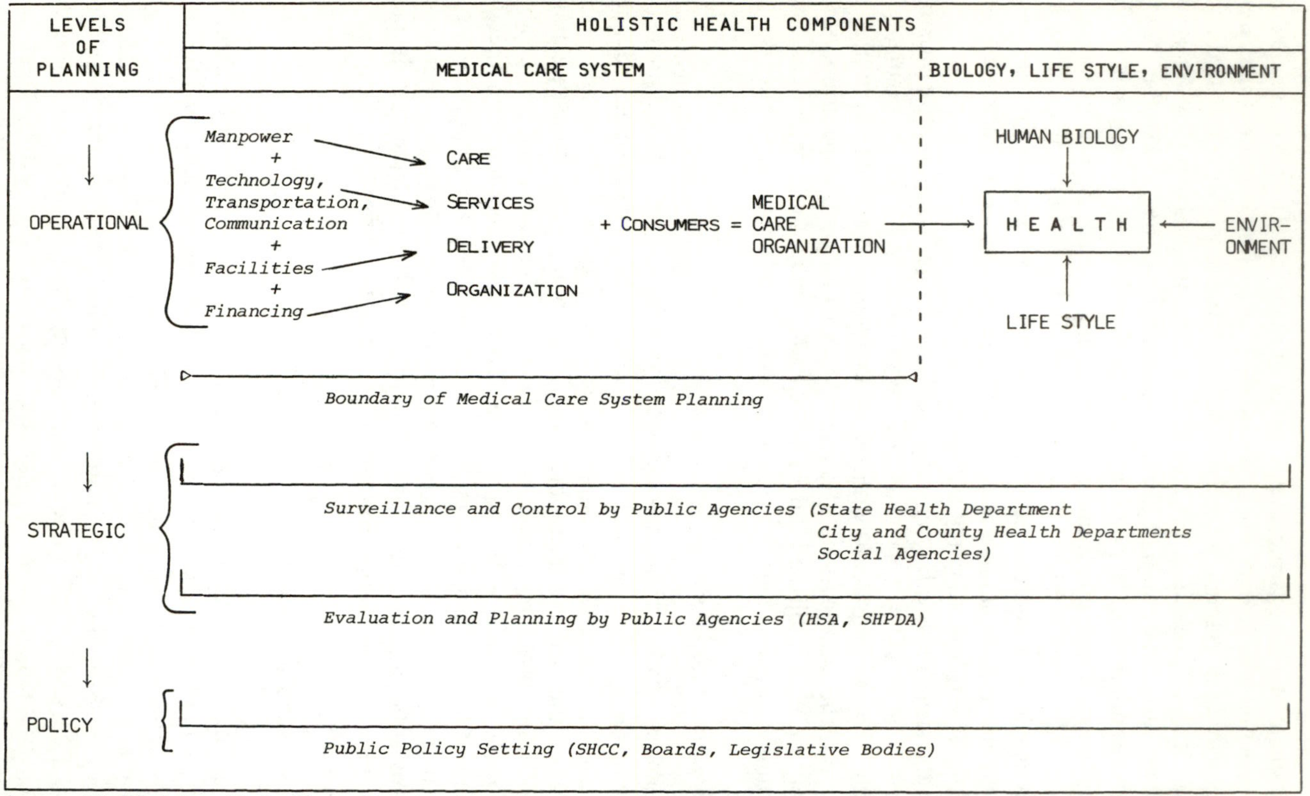

Source: Modified from H. L. Blum, *Planning for Health: Development and Application of Social Change Theory* (New York: Human Sciences Press, 1974), p. 278.

"will" ensure operational planning of the medical care system, we are just beginning to let go of the concepts of "can" and "ought to" for life style, environment, and biology. We have been stuck in our "tunnels" about the medical care system. To achieve holistic health, we will have to let go of the hope of "can" and "ought," operationalize all the components of holistic health, and move to the "will" level.

As we proceed from the broad area of policy planning to specific operational plans, we must focus on the details of how a change will be effected. Public policy setting (policy planning) deals with the broad goals of society. Strategic planning deals with specific objectives expressed in terms of what should be achieved. Operational planning deals with the mechanics of implementing the strategic plans.

In developing plans at all three levels, guidelines for health planning suggested by WHO may be useful in developing a holistic approach:

1. Planning should be population-based; that is, the population base or denominator must be appropriate.
2. Epidemiology and social studies are the fundamental health planning sciences, dealing with the behavior of diseases, individuals, and groups.
3. Indicators and proxy measures should be used for attributes and events that are not easy to measure directly.
4. Needs, resources, and uses must all be balanced, with attention paid to tradeoffs and system dynamics.
5. Health is conceived as "the essence of productive life." All sectors of society affect health.
6. Other sectors can substitute for the health sector in improving the health status of the population.
7. Resources within the health sector can be substituted for otherwise scarce resources (for example, a nurse providing primary health care).
8. Improvement in either productivity or efficiency is of little value if outcomes are not clearly beneficial.
9. Effectiveness must be measured in relation to target groups.
10. Objective evidence of benefits is necessary in assessing the efficacy either of intervention in treatment or of doing nothing.
11. Services must be appropriate to the existing circumstances, adequate, and acceptable.
12. What to do is more important than how to do it.
13. There must be clear ordering of means and ends.[34]

If these guidelines are combined with careful consideration of the planning aspects (policy, strategic, operational) and of the organization for which a plan is created, and if a systems design approach is followed, the developed plan should produce desired results.

APPLICATION OF THE PLANNING PARADIGM TO WELLNESS AND HOLISTIC HEALTH

Planning for Change

By applying Jantsch's planning model to the concept of high-level wellness in a community health care system, we can illustrate the systems design approach to health planning (Figure 3-3). The full development of the planning model through the various levels can produce the design of a health care system that reflects society's values. In the Figure 3-3 model, we find that people value a high quality of life, an opportunity for a productive life, wellness, and freedom from sickness. The associated norms of reduced morbidity, disability, mortality, and of increased levels of wellness become expectations in the model. At the policy level, anticipations of high-level wellness proceed dynamically through appropriate functions toward being and the achievement of a high-level wellness society. This holistic design leads to the creation of an institution called a "community health care system." In the second phase of planning, strategies that closely parallel the policy phase are determined. For example, anticipations of high-level wellness evolve to strategies of physical exercise, nutritional awareness, stress management, and self-responsibility. At this operational phase of the planning process, the activities become running, swimming, cycling, consumption of vitamins and healthful foods, and the development of coping skills. As actions, these activities put high-level wellness into day-to-day living and point up the need for individual responsibility and authority in the management of one's health. By developing a health care system reflecting these values, we have greater potential to meet the needs of society.

In contrast, the current health care system breaks down because it ignores the comprehensive interdependencies and feedback in the model. Note (Figure 3-4) the isolated boxes of system dynamics, system design, and health care system. Here we have what Jantsch calls the "technocratic type" of action[35] in which the emphasis is on technology's ability to accomplish all things and to cure all of society's ills (heart transplants, life-sustaining machines, pills, immunizations, bionics). The mere fact that we can do something implies that we ought to do it. No attention is paid to societal values; norms and anticipations depend only upon the technological ability to accomplish something.

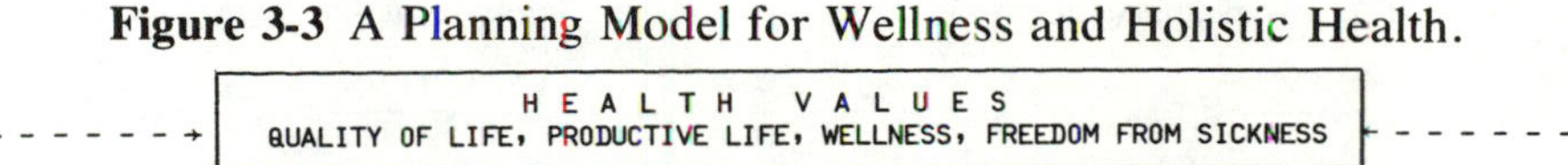

Figure 3-3 A Planning Model for Wellness and Holistic Health.

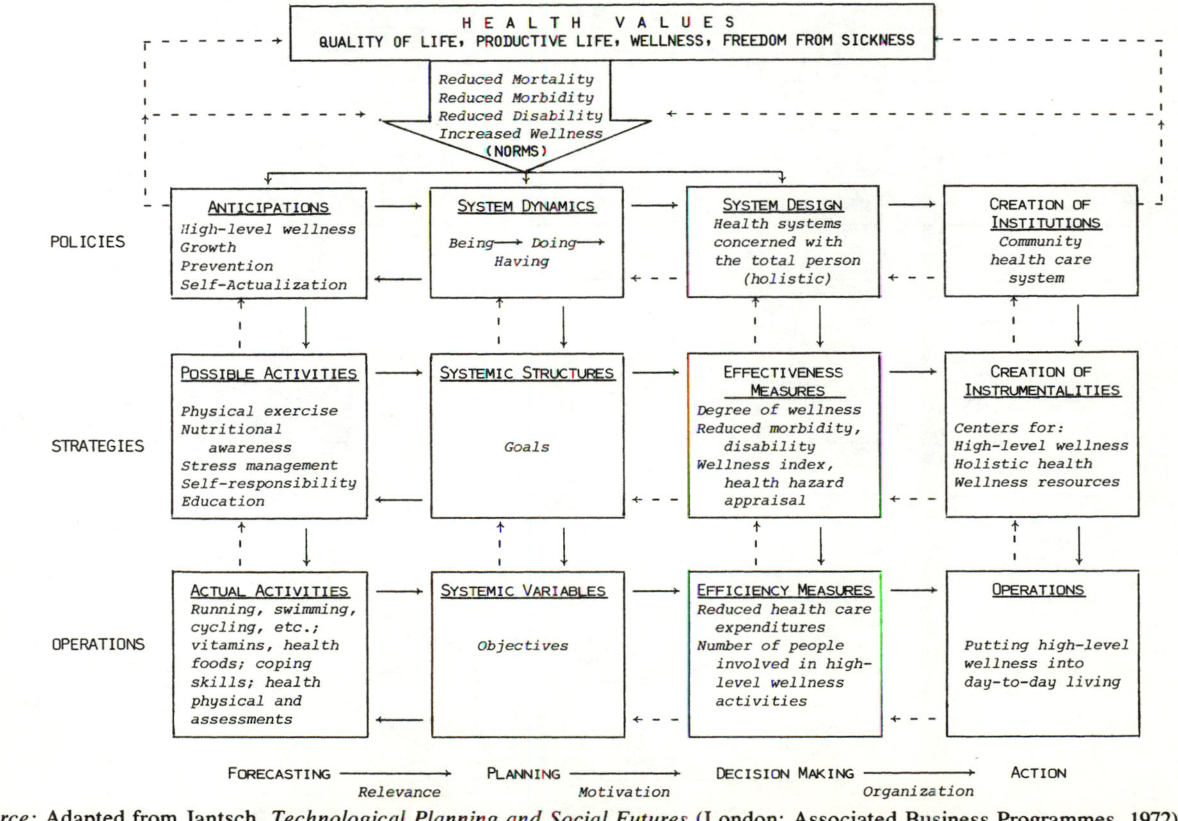

Source: Adapted from Jantsch, *Technological Planning and Social Futures* (London: Associated Business Programmes, 1972), p. 16.

Figure 3-4 The Traditional Planning Model for Medical Care

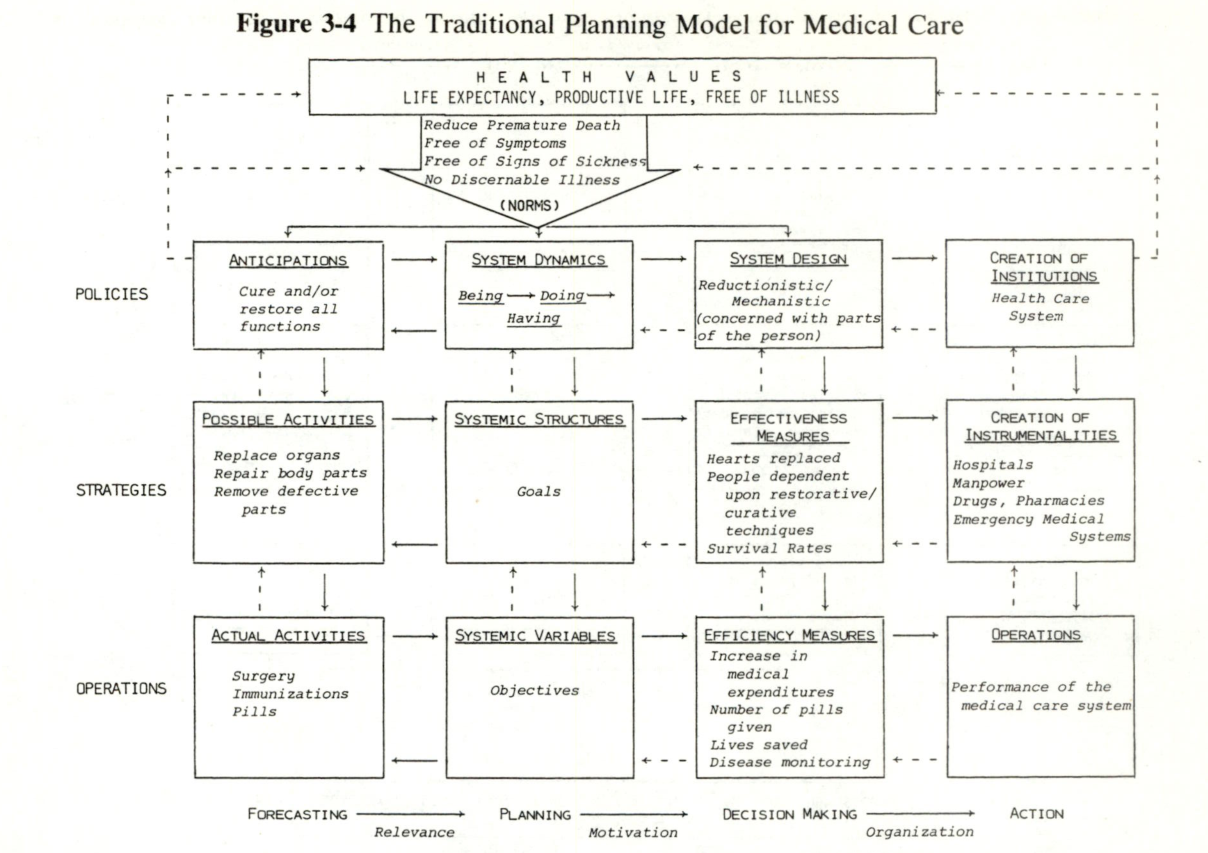

Source: Adapted from Jantsch, *Technological Planning and Social Futures* (London: Associated Business Programmes, 1972), p. 16.

Clearly, now is the time to plan for health from the holistic point of view, as outlined in the planning model for wellness and holistic health (Figure 3-3). Planning for change is the first major step toward the adoption of a holistic health plan.

Evaluation—Accounting for Change

The second step toward holistic health planning is evaluation or accounting for change.[36] Evaluation is essentially the ascertainment of the value or amount of success in achieving specific objectives. The actual processes of establishing objectives involve several facets, depending on the level of planning and operation as outlined in the previous section. Goals and objectives should be stated as comprehensively as necessary. The use of a holistic model to emphasize the interrelated aspects of environment, life style, human biology, and system of health care delivery requires the design of a system capable of reaching goals. Thus, the emphasis is on a comprehensive health policy which reflects desired program objectives.

Setting Realistic Objectives

The development of a comprehensive health policy requires data analysis and the use of the political process. Data analysis examines existing conditions, trends, and forecasts to determine community needs. An essential condition is the establishment of baseline or benchmark measures. This may be accomplished in either of two ways:

1. If prior knowledge or available data on the health status of the population being investigated are lacking, collect data for the first year of operation to establish a baseline for the following years.
2. If data are available, develop baseline or benchmark studies to establish past and present levels, making it possible to set realistic objectives to be attained at single and multiyear intervals. Essential to this analysis is regional access to timely, accurate, and reliable community-based data.

At this point, we must ask two very critical questions: What kinds of objectives should we select for inclusion in the health plan? and, How do we determine what level of attainment of objectives would be realistic?

The answer to the first question is a direct consequence of the adopted holistic health policy. If the health policy is broad and includes elements of the environment, biology, life style, and system of health care delivery, the objectives should reflect such a policy. Nontraditional as well as traditional objectives which have a decided impact on changing disease patterns should be identified. A parallel approach would be to identify the disease patterns (specific program problems) for each community—an obvious requirement but not always met.

As to the second question, the level of attainment of objectives may be derived from realistic assumptions (value-derived standards of expectations) or it may be determined quantitatively (by applying general, promulgated standards). In addition to baseline or benchmark measures, trends or standards for specified health-status measures must be determined as a basis for setting goals. For example, the reduction of the rate of infant mortality by 20 percent within the next year may be a totally unrealistic objective in light of the fact that the rate has been reduced by only 2 percent per year over the last ten years and is already below the national level. Thus, a review of past trends and promulgated standards can reveal appropriate targets or standards for the attainment of objectives. Another question to be considered is, What will happen if one does nothing? Will infant mortality continue to decrease by 2 percent anyway? If so, possibly a 3 percent decrease might be expected if a new program were implemented.

When setting objectives, remember that rates may change within certain probability limits. Accounting for such variations is another way to set realistic objectives. Readjustment of objectives is always feasible in the light of unforeseen issues which may surface to produce an impact on the program.

The political process recognizes the trade-off between the virtually unlimited needs and desires of a community and the scarcity of available resources. The objectives of any health improvement program must therefore be guided by the need to provide the greatest benefit at the least cost. More than likely, resources available to communities will decrease further in the 1980s, making it imperative to develop efficient and cost-effective programs. Data analysis will provide the framework for decision making, but ultimately the political process will participate in the determination of appropriate resource allocation based on a range of alternatives.

Types of Evaluation

Evaluation is impossible to achieve unless goals are related to the questions of what, how much, who, where, and when. Evaluation determines changes in health in terms of programmatic effects. The results become an input to the continuing process of planning, budgeting, and evaluation. Within the evaluation component are three areas of concern: costs, activities, and outcomes. These are more commonly called fiscal, process, and outcome evaluation:

- Fiscal evaluation focuses on and determines cost accountability.
- Process evaluation determines program activity in terms of (1) the population receiving the program, by age, sex, race, or other demographic variables; (2) the program organization, staffing, and funding; and (3) the program location and timing. Process evaluation is a measure of program efforts or proposed activities rather than program effects.
- Outcome evaluation delineates program objectives in terms of effects to determine if a change in health status has occurred as a result of the program.

The following observations are relevant to program evaluation:

1. Most management decisions are based on intuition rather than facts.
2. The purpose of evaluation is to answer the practical questions of administrators who want to know whether to continue a program, to extend it to other sites, to modify efforts, or to close it down.
3. Evaluation is more productive when it is a continuous process, with a continuous feedback loop to those administrators, supervisors, and program managers who make decisions. Routine evaluation reports should inform administrators about the efforts of policy and program decisions. They should alert supervisors to service delivery trends and point to problems calling for corrective action.

Comprehensive health program assessments are lacking. Perhaps this reflects a fear that programs will prove inadequate. Indeed, administrators, supervisors, and program managers may well perceive evaluation as a risky process, since it presumes that positions and programs may be reduced as well as increased.

Sometimes evaluation is undertaken for inappropriate reasons. Program decisionmakers may turn to evaluation to delay a decision ("Let's have a study!") or to legitimize a decision already made. Another problem is that most state agencies' information systems are not designed to provide the data needed for effective program evaluation. As less tangible performance objectives are addressed and outcome measurement criteria in certain areas become much less direct than economic factors, evaluation problems are compounded. Thus, failure to conduct program evaluation studies results, in large measure, because agencies feel threatened by such studies and because available data are inadequate for the purpose.

Too often, programs claim success because they completed proposed activities, such as testing or screening clients and providing specific hours of therapy (process evaluation), rather than because they showed demonstrable health improvements among the people being served (outcome evaluation). Health programming is characterized largely by evaluation of effort (process evaluation) rather than by assessing whether or not program services were effective in decreasing the negative consequences of disability, morbidity, and mortality (outcome evaluation).

The introduction of fiscal, process, and outcome evaluation objectives into an organization will produce the following changes:

1. Program planning will be improved as administrators formulate program objectives more precisely, specify plans to achieve objectives, and monitor progress toward accomplishing objectives.
2. Management practices will be improved as administrators, supervisors, and health program managers have greater access to evaluation and control data to assist them in the planning and direction of their own work as well as in assessing the work of others.
3. Information provided by evaluation allows state and other health agencies to make more timely and relevant reports to the general public and to legislative bodies. This information is becoming more and more critical; legislators are becoming increasingly suspicious of programs that rely on appeals to sympathy and humanitarian concerns but fail to demonstrate concrete accomplishments.

An Evaluation Model for Community Health Agencies

The key components of an evaluation model for community health agencies are (1) monitoring results (fiscal and process evaluation) and (2) assessing change (outcome evaluation). In the context of the planning model previously presented, the evaluation process focuses on the system's relationship to societal values and on the full interdependencies of the system.

Monitoring Results

The first level of evaluation looks at the details of operations. The concern here is with inputs and processes. Two types of evaluation are relevant: process and fiscal. The relationship of the planning model for wellness and holistic health to the evaluation process is shown schematically in Figure 3-5. In this model, social values are used to establish specific health status goals. The goals consist of broad statements relating

Figure 3-5 A Schematic Showing the Relationship of the Planning Model for Wellness and Holistic Health to the Evaluation Functions

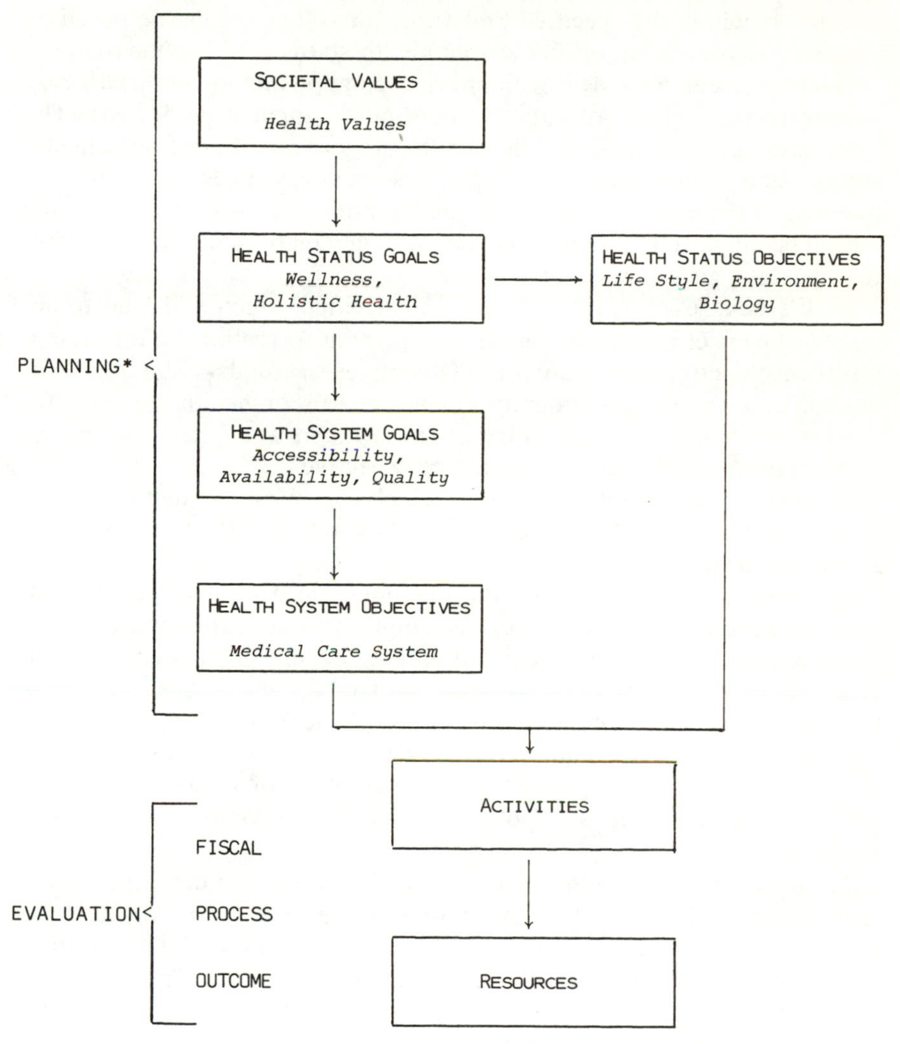

*See Figure 3-3 for the complete Planning Model for Wellness and Holistic Health.

to the long-range objectives of the planning model for wellness and holistic health—reduced mortality, morbidity, and disability, and increased wellness. Within the health system, these goals incorporate major inputs of specific health status and health system objectives. Health status objectives include short-range desired changes in a population's health status, for example, a 2 percent reduction in infant mortality or a 30 percent increase in participation in a physical exercise program. The objectives must take into account the population's present health status and be achievable within the specified time frame, and they should be based on long-term achievement of the desired health status goal (wellness).

Health system goals deal with specific components of the health care system (accessibility, availability, continuity, quality, and cost). The basic assumption must be that the health care system influences the health status of the population. Although this has not always been true, it is more likely to be the case if we have designed our health care system through a logical planning and system design process, guided by social values rather than technological brilliance.

At the next level, activities must be specified which will lead to accomplishment of the objectives. It is important to realize the distinction between objectives and activities. Objectives are ends—statements of desired changes in a community's health status or health system. Activities are specific actions which must be taken to achieve objectives; they represent the process of obtaining objectives.

At the final level are the resources which must be expended to accomplish activities. These may consist of dollars, human effort, or any other method of producing activity.

Proceeding upwards through the planning and evaluation levels, one can perceive certain underlying assumptions: the expenditure of resources will cause activities to occur and the occurrence of activities will cause objectives to be accomplished. Part of the evaluation process is concerned with ascertaining the validity of these assumptions.

At the first level of evaluation, we are concerned with the bottom two steps in the evaluation process, the expenditure of resources and the performance of activities, involving two different kinds of evaluation: fiscal and process.

Fiscal evaluation asks these questions: (1) Were resources expended in a planned manner? (2) Did the expenditure of these resources result in the occurrence of planned activities? (3) Was the expenditure of the resources the most efficient means of assuring the desired activities? The first question is the easiest to answer. The answer is obtained by comparing planned or budgeted expenditures with actual expenditures. Although one of the easiest methods of fiscal evaluation, it is most often overlooked. The key to this evaluation step is that resources have been expended for planned activities and not for extraneous purposes, that is, that other miscellaneous items do not draw upon resources budgeted to achieve the specified activities. The second question looks at whether or not activities occurred as a result of the expenditure of resources. Here it is important to separate activities that would have occurred regardless of expenditures and those that resulted directly from planned expenditures. Further evaluation of such activities will occur at the process level. The third question addresses both the actual cost of accomplishing activities and alternative costs. A commonly used measure here is the cost per unit of activity, for example, the cost per patient served.

Process evaluation deals with activities that are planned to occur. Results are determined by comparing these planned activities with accomplished activities, as in the ratio: Actual activities/Planned activities × 100 = Percentage attainment of activities.

Process evaluation is the most frequently conducted evaluation, possibly because of its basic simplicity. It assumes that planned activities will result in achieving objectives (which must be separately addressed in outcome evaluation). Process evaluation is conducted for two basic reasons: (1) as a means of monitoring results continuously during the duration of a program, thus providing evidence of program operation and a method of program control; and (2) because it can be easily accomplished and, if causal assumptions are correct, can serve as an early indicator of program outcome.

Several examples of process evaluation are available in the recent literature. For example, Barbas and McGill report on an evaluation of a referral monitoring process in EPSDT screening:[37] Three different groups of children in a Texas health program were identified. Group I children were selected from referrals made in a period prior to the project's beginning. Group II children were screened immediately following the project start-up, with welfare workers assisting clients in initiating the diagnosis and treatment indicated in the screening. Group III children were drawn from another project area that was essentially the same as that of Group II except that welfare workers assisted continuously from initiation of referral through completion of treatment. Results indicated that children in Groups II and III were more likely to reach treatment than those in Group I. No significant differences, however, could be detected in the continuing treatment process. This lead the authors to conclude that, once the treatment state is reached, a child is likely to complete treatment regardless of continuous care monitoring. These results indicate that the additional time and expense of care monitoring may not be cost-effective.

Assessing Change

After monitoring results to achieve process and fiscal evaluation, the next stage of evaluation is the assessment of change. Here we are concerned with program outcomes and with the testing assumptions that resources and activities have accomplished objectives. The first step at this level of evaluation is to determine the outcomes desired from a program. From this point, planned accomplishments can be compared to actual accomplishments. Program goals at this stage must be specific, a requirement that is not always met. Unless specific goals are established, however—either explicitly or implicitly—evaluation is impossible; if nothing is planned, there is simply nothing to evaluate.

Weiss[38] has proposed certain steps in conducting outcome evaluations:

1. *Formulate program goals.* Goals must be clear, specific, and measurable; and they must address program consequences or outcomes.
2. *Choose specific goals to evaluate.* Choices are guided by: (1) usability and practicality (Will the evaluation of a goal prove usable to the community or organization, and is evaluation of the goal possible?); (2) relative importance (Is attainment of a goal important enough to a community to make it worthwhile to spend valuable resources in an evaluation study?); (3) incompatibilities (Are the goals to be evaluated compatible with each other? Or is the desired outcome of one goal the opposite of that for a second goal?); (4) short-term or long-term goals; evaluation of long-term impacts is clearly desired, although there may be an immediate need for evaluation based on short-term results.
3. *Establish measurement yardsticks.* What yardstick will measure successful achievement of a goal? Will 2 percent reduction in mortality be sufficient, or must 10 percent be the goal?
4. *Determine unanticipated outcomes.* Unplanned program effects are very likely to occur and may be either negative or positive. All unplanned effects are not necessarily bad, however; many desirable unplanned achievements may result from specific programs.
5. *Develop indicators of outcomes.* What will measure outcome achievements? Here several issues arise: (a) The development of measures. What is the appropriate means of measuring an outcome or indicator of income? (b) Multiple measures. Several indicators should be measured to gain a better understanding of outcomes. These can then be continued to indicate overall program success. (c) Proximate measures. When goals are very long range, it is often necessary to use proxy measures to evaluate short-range outcomes with the assumption that achievement of these short-range goals will result in the achievement of long-range results. (d) Types of measures. Effects may be measured (1) on the persons served (measurement of changes in patient health status, attitudes, values, and skills must reflect the goals of the organization); (2) on agencies (assessing the effect of goals that seek to change institutions, for example, by

making them more responsive or by offering specific services); (3) on larger systems (some goals seek to change relationships within a network of agencies or an entire community; assessment of such goals must be made at this level); or (4) on the public (if the program goals are to change public opinion, public opinion surveys are appropriate).

Hatry et al. specify some guidelines to identify program objectives, evaluation criteria, and client groups for evaluation at this level:

1. Identify objectives and evaluation criteria that are people-oriented. The impact on a community's citizens should be the first concern of any evaluation. The evaluation should cover the public conditions which the program is designed to change. Exhibit 3-1 suggests characteristics that evaluation criteria should address.
2. Explicitly consider potential ''unintended'' consequences of programs, particularly negative effects. Nearly all programs have some negative effects. These should be explicitly identified and, if possible, eliminated. If it is not possible to eliminate them, careful consideration of their negative effects will at least help to put the overall worth of a program into perspective.
3. Consider more than one objective and one evaluation criterion. Since a program will normally have several purposes, the full effects of the program must be considered. Rarely will a program be adequately described with a single objective, and rarely can a single evaluation criterion measure a program impact.
4. Do not reject evaluation criteria because of apparent difficulties in measuring them. It is more important to identify the criteria for evaluating a program and then to deal with problems of measurement as the evaluation proceeds.
5. Too many objectives and criteria are better than too few. Often it is difficult to determine which objectives or criteria may be important as the evaluation proceeds.
6. Specify client groups on whom the analysis should attempt to estimate program impacts. Target groups for whom the program is designed must be specified and effects evaluated for these specific groups. Typical client group classifications are: residence location, sex, age, race, education, employment status, income, family size, and handicap groups.
7. Always include dollar costs as one criterion. All resource expenditures should receive fiscal evaluation.[39]

Exhibits 3-2 and 3-3 provide guidelines to identify evaluation criteria and to select the final set of measures.

Exhibit 3-1 Characteristics That Evaluation Criteria Should Address

1. To what degree does the service meet its intended purposes, such as improving health, reducing crime, or increasing employment?
2. To what degree does the program have unintended adverse or beneficial impacts? For example, does a new industry increase water and air pollution or cause inconvenience to citizens?
3. Is the quantity of the service provided sufficient to meet the needs and desires of citizens? What percent of the eligible "needy" population is actually served?
4. How fast does the program respond to requests for service?
5. Do government employees treat citizens who use the service with courtesy and dignity?
6. How accessible is the service to users?
7. Do citizens who use the service, or who might use the service, view it as satisfactory?
8. How much does the program cost?

Source: Reprinted from *Program Analysis for State and Local Governments* by Harry Hatry et al., by permission of the Urban Institute, copyright 1976, Washington, D.C., p. 38.

Exhibit 3-2 Questions to Help Identify Objectives, Evaluation Criteria, and Client Groups

1. What are the purposes of the program? Why was it (or should it be) adopted?
2. What is to be changed by the program, in both the immediate future and the long run? How would the program manager know if the program was working or not working? What would be accepted as evidence of success?
3. Who are the targets of the program? Is the community as a whole likely to be affected either directly or indirectly? Who else might be affected by the program?
4. What are possible side effects, both immediate and long-run?
5. What would be the likely consequences if the new program were introduced or if an existing program were discontinued? What would be the reaction of citizens in the community? Who would complain? Why would they complain? Who would be glad? Why?

Source: Reprinted from *Program Analysis for State and Local Governments* by Harry Hatry et al., by permission of the Urban Institute, copyright 1976, Washington, D.C., p. 48.

Exhibit 3-3 Criteria for Selecting Final Set of Measures

Importance

Does the measure provide useful and important information on the program which justifies the difficulties in collecting, analyzing, or presenting the data?

Validity

Does the measure address the aspect of concern? Can changes in the value of the measure be clearly interpreted as desirable or undesirable, and can the changes be directly attributed to the program?

Uniqueness

Does the information provided by the measure duplicate or overlap with information provided by another measure?

Accuracy

Are the likely data sources sufficiently reliable or are there biases, exaggerations, omissions, or errors which are likely to make the measure inaccurate or misleading?

Timeliness

Can the data be collected *and analyzed* in time for the decision?

Privacy and Confidentiality

Are there concerns for privacy or confidentiality which would prevent analysts from obtaining the required information?

Costs of Data Collection

Can the resource or cost requirements for data collection be met?

Completeness

Does the final set of measures cover the major aspects of concern?

Source: Reprinted from *Program Analysis for State and Local Governments* by Harry Hatry et al., by permission of the Urban Institute, copyright 1976, Washington, D.C., p. 48.

EVALUATION DESIGNS

Figure 3-6 presents five evaluation designs for identifying and quantifying program effects brought about by the program. The figure also includes procedures and applications in using the designs.[40 41]

Design 1.—Before versus After Program Comparison

Purpose

This design compares program results of the same geographical area, measured at two points in time—before the program begins and after its implementation. Though this is a common design, it is often difficult to separate the effects of program activities from other influences. The design is very practical for the health agency because of time availability and personnel limitations. Next to Design 5, it is the simplest and least expensive evaluation. The agency should use this design extensively in its annual implementation plan.

Procedures

1. Identify appropriate goals, objectives, and evaluation criteria.
2. Obtain the values of these criteria at a point before the program begins and after it is implemented.
3. Compare "before" and "after" program data to estimate changes brought about by the program.

Applications

This design is appropriate when the duration of program is short and of narrow scope (for example, an intensive health promotion campaign, physical exercise program). It is also appropriate when conditions are stable over time (that is, it should not be distorted by seasonal changes, such as immunizations or influenza would be).

Design 2.—Time Trend Projection of Preprogram Data versus Actual Postprogram Data

Purpose

This design compares actual postprogram data to estimated data from a number of time periods prior to the program. Changes are identified as actual differences versus what they are estimated to be by the projections. To utilize this design in an HSA, the following should be considered:

Figure 3-6 Five Evaluation Designs to Identify and Quantify Program Effects

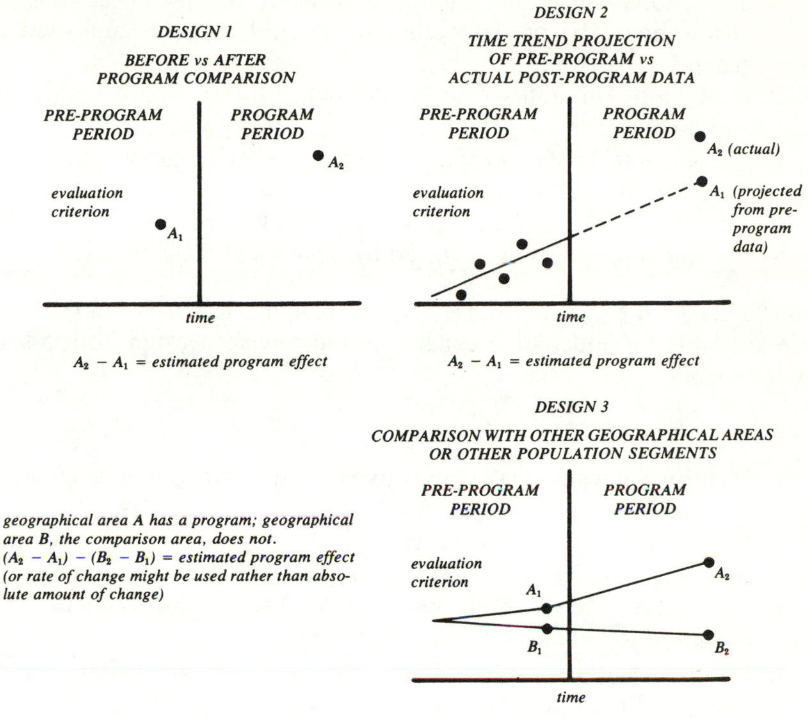

DESIGN 4

CONTROLLED EXPERIMENTATION
COMPARISON OF PRE-ASSIGNED SIMILAR GROUPS
ONLY ONE OF WHICH IS SERVED BY THE PROGRAM

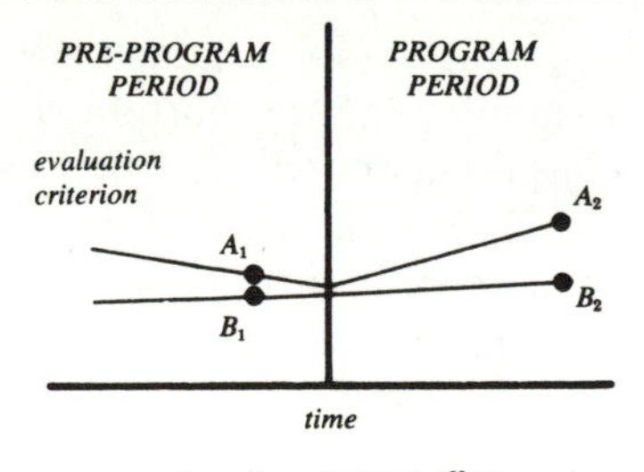

$A_2 - B_2$ = program effect

DESIGN 5

PLANNED vs ACTUAL PERFORMANCE

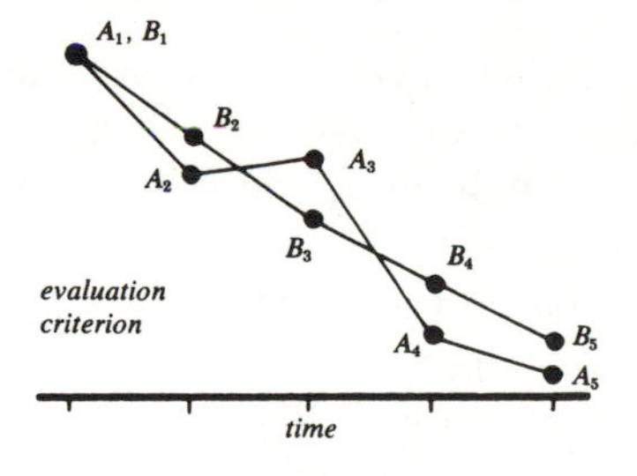

planned performance (B)
actual performance (A)
(A/B) X 100 = percent of performance level achieved or percent of objectives targeted

Source: Adopted and reprinted from *Practical Program Evaluation for State and Local Government Officials* by Harry Hatry et al., by permission of the Urban Institute, copyright 1973, Washington, D.C., p. 42.

1. The statistical variations in the data must be accounted for by aggregating time periods or geographical areas. If not accounted for, projections will be misleading or possibly invalid. That is, several years should be used together or several counties analyzed as a group.
2. Projections, in addition to being linear ($Y = a + bX$), may also be curvilinear ($Y = ab^X$, $Y = aX^b$).
3. Statistical tests of significance can help verify the appropriateness of the projections.
4. Added data collection for prior years will be required.
5. Technical expertise is required for statistical projections.

The health agency can use Design 2 if technical expertise and resources are available for added data collection. Otherwise, Designs 1 or 5 should be followed.

Procedures

1. Identify relevant goals, objectives, and corresponding evaluation criteria.
2. Obtain data on each of the criteria at several intervals prior to the program and after implementation.
3. Using statistical methods and the data, make projections to the end of the period covered by the evaluation.
4. Compare actual and projected estimates of numerical changes resulting from the program.
5. Look for other plausible explanations for the changes.

Applications

This design is very useful for health programs demonstrating underlying long-term trends (up or down), for example, infant mortality, major causes of mortality, and hospital needs assessment (that is, bed needs). The design's projections need not be based only on time trends but can also be based on changing demographics and disability dysfunctions for special social groups. An example is the changing distribution of age, sex, and racial characteristics in urban and rural settings.

Design 3.—Comparison with Other Geographical Areas or Population Segments Not Served by the Program

Purpose

This design compares evaluation criteria by utilizing data from two geographical areas or population groups, that is, where the program is operating and where it is not operating. It is necessary to identify similar areas or groups and to collect comparable data from the two geographical areas or population groups. These segments must be matched as closely as possible to reduce the effects of the evaluation criteria on the program.

Procedures

1. Identify relevant goals, objectives, and corresponding evaluation criteria.
2. Select other similar geographical areas or population groups within the same geographical area where the program is not operating.
3. Obtain data on each of the evaluation criteria for the geographical areas or population groups. Do this from a point before implementation of the program to the time of evaluation.
4. Compare the rate and magnitude or amount of change for the geographical areas or population groups.
5. Look for plausible explanations for changes or criteria other than the program.

Applications

This design is very useful for HSA evaluation and for evaluation of state health programs. One can compare program effects for one county or service area compared to another, or for similar population groups compared to each other within the same county. It is recommended that this design be used in association with Designs 1 and 5 to ensure reliable measures of program efforts. That is, the health agency should concentrate on Designs 1 and 5 and then employ Design 3, using standardized and available data sources (infant mortality, utilization rates, physician ratios, and so forth).

Design 4.—Controlled Experimentation

Purpose

This design compares preselected, similar groups, some of whom are served and some of whom are not served. The critical aspect is that the comparison groups be randomly assigned before program implementation so that the groups are as similar as possible except for the program treatment. The reason for this is that members may respond differently if they know they are part of the experiment (the Hawthorne effect). Also political problems or pressures may make it difficult to provide a service to one group and not to another. An HSA will rarely do this kind of controlled experimentation.

This design is the best of the five presented. It is also the most difficult and costly to undertake. It is *not* highly recommended for use by HSAs.

Procedures

1. Identify relevant goals, objectives, and corresponding evaluation criteria.
2. Select the groups to be compared (control and experimental groups) through a random probability sample.
3. Measure the preprogram performance of each group.
4. Apply the program to the experimental group.
5. Monitor the experiment to see if any actions distort the findings.
6. Measure the postprogram performance of each group.
7. Compare the prechanges versus postchanges in the evaluation criteria for these groups.
8. Look for plausible explanations for differences between the two groups.

Applications

This design is used typically in evaluation of clinical research and community medicine programs. It can be used when a program is introduced into only one county or area and not into others. It presents a variation for the HSA when comparing different geographical areas or counties within a community under controlled circumstances. Government programs, however, frequently are presented in limited areas because of limited resources that must be allocated on a priority basis.

Design 5.—Comparison of Planned versus Actual Performance

Purpose

This design compares preprogram planned targeted objectives to the actual program performance. It requires that realistic goals or targets be established for the evaluation criteria. Thus, the establishment of targets is likely to become an important issue. The design assumes that the targets that are set are the best available. If, however, the evaluation is not seriously applied, such goalsetting may not be taken seriously.

Procedures

1. Identify relevant goals, objectives, and corresponding evaluation criteria.
2. Set specific goals or targets for these criteria for specific time periods.

3. Obtain data on actual performance after the time period (quarterly).
4. Compare the actual performance to the planned targets.
5. Look for plausible explanations for changes in the criteria other than the program.

Applications

This design establishes targets that are the best available indicators of what actual accomplishments should be. It can be used widely and regularly once provision is made for regular collection of the data needed (for example, monthly health program activity reporting) in process evaluation.

Evaluation Overview

To summarize, Designs 1, 3 and 5 are the most practical for a health agency and should be used regularly and extensively. Each of these designs may be applied with limited resources and minimal personnel, or they may be used in combination to estimate the net efforts of a program. Design 2, although practical, requires more sophistication and expertise than a small health agency staff would have available. Design 4 is the best of the five, but it is the least appropriate for health agency application because such agencies rarely do programs of controlled experimentation.

As a health program management tool, evaluation must demonstrate its worth. It must lead to reduced costs or increased benefits (fiscal evaluation), improved effectiveness (process evaluation) and be related to changed health status (outcome evaluation). Seldom can one be absolutely positive a change in health status has been due to a program's effects, but effective evaluation may resolve uncertainties.

SUMMARY

Typically, planning for one institution or for one dimension of health without acknowledging the interrelationships with other areas—such as life style, environment, and biology—results in a very atomistic or reductionistic approach to the problem. The planning model presented in this chapter recognizes the shortcomings of the single-shot effort. Consequently, it represents a systematic approach to the achievement of our norms of reduced disability, morbidity, and mortality and of increased levels of wellness. In this way, the assessment of change (what needs to be done) becomes a major steppingstone to change and to further accounting for change (evaluation). Some researchers hold out little hope for wellness and holistic health. These individuals are too hasty in their judgment. The movement and acceptance of wellness into our daily life styles is a long-term diffusion process. No one can expect all individuals to adopt wellness practices when their belief systems provide them with conflicting values.

Thus, the changing of belief systems is a long-range goal, and one should be willing to let this process be slow and insidious. After all, the present diseases are just that—their onset is slow and insidious. We must have faith. We are trying to turn around behavior patterns which have been established for years, and thus it will take years to develop change. Let's not leave this wellness tunnel before we get to the cheese. Let's not be judgmental and make what we are doing right and what others do, wrong. That would be a sure and direct route to failure. Of course, this does not mean all wrong behaviors are to be given carte blanche. If the cheese is in the tunnel, individuals will find it.

NOTES

1. John P. Van Gigch, *Applied General Systems Theory* (New York: Harper and Row, 1974), p. 2.

2. Russell L. Ackoff, "Towards a System of System Concepts," *Management Science* 17, no. 11 (July 1971): 661–671.

3. WHO, *International Collaborative Study of Medical Care Utilization, Health Services: Concepts and Information for National Planning and Management* (Geneva: World Health Organization, 1977).

4. Henrich L. Blum, *Planning for Health: Development and Application of Social Change Theory* (New York: Human Sciences Press, 1974), p. 622.

5. William Shonick, *Elements of Planning for Area Wide Personal Health Services* (St. Louis: C. V. Mosby Co., 1976), p. 227.

6. Herbert H. Hyman, *Health Planning—A Systematic Approach* (Germantown, Md.: Aspen, 1975), p. 460.

7. A. D. Spiegel and H. H. Hyman, *Basic Health Planning Method* (Germantown, Md.: Aspen, 1978), p. 500.

8. A. Donabedian, *Aspects of Medical Care Administration—Specifying Requirements for Health Care* (Cambridge, Mass.: Harvard University Press, 1973), p. 649.

9. Blum, *Planning for Health*, pp. 251–344.

10. N. T. J. Bailey, "Systems Modelling in Health Planning," in *Systems Aspects of Health Planning*, N. T. J. Bailey and M. Thompson, eds. (Amsterdam: North Holland Publishing Co., 1975), pp. 7–11.

11. Shonick, *Elements of Planning*, p. 227.

12. Hyman, *Health Planning*, pp. 371–416.

13. Erich Jantsch, *Technological Planning and Social Futures* (London: Associated Business Programmes, 1972), p. 14.

14. *Ibid.*
15. Van Gigch, *Applied General Systems Theory,* p. 2.
16. Hyman, *Health Planning,* p. 67.
17. Bailey, "Systems Modelling in Health Planning," p. 9.
18. *Ibid.*
19. Jan Kostrzewski, "Uses of Epidemiology in the Planning and Evaluation of Health Care Systems," in Bailey and Thompson, eds., *System Aspects of Health Planning,* pp. 227–237.
20. *Ibid.,* p. 233.
21. Blum, *Planning for Health,* pp. 2–11.
22. J. N. Morris, *Uses of Epidemiology,* 3rd ed. (Edinburgh: Churchill Livingstone, 1975), pp. 173–180.
23. M. Lalonde, *A New Perspective on the Health of Canadians* (Ottawa: Office of the Canadian Minister of National Health and Welfare, April 1974), p. 76.
24. G. E. A. Dever, "An Epidemiological Model for Health Policy Analysis," *Social Indicators Research* 2 (1976): 453–466.
25. Blum, *Planning for Health,* p. 89.
26. Community Action Studies Project, *Action Planning for Community Health Services* (Washington, D.C.: Public Affairs Press, 1967), p. 21.
27. Robert M. Sigmond, "Health Planning," in *Dimensions and Determinants of Health Policy,* William L. Kissick, ed., Milbank Memorial Fund Quarterly 46, no. 1, pt. 2 (January 1968): 91–117.
28. Jantsch, *Technological Planning and Social Futures,* p. 18.
29. *Ibid.,* p. 19.
30. Blum, *Planning for Health,* p. 5.
31. Sigmond, "Health Planning," p. 92.
32. Blum, *Planning for Health,* p. 5.
33. Sigmond, "Health Planning," p. 95.
34. WHO, *International Collaborative Study,* pp. 108–114.
35. Jantsch, *Technological Planning and Social Futures,* p. 20.
36. G. E. A. Dever and Charles M. Plunkett, "Evaluation in Community Health—An Overview," in *A Companion to the Life Sciences,* S. B. Day, ed. (New York: Van Nostrand Reinhold, 1979), pp. 93–97.
37. Nancy Barbas and Laurilynn McGill, "An Exploratory Study of the Effects of Monitoring Referrals in EPSDT Screening," *American Journal of Public Health 68,* no. 10 (Oct. 1978): 1021–1023.
38. Carol H. Weiss, *Evaluation Research: Methods of Assessing Program Effectiveness* (Englewood Cliffs, N.J.: Prentice Hall, 1972), pp. 24–59.
39. Harry Hatry et al., *Program Analysis for State and Local Governments* (Washington, D.C.: The Urban Institute, 1976), pp. 37–55.
40. Harry Hatry et al., *Practical Program Evaluation for State and Local Government Officials* (Washington, D.C.: The Urban Institute, 1973), pp. 39–70. Adopted with permission.
41. S. M. Shortell and W. C. Richardson, "Evaluations Designs," *Health Program Evaluation* (St. Louis: C. V. Mosby Company, 1978), pp. 38–73.

Chapter 4

Basic Statistical Measures for Community Health Analysis

THE ROLE OF STATISTICS IN COMMUNITY HEALTH ANALYSIS

Statistics is the science of measuring population characteristics. It is the means of establishing baseline characteristics, measuring change, or testing hypotheses. It forms the cornerstone of quantitative evaluation techniques. Above all, it allows inferences to be made to a large population from a small sample of the population through application of probability concepts and distributional characteristics. Today, statistics is playing an increased role in all aspects of community health, including planning and evaluation, as well as in epidemiology and the other health sciences. Statistics is the tool for community health analysis.

In this chapter, basic concepts and applications of statistical methods are presented, with particular application to community health analysis. The reader is referred to the many excellent statistical texts on the market for detailed discussion of specific techniques.

Descriptive Statistics

"The major emphasis of statistical descriptive techniques is to take a large mass of useful but poorly organized information [health] data and condense it so that the basic characteristics of the data are clearly evident."[1] Descriptive measures form the basis for establishing the characteristics and describing the health status of a population. Several basic concepts must be understood before such analysis is undertaken. In this section, the most commonly used descriptive measures are presented, together with a discussion of the underlying concepts important to these measures.

The Frequency Distribution

The frequency distribution is a table in which all scores are listed in one column and the number of individuals or events receiving each score appear as frequencies in the second column. The result is a simple frequency distribution, where the score range is ranked from high to low in one column and the frequencies are listed in the second column. A grouped frequency distribution establishes class intervals of equal width in one column, and the corresponding frequencies are listed in another column. The rules for constructing class intervals in a grouped frequency distribution are these:

1. In general, there should be between 10 and 20 class intervals based on the optimal number that will efficiently summarize the data without distorting its shape. Too few intervals compress the data, concealing meaningful changes in its shape; too many stretch out the data, creating unnecessary gaps.
2. The width of the class interval is a function of the range of the raw scores and the number of class intervals desired. To illustrate, if the raw score range were $75 - 15 = 60$, and the researcher wants about ten class intervals, then: $60 \div 10 = 6$. Thus, a class interval width of six is obtained.

As an example, for a count of live births in a community, Table 4-1 shows a frequency distribution by age of mother. We can see that the largest number of births occurred in the age group 20–24 and the next largest number in age group 25–29, and so on. This kind of information

Table 4-1 Frequency Distribution of Live Births by Age of Mother

Age of Mother	Number of Live Births
10–14	607
15–19	18,071
20–24	27,419
25–29	21,246
30–34	8,566
35–39	2,420
40–44	536
45 up	28

Source: Georgia Vital and Health Statistics, 1976, Division of Physical Health, Georgia Department of Human Resources, p. 140.

would not be available from raw data. A graphic technique to show this distribution would mark off class intervals on a horizontal axis and frequencies on a vertical axis, as demonstrated in Figure 4-1.

One of the most common frequency distributions is the normal distribution, which forms the basis for statistical inference and hypothesis testing. Figure 4-2 illustates normal, positively skewed, negatively skewed, and uniform distributions.

Measuring Distributions

All distributions can be described by measures of central tendency and dispersion.

Figure 4-1 Frequency Distribution of Live Births by Age of Mother

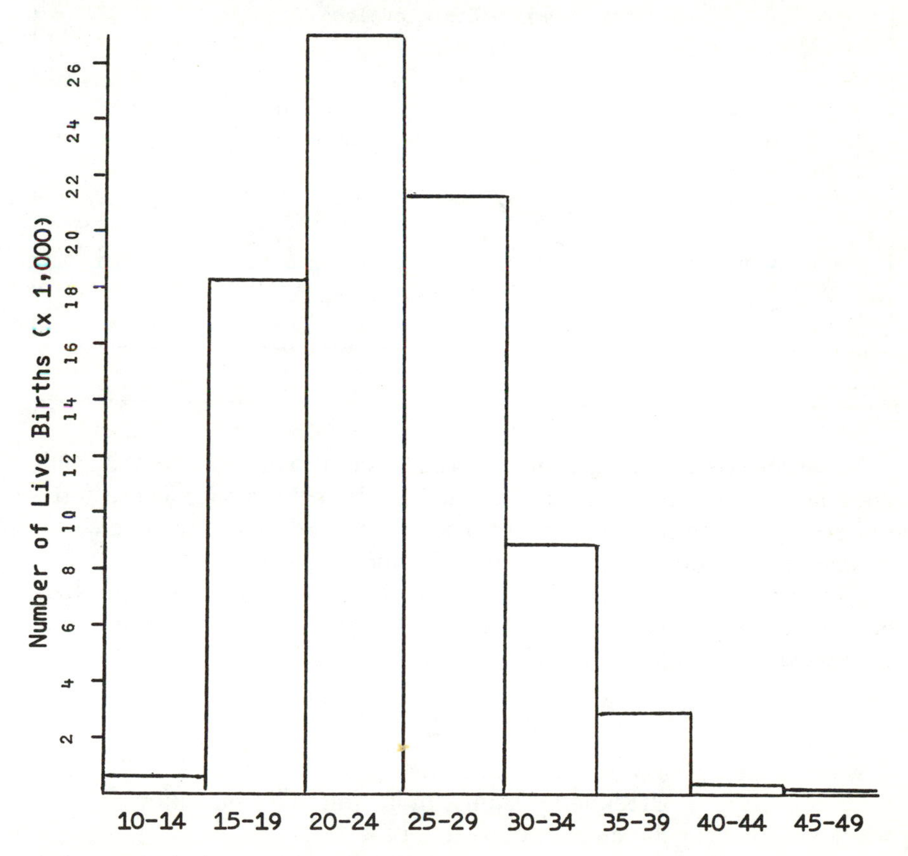

Source: Author's adaptation of Table 4-1.

Figure 4-2 Types of Frequency Distributions

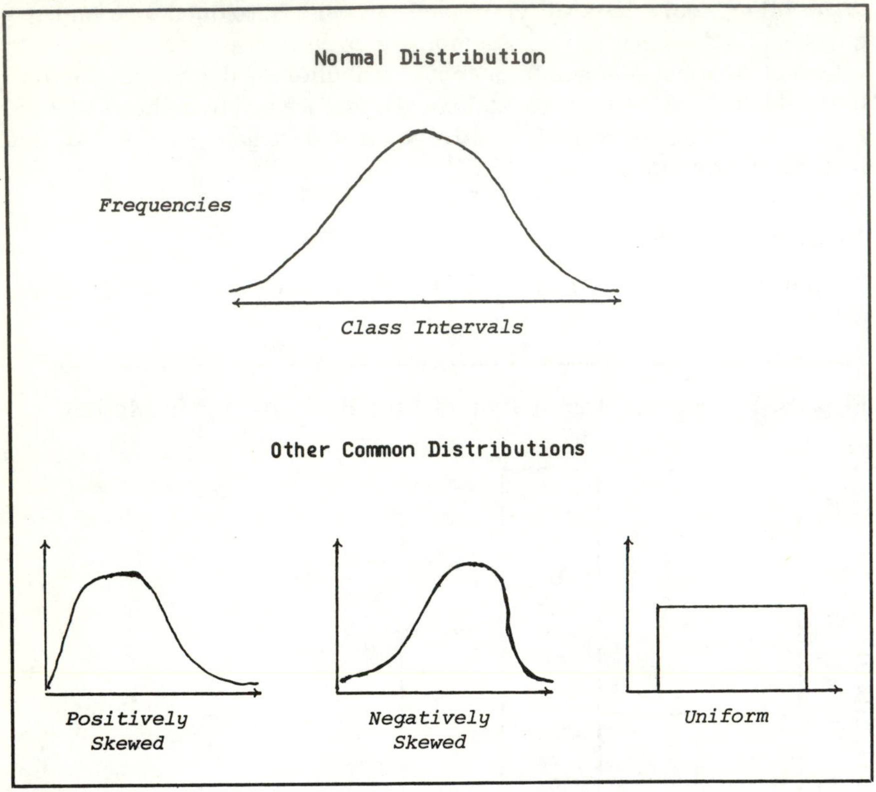

Normal Distribution

Frequencies

Class Intervals

Other Common Distributions

Positively Skewed

Negatively Skewed

Uniform

Measures of Central Tendency. Three basic measures of central tendency are the arithmetic mean, the median, and the mode. These three measures are the most commonly used, although there are others, for example, the geometric mean and the harmonic mean.

The arithmetic mean is often referred to as the simple average. It is computed by summing the values of all observations and dividing by the number of observations. Thus:

$$\langle X \rangle_{av} = \sum X/n$$

where: $\langle X \rangle_{av}$ = arithmetic mean or average (*av*)
$\sum$ = Greek letter sigma, indicating the summation
n = the number of values of X
$\sum X$ = sum of the n values of X

For example, suppose we had the following mortality rates for a group of ten census tracts or counties: 16.0, 12.0, 14.0, 6.0, 8.0, 9.0, 9.0, 10.0, 11.0, 10.0. Then:

$$\sum X = 16.0 + 12.0 + 14.0 + 6.0 + 8.0 + 9.0 + 9.0 + 10.0 + 11.0 + 10.0 = 105$$

$$n = 10$$

$$\langle X \rangle_{av} = 105/10 = 10.5$$

The value 10.5 is the arithmetic mean of the distribution of mortality rates.

An alternative way of determining the mortality rates for the census tracts would be to determine the total number of deaths for the ten tracts, divide by the population at risk, and multiply by a constant. The result is a mortality rate per 1,000 population for the ten census tracts. However, much of the data that health planners are able to collect requires calculating the average rate for an aggregate number of geographical units or time periods.

In the normal frequency distribution, the mean is the center of the distribution. In the skewed or nonnormal distribution, the mean is shifted by the large number of low or high value observations.

The median is the midpoint of a distribution. Like the mean, it represents an average value; but unlike the mean, the median is not influenced by the values of each observation. The median is constructed so that one-half the observations are above it and one-half below. Thus, in the distribution of mortality rates above, we would find the median by ordering the observations from low to high: 6.0, 8.0, 9.0, 9.0, 10.0, 10.0, 11.0, 12.0, 14.0, 16.0. Since we have ten values, the median would lie between the fifth and sixth values. In this case, it would be equal to ten.

The mode represents the most frequently occurring value in a distribution. In the previous example, the mode would be nine or ten, since each appears twice (a bimodal distribution) and no other value appears more than once. The planner should be aware that, in the normal distribution, the mean, median, and mode are all equal.

Isaac[2] has the following suggestions for selecting the appropriate measure of central tendency:

1. Compute the arithmetic mean when any of the following conditions apply:
   a. "The greatest reliability is wanted. The mean usually varies less from sample to sample when they are drawn from the same population."

b. "Other computations, such as finding measures of variability, are to follow."

c. "The distribution is symmetrical about the center, and especially when it is approximately normal."[3]

2. Compute the median when any of the following conditions apply:

a. "There is not sufficient time to compute the mean."

b. "Distributions are markedly skewed. This includes the case in which one or more extreme measurements are at one side of the distribution."

c. "We are interested in whether cases fall within the upper or lower halves of the distribution and not particularly in how far from the central point."

d. "An incomplete distribution is given."[4]

3. Compute the mode when any of the following conditions apply:

a. "The quickest estimate of central value is wanted."

b. "A rough estimate of central value will do."

c. "We wish to know the typical case."[5]

Measures of Dispersion. Although measures of central tendency provide some indication of the average value of a distribution, we gain no information about how values are distributed about this mean. Values may be clustered very closely to the mean, or they may be scattered over a broad range. In other words, we do not know how representative the mean may be of the distribution. When values cluster closely about the mean, it is an effective representation of the distribution; when values are scattered broadly, it is less representative. The range, standard deviation, and coefficient of variation are three measures of dispersion in a distribution.

The range is the simplest measure of dispersion to compute. It measures the difference between the lowest and the highest values in the distribution. It is computed by subtracting the lower value from the higher value. It is thus based only on the extreme values of the distribution.

The standard deviation, the most important measure of dispersion about the mean, forms the basis for most statistical analysis. It consists of the square root of the sum of the squared deviations of each value from the mean, divided by the number of observations, or:

$$S = \sqrt{[}\sum_{i=1}^{n} (X_i - \langle X \rangle_{av})^2]/n$$

where: S = standard deviation

$(X_i - \langle X \rangle_{av})^2$ = the mean value $\langle X \rangle_{av}$ from the value of X_i, then squared

n = number of observations

The standard deviation indicates the degree of dispersion about the mean value of a distribution. One unique property of the standard deviation in the normal distribution is that 68 percent of the observed values will fall within one standard deviation on either side of the mean, 95 percent within about two standard deviations, and 99 percent within three standard deviations. As we shall see later, this property has important consequences for testing hypotheses and significance levels through statistical analysis.

The coefficient of variation is appropriate when comparisons are being made between two populations with differing means. This measure of dispersion adjusts the standard deviation for the mean value and is computed as follows:

$$CV = S/\langle X \rangle_{av}$$

where: CV = coefficient of variation
S = standard deviation
$\langle X \rangle_{av}$ = mean

The coefficient of variation is often expressed as a percentage by multiplying the computed value by 100.

Inferential Statistics

When measuring a population rate, such as an infant mortality rate, we would like to estimate the true rate for the population. Since we are unable to measure every value in the population, however, we take some smaller number of measurements, and from these we estimate the true mean. Thus, when we wish to determine a population mean or some other population parameter, we usually take a small sample of the total population and estimate the true population mean from the sample. If we were to take all possible samples of a given size from the same population, we would get a distribution of sample means with the shape of a normal distribution. Regardless of the shape of the population distribution, however, the distribution of the sample means will be about normal. This is expressed in the *central limit theorem,* which states that for almost all populations the sampling distribution of the means will be about normally distributed, given a sufficient sample size. Sufficient sample size is generally considered to be 30 or more elements. This theorem allows inferences to be drawn about population means and mortality rates from information extracted from samples in time or space.

Like a population distribution, a distribution of sample means has a variance associated with it. The *variance of the sample mean* is equal to the variance calculated from a sample divided by the size of the sample used to calculate the variance, or:

$$S_{\langle X \rangle av}{}^2 = S^2/n$$

The square root of the variance of the sample mean is called the *standard error of the mean* and is denoted with the symbol $S_{\langle X \rangle av}$

$$S_{\langle X \rangle av} = \sqrt{S^2/n)} = S/\sqrt{(n)}$$

where: $S_{\langle X \rangle av}$ = standard error of the mean
S = standard deviation
$\sqrt{}$ = square root
n = number of observations

The standard error of the mean is the statistic that permits statements to be made regarding population estimates of the true mean with specified levels of confidence. For example, suppose we took a sample of 100 people at a health clinic and asked them how long they had been waiting before receiving service. We may have found a mean waiting time of 15 minutes, with a standard deviation of 5 minutes. The standard error would be calculated:

$$S_{\langle X \rangle av} = S/\sqrt{(n)} = 5/\sqrt{(100)} = 5/10 = \tfrac{1}{2}''$$

where:

$S_{\langle X \rangle av}$ = standard error
S = sample standard deviation
n = sample size

Using the standard error, we can calculate that if we took all possible samples of size 100 from the population of clinic patients, 68 percent of the sample means would be within ±½ minute of the true mean, and 95 percent would be within ±1 minute [2 × (½)] of the true mean.

Estimating Population Parameters—A Computing Guide

In this section, a computing guide is offered to enable one to construct confidence intervals in estimating population parameters. The interested reader is advised to consult elementary statistics texts for a complete discussion of each topic covered. The following material has been excerpted from several sources.[6 7 8]

Confidence Interval Estimate of the Mean

If we take a sample and compute its mean, we have a point estimate of the population mean. Though we do not have the true population mean, we do know that about 95 percent of all possible sample means will lie between ±2 standard deviations of the true mean. Given this information, we would like to estimate the range within which the true population mean lies. This range is called the confidence interval. If we compute the confidence interval about the sample mean, $CI = \langle X \rangle_{av} \pm 2\,(S_{\langle X \rangle_{av}})$, we can be 95 percent confident that the true mean lies within this interval. This implies that 5 percent of the time the true mean will be outside this range. If a 5 percent error is not acceptable, we can move out to ±3 standard errors from the sample mean and gain a 99 percent confidence interval.

If we have a narrow confidence interval, we can say that the sample mean is close to the population mean under consideration. For example, suppose we had a population sample size of 100 for which the mean $\langle X \rangle_{av} = 10$ and the standard deviation = 3. The 95 percent confidence interval would be:

$$CI = \langle X \rangle_{av} \pm 2\,(S_{\langle X \rangle_{av}})$$

$$S_{\langle X \rangle_{av}} = S/\sqrt{(n)} = 3/\sqrt{(100)} = 3/10 = .333$$

$$\langle X \rangle_{av} \pm 2\,(S_{\langle X \rangle_{av}}) = 10 \pm 2(.333) = 10 \pm .667$$

$$95\%\ CI = 9.333 \text{ to } 10.667$$

where:
$\langle X \rangle_{av}$ = sample mean
$S_{\langle X \rangle_{av}}$ = standard error of the mean
S = sample standard deviation
n = sample size
CI = confidence interval

Thus, we are 95 percent confident that the true mean lies within the interval (9.333, 10.667).

Confidence Intervals for a Population Rate

Method 1. If we have computed a rate for a population at a point in time, we can consider this rate as a sample estimate of the true rate or as a sample in time or space, thereby allowing us to use confidence interval estimations. An estimate of the true rate reflects the true rate plus random error. To construct a confidence interval for the rate, we use the following formula:[9]

$$\text{95\% confidence limits:}$$
$$\text{Upper limit} = 1{,}000/n\,[d + 1.96\sqrt{(d)}]$$
$$\text{Lower limit} = 1{,}000/n\,[d - 1.96\sqrt{(d)}]$$

where: d = number of deaths upon which rate is based
n = denominator of rate (i.e., the target population)

The step-by-step procedure is shown in Exhibit 4-1.

If the death rate is greater than 100 per 1,000, replace $\sqrt{(d)}$ with $\sqrt{d[1-(d/n)]}$. If the rate is of some base other than 1,000 (10,000 or 100,000), exchange this base for 1,000 above. The procedure for calculating 95 percent confidence intervals using Method 1 is illustrated in Exhibit 4-2.

Exhibit 4-1 Steps in Calculating a Confidence Interval for a Population Rate

1.	Find the square root of *d*.	$\sqrt{d}$
2.	Multiply the square root of *d* by 1.96.	$1.96 \times \sqrt{d}$
3a.	For the upper limit, add *d* to $1.96\sqrt{d}$.	$d+1.96\sqrt{d}$
b.	For the lower limit, subtract $1.96\sqrt{d}$ from *d*.	$d-1.96\sqrt{d}$
4.	Divide 1,000 by *n*.	$1{,}000/n$
5a.	Multiply the quotient in #4 ($1{,}000/n$) by the sum in #3a ($d+1.96\sqrt{d}$) to get the *upper limit*.	
b.	Multiply the quotient in #4 ($1{,}000/n$) by the difference in #3b to get the *lower limit*.	

Exhibit 4-2 Method 1. Procedure for Calculating 95 Percent Confidence Intervals for a Population Rate

The 95 percent confidence intervals for a Bryan County birth rate (1973–1976) of 21.0 are:

$$CI = 1{,}000/n\,[d \pm 1.96\sqrt{(d)}]$$

Number of births on which rate is based = 632 (4 years) (d)

1-year population = 7,800

Estimated 4-year population = 31,200 (n)

Rate = $d/n \times 1{,}000$ (Use the constant which is appropriate: 1,000, 10,000, 100,000)

Exhibit 4-2 continued

1. $\sqrt{(632)} = 25.13961$
2. $25.13961 \times 1.96 = 49.273636$
3a. $632 + 49.273636 = 681.273636$ (+ for high limit)
 b. $632 - 49.273636 = 582.723636$ (− for low limit)
4. $1{,}000/31{,}200 = .0320513$
5a. $.0320513 \times 681.273636 = 21.8$ (rounded to nearest tenth)
 b. $.0320513 \times 582.72636 = 18.7$ (rounded to nearest tenth)
 c. $CI = 18.7$ to 21.8 (95%)

The confidence interval values of 18.7 and 21.8 tell us that 95 percent of the time we can expect the rate to lie between these two values.

Method 2. A 95 percent confidence interval for over 30 observations can be derived from the following formula. That is, the formula will give two specified limits (confidence limits) in which the probability is 95 percent that the true value lies between these limits:

$$95\% \text{ confidence interval or } CI = \pm\, 1.96 \sqrt{[(p \times q)/n]}$$

where: p = the rate
$q = (1-p)$
n = the population for the rate

To calculate the confidence interval:

1. Multiply the rate (p) by one minus the rate (q): $p \times q$. This puts the rates on a per-person basis.
2. Divide the product of $p \times q$ by the population for the rate (n): $(p \times q)/n$.
3. Find the square root for the preceding quotient: $\sqrt{[(p \times q)/n]}$.
4. Multiply the preceding square root by 1.96. That is: $1.96 \times \sqrt{[(p \times q)/n]}$. (Multiply the product by the number used to get the rate to a per-person basis.)
5. To find the two specified confidence limits, add the preceding product to the real rate for the high limit and subtract the product from the real rate for the low limit. Thus, the Standard Rate $= \pm\, 1.96 \sqrt{[(p \times q)/n]}$.

The procedure for calculating 95 percent confidence intervals using Method 2 is illustrated in Exhibit 4-3.

Exhibit 4-3 Method 2 Procedure for Calculating 95 Percent Confidence Intervals for Population Rates

The 95 percent confidence intervals for a Bryan County birth rate (1973–1976) of 20.3 are:

$$CI = \pm 1.96 \sqrt{[(p \times q)/n]}$$

Crude birth rate = 20.3 per 1,000 population
1-year population = 7,800
Estimated 4-year population = 31,200
(To get the rate on a per-person basis, change 1,000 to 1. This is done by dividing 20.3 by 1,000 = .0203.)

1. .0203 × .9797 = .019888
   (.9797 is obtained by subtracting .0203 from 1, as defined for q.)
2. .019888/31,200 = .0000006
3. $\sqrt{.0000006}$ = .0007746
4. 1.96 × .0007746 = .0015182 (× 1,000) = 1.5
   (Multiply by 1,000 to return the rate limits to a per-1,000 basis.)
5. 20.3 + 1.5 = 21.8 (high limit)
   20.3 − 1.5 = 18.8 (low limit)

The confidence interval values of 21.8 and 18.8 tell us that 95 percent of the time we can expect the rate to lie between these two values.

Confidence Intervals for Mortality Indexes

Before confidence intervals are constructed it is obviously necessary to calculate the mortality index values. The resulting index values may require the estimation of confidence intervals. Consequently, confidence intervals can also be constructed for adjusted mortality indexes,[10] using the general formula:

$$I \pm 1.96\, S_I$$

where:
I = mortality index
1.96 = standard deviation for 95% confidence interval
S_I = standard error of the index

The standard error is computed for each of the following indexes:

Standardized Mortality Ratio.[11]

$$S_{smr} = \sqrt{(d)}/[(1/1,000)\ (\sum M_a\, p_a\ )]$$

where: d = number of deaths
M_a = standard age-race-sex specific rates per 1,000
ρ_a = area population in age-race-sex group a
$\sum$ = sum over all age-sex-race groups

Comparative Mortality Figure.[12]

$$S_{cmf} = \sqrt{\{\sum 1{,}000 m_a/\rho_a (P_a/P)^2\}}/\sum (M_a)(P_a/P)$$

where: $m_a = d_a/\rho_a \times 1{,}000$ = area's age-specific death rate per 1,000
ρ_a = area population in age group a
P_a = standard population in age group a
P = total standard population = $\sum P_a$
M_a = standard age-specific death rates

Years-of-Life-Lost (YLL) Index.[13]

$$S_{y11} = \sqrt{\sum d_a (70-y_a)^2}/1/1{,}000 \{\sum M_a \rho_a (70-y_a)\}$$

where: d_a = deaths in each age group a
M_a = standard age-specific death rates
ρ_a = area population in age group a
y_a = the midpoint of each age interval a

Suppose we had calculated a YLL Index of .851 for DeKalb County, Georgia, based on the data in Table 4-2.[14] Since the formula for YLL extends only to age 70, we will use the age group 55–64 as the last one in the computation. Therefore:

For $d_a(70-y_a)^2$ we have:

$$64\,(69.5)^2 = 64\,(4{,}830.25) = 309{,}136$$
$$12\,(67)^2 = 12\,(4{,}489) = 53{,}868$$
$$13\,(60)^2 = 13\,(3{,}600) = 46{,}800$$
$$31\,(50)^2 = 31\,(2{,}500) = 77{,}500$$
$$41\,(40)^2 = 41\,(1{,}600) = 65{,}600$$
$$68\,(30)^2 = 68\,(900) = 61{,}200$$
$$155\,(20)^2 = 155\,(400) = 62{,}000$$
$$235\,(10)^2 = 235\,(100) = 23{,}500$$

$$\sum d_a (70-y_a)^2 = 699{,}604$$
$$\sqrt{\sum d_a (70-y_a)^2} = 836.42$$

Table 4-2 Years-of-Life-Lost Data

a (Age Group)	p_a (Population)	d_a (Deaths)	y_a (Midpoint)	m_a (Mortality Rate/ 1,000)	$M_a \rho_a$* (Expected Deaths)
< 1	3,325	64	.5	19.25	70.26
1–4	12,669	12	3	.95	10.64
5–14	38,883	13	10	.34	18.18
15–24	29,136	31	20	1.06	49.82
25–34	27,383	41	30	1.50	48.47
35–44	24,223	68	40	2.81	83.33
45–54	20,201	155	50	7.67	178.37
55–64	11,128	235	60	21.12	245.15
65 +	7,103	520	75	73.21	235.74
Total	173,051	1,139			

*M_a is the U.S. age-specific death rate.

Source: Joel C. Kleinman. "Mortality," *Statistical Notes for Health Planners,* National Center for Health Statistics, DHEW, Washington, D.C., February 1977, p. 9.

And for 1/1,000 $M_a \rho_a (70-y_a)$ we have:

$$
\begin{aligned}
70.26\ (69.5) &= 4{,}883.07 \\
10.64\ (67) &= 712.88 \\
18.18\ (60) &= 1{,}090.8 \\
49.82\ (50) &= 2{,}491.0 \\
48.47\ (40) &= 1{,}938.8 \\
83.33\ (30) &= 2{,}499.9 \\
178.37\ (20) &= 3{,}567.4 \\
245.15\ (10) &= 2{,}451.5 \\
\hline
\sum M_a \rho_a (70-y_a) &= 19{,}635.4
\end{aligned}
$$

Since:

$$S_{y11} = \sqrt{\sum d_a (70-y_a)^2}/1/1{,}000 \{\sum M_a \rho_a (70-y_a)\}$$

Therefore:

$$S_{y11} = \sqrt{699{,}604}/19{,}635.4 = 836.423/19{,}635.4 = .0426$$

Given the standard error for YLL is .0426, and the 95 percent confidence interval is:

$$
\begin{aligned}
I \pm 1.96\ (S_{y11}) &= .851 \pm 1.96\ (.0426) \\
&= .851 \pm .083 \\
&= (.768,\ .934)
\end{aligned}
$$

Thus, we can expect that the YLL index for DeKalb County will be between .768 and .934, 95 percent of the time.

In health planning, the YLL index appears to be the most useful of the three presented. Essentially, the data is readily available to compute the index and the confidence intervals. In addition, this index may be used to compare different areas. However, a slightly modified formula is required where the ratio of the index values is used. Finally, the health planner is not restricted to an index based on total values or all ages, but the index may be used for portions of the age range, e.g., groups 15–44.

Summary

A confidence interval should always be constructed when presenting data derived from a sample of a population or when presenting rates for a population. The reason is that death rates are often based on relatively low numbers of deaths, and the width of the confidence interval will take this into account. If a small number of deaths is used, the confidence interval will be quite wide. With a large number of deaths, the confidence interval is narrower, indicating that a better estimate of the true population rate has been obtained.

Synthetic Estimation

Quite often, in dealing with health data, we may not have information available for a county, city, or state. This is especially true when dealing with morbidity, disability, utilization, life style, and environmental factors. In such cases, we may still want to compute an estimate for the area of interest based on available data (either national, regional, or state). Synthetic estimation provides a means of doing this.[15]

Synthetic estimation converts rates or means into frequency counts. This technique can sometimes provide us with rough usable estimates about population characteristics when we have no data for our specific population.

National survey data provide estimated rates for many health-related phenomena. They also provide some estimates for regions of the United States and for selected metropolitan areas. They are not designed, however, to yield state or local estimates. Yet local planners often need an estimate of the magnitude of a problem which takes into account such things as the age, sex, race, or education distribution of the local population. Synthetic estimation is a way of using national rates to obtain an estimate of the size of a target group.

A synthetic estimate is not a true estimate. It does not reflect intragroup differences between the target area and the United States as a whole. Special events, such as an outbreak of contagious disease, are not taken into account. A synthetic estimate, however, can provide for planning purposes a useful provisional estimate for a relatively stable characteristic not influenced by local events.

Table 4-3 presents an example of synthetic estimation that could be for a county census tract or service area. We do not know if the estimate of 10.4 percent is correct. This is lower than the national average because this census tract has a relatively young population. The critical assumption is that the age-specific rates or proportions are the same in both the small and large areas from which estimates were derived. The percentage

Table 4-3 An Example of Synthetic Estimation

Census Data
Number of Persons

	Male	*Female*
Total	116,182	117,921
Under 17	34,037	32,559
17–44	60,077	59,531
45–64	16,662	17,626
65 and over	5,406	8,206

National Health Interview Survey Data
Percent of Persons with High Cholesterol Levels

	Male	*Female*
Under 17	3.2	2.6
17–44	9.0	6.8
45–64	21.9	19.2
65 and over	47.2	41.2

Synthetic Estimates
Number of Persons with High Cholesterol Levels

	Total	*Male*	*Female*
Total	24,353 (10.4%)*	12,695	11,658
Under 17		1,089 (3.2 × 34,037)	846 (2.6 × 32,559)
17–44		5,406 (9.0 × 60,077)	4,048 (6.8 × 59,531)
45–64		3,649 (21.9 × 16,662)	3,384 (19.2 × 17,626)
65 and over		2,551 (47.2 × 5,406)	3,380 (41.2 × 8,205)

*Percentage for the U.S. as a whole is 24,353/234,103 = .1040 × 100 = 10.4%.

Source: R. Zemach and T. R. Ervin. *The Use of Statistical Data and Techniques in Health Programs,* Applied Statistics Training Institute, Denver, Colorado, August 12–16, 1974 (not numbered).

difference comes from applying these rates to the age distribution of the smaller area.

Testing for Significance

A test of differences between hypothetical population parameters and estimates derived from samples is frequently desired. This requires a direct extension of the concept of a confidence interval. In health analysis, we are interested most often in comparing rates of two different areas or of two different times for the same area. The objective is to determine if a significant difference exists between the rates or if the difference is due solely to random effects. Several commonly used methods to test such differences in health data follow.

Testing the Differences Between Two Means for Large Samples ($n > 30$)

We have two mean values derived from two samples. We would like to know whether the two samples were drawn from the same population or if they were drawn from two populations, that is, are they significantly different? The Z test is the appropriate test to use. Z is the value of the standard normal deviation, corresponding to a standard deviation on a standard normal distribution (95 percent of values with ± 1.96 standard deviation). Values are obtained from a table of Z values available in most statistics texts. The formula is:

$$Z = (\langle X \rangle_{av1} - \langle X \rangle_{av2})/\sqrt{(S_{x\ 1}^{2}/n_{x_1}) + (S_{x\ 2}^{2}/n_{x_2})}$$

where: $\langle X \rangle_{av1}$ = mean from sample 1
$\langle X \rangle_{av2}$ = mean from sample 2
$S_{x\ 1}^{2}$ = variance from sample 1
$S_{x\ 2}^{2}$ = variance from sample 2

A critical value (μ) is selected from a table for the normal distribution. Three commonly used values are:

μ	90%	95%	99%
Z	1.65	1.96	2.33

For example, suppose we had computed that the average number of miles jogged per month by 50 persons from Atlanta is 69.5 miles, with a standard deviation of 2.5 miles. In a group of 60 people from a second city, the average is computed as 70.1 miles, with a standard deviation of 2.3 miles.[16]

$$Z = \frac{70.1 - 69.5}{\sqrt{[(5.29)/(60)] + [(6.25)/(50)]}} = 1.29$$

Thus, we can conclude that the two cities are not significantly different in jogging habits at the 90 percent level.

Testing the Difference Between Two Means for Small Samples (n < 30)

This case is the same as the Z test above, but, because of small sample sizes, the distribution of the sampling statistic is more closely approximated by the t distribution. The formulae are:[17]

and $t = |\langle X \rangle_{av} - \langle Y \rangle_{av}| / S\sqrt{[(1)/(n_x)] + [(1)/(n_y)]}$

$$S = \sum(X_1 - \langle X \rangle_{av})^2 + \sum(Y_1 - \langle Y \rangle_{av})^2 / n_x + n_y - 2$$

where:

S	= pooled estimate of the standard deviation
$\langle X \rangle_{av}$	= mean of first sample
$\langle Y \rangle_{av}$	= mean of second sample
n_x	= number of observations in first sample
n_Y	= number of observations in second sample
$\sum(x_1 - \langle X \rangle_{av})^2$	= sum of the squared deviation of the first sample observations from $\langle X \rangle_{av}$
$\sum(Y_1 - \langle Y \rangle_{av})^2$	= sum of the squared deviation of the second sample observations from $\langle Y \rangle_{av}$

The critical value is found in a table of the t distribution and is dependent upon the number of values in the sample. The t table is entered at the desired level of significance and degrees of freedom. Degrees of freedom, in this case, are equal to the sum of the sample sizes less two ($n_x + n_y - 2$). For example, suppose one group of children was instructed to take multivitamins and another group to take vitamin C. The research hypothesis predicts that vitamin C is important to the prevention of colds. We can test for the significance, using the t test:

	Multivitamin Group	*Vitamin C Group*
Number of Observations	$n_x = 10$	$n_y = 10$
Average number of	$\langle X \rangle_{av} = 25.5$	$\langle Y \rangle_{av} = 22.0$
colds in a year	$\sum(X_1 - \langle X \rangle_{av})^2 = 168.5$	$\sum(Y_1 - \langle Y \rangle_{av})^2 = 178.0$

$$S = \sqrt{[(168.5 + 178.0)/(10 + 10 - 2)]} = \sqrt{19.25} = 4.39$$

$$t = (25.5 - 22.0)/4.39\sqrt{[(1/10) + (1/10)]} = 3.5/1.96 = 1.786$$

The t value for a 95 percent significance level at $(10 + 10 - 2)$ 18 degrees of freedom with a one-tail test is 1.72. Since $1.786 > 1.72$, we can conclude that the mean for the group using multivitamins is significantly higher than the mean for the group using vitamin C. Thus, vitamin C potentially is a preventive measure for the common cold when compared to the multivitamins.

Testing for the Differences Between Two Sample Variances—the F Test

Once we have computed the variances from two samples, we may be interested in determining whether the two are significantly different. The appropriate test in this case is the F test. The value of F is calculated by dividing the variance of the first sample by the variance of the second, or:

$$F = S_1^2/S_2^2$$

Normally, the larger of the two variances is placed in the numerator so that the values of F will exceed one. In fact, if the two variances are exactly equal, the value of F will equal one. The F test for significance tells us whether, given the sample sizes, the computed F value is significantly larger than one, indicating that the two variances are unequal.

Suppose we had computed the sample variance of Group A, nonsmokers who could run two miles ($n = 40$, $S_1^2 = 8.4$), and the sample variance of Group B, smokers of two packs per day who could run two miles ($n = 30$, $S_2^2 = 4.5$):

$$F = 8.4/4.5 = 1.867$$

Using a table of F at the 95 percent confidence level, for 39 $(n-1)$ degrees of freedom in the numerator and 29 $(n-1)$ in the denominator, we find a critical value of $F = 1.64$. Since the calculated F value of 1.867 exceeds the critical value, we can state that the two variances are not equal but significantly different. Alternatively, there is a significant difference in the variances of smokers and nonsmokers who could run two miles.

Testing for the Differences Between a Sample Variance and a Population Variance–the χ^2 Test

If we wish to determine if a calculated sample variance is significantly different from a known population variance, the χ^2 (chi square) test is used. As in the F test, we calculate the χ^2 value as the ratio between two variances, but this time the sample variance is divided by the population variance:

$$\chi^2 = (n - 1) S^2/\sigma^2$$

The analysis proceeds as for the F test, except that this time we use the critical value from the table of χ^2 to determine the degrees of freedom from the sample $(n-1)$.

Testing for the Difference Between Two Rates

When Rates Are Independent. When comparing rates from two communities or areas, or when comparing rates from the same community at different points in time, we would like to answer the question, Is there a significant difference between the two independent rates? To answer this question, we use the confidence interval for the ratio between the two rates or the difference between the two independent rates.[18] The ratio between two rates is defined as:

$$R = r_1/r_2$$

where: r_1 = death rate for community 1
r_2 = death rate for community 2

The 95 percent confidence interval for R is defined as:

$$R \pm 1.96\, R\sqrt{[(1/d_1) + (1/d_2)]}$$

where: d_1 = number of deaths in community 1
d_2 = number of deaths in community 2

In order to establish a significant difference, one must determine whether the confidence interval contains one. If it does not, we can state that the two rates are significantly different. If the interval does contain one, we cannot conclude that a significant difference exists.

Kleinman gives the following example:[19]

Years	Number of Infant Deaths	Number of Live Births	Infant Mortality Rate per 1,000 Live Births
1961–65	200	5,000	40
1966–70	100	4,000	25

$$R = 40/25 = 1.6$$

$$1.96\, R \sqrt{[(1/d_1) + (1/d_2)]} = 1.96(1.6)(.1225) = .384$$

Upper limit: $1.6 + .384 = 1.984$
Lower limit: $1.6 - .384 = 1.216$

Thus, the rate in 1961–65 can be said with 95 percent confidence to be from 1.22 to 1.98 times the 1966–70 rate. Since the interval does not contain one there is a statistically significant decrease in the area's infant mortality rate. An alternate form of computing the confidence interval for the ratio between two rates is:

$$R \pm R\sqrt{\{[(CL_1/r_1)^2] + [(CL_2/r_2)^2]\}}$$

where: CL_1 = confidence level for rate 1
CL_2 = confidence level for rate 2
r_1, r_2 = rates for areas 1 and 2, respectively

Kleinman points out that the procedure for using the ratio of two rates requires that the two rates be independent, that is, a death included in one rate should not be included in a second rate. Thus, overlapping time periods (for example, from 1960–70 and 1965–75) or from a geographical hierarchy (for example, comparing a town's rate to the rate for the county it is in) are not valid. Moreover, this formula is valid only when the number of deaths used to calculate the rate in the denominator exceeds 100.

The confidence level for the difference between two rates ($D = r_1 - r_2$) is given by:

$$D \pm \sqrt{(CL_1^2 + CL_2^2)}$$

where: D = difference between two independent rates
CL_1, CL_2 = confidence level for rates 1 and 2, respectively
and CL = $1.96\sqrt{d}$ (where d = number of deaths)

In this case, if the interval includes zero, we cannot conclude that the difference between the two rates is significant.

Kleinman presents the following example:[20]

	Santa Cruz, Calif.	DeKalb County, Ga.
Population (n), white males 45–54	6,051	20,201
Number of deaths (d)	63	155
Death rate per 1,000	10.41	7.67

Substituting in the formula from Method 1, we have:

$$\text{Santa Cruz: } \frac{1{,}000}{6{,}051}(63 \pm 1.96\sqrt{63}) = 10.41 \pm 2.57$$

$$\text{DeKalb: } \frac{1{,}000}{20{,}201}(155 \pm 1.96\sqrt{155}) = 7.67 \pm 1.21$$

The confidence interval for the difference between the two rates is:

Difference: $D = 10.41 - 7.67 = 2.74$

$$\begin{aligned}\text{Confidence level} &= D \pm \sqrt{(CL_1^2 + CL_2^2)} \\ &= 2.74 \pm \sqrt{(2.57^2 + 1.21^2)} \\ &= 2.74 \pm \sqrt{8.0690} \\ &= 2.74 \pm 2.84\end{aligned}$$

Thus, the 95 percent confidence interval would be (–.10 to 5.58). Since the interval includes zero, we can conclude that the rates for the two counties are not significantly different.

When Rates Are Not Independent. When comparing a rate to a standard rate (that is, when rates may not be independent), a slightly more complex formula is needed:

$$\mu = (r-s)\ \sqrt{[n/(s-s^2)]}$$ [21]

where: r = the observed rate or rate to be compared
s = the standard rate (state, region, nation, etc.)
n = the denominator (population) on which the rate is based

This formula is calculated as follows:

1. Square (multiply by itself) the standard rate, s: $(s \times s = s^2)$. Change all rates to a per-person basis (divide by the rate's denominator).
2. Subtract the square of s from s: $s-s^2$.
3. Divide the denominator on which the rate is based, n, by the difference of $s-s^2$: $n/(s-s^2)$.
4. Find the square root of the quotient from the last step: $\sqrt{[n/(s-s^2)]}$.
5. Subtract the standard rate s from the observed rate, r: $r-s$.
6. Multiply the square root in the fourth step by the difference in the fifth step: $\mu = (r-s)\ \sqrt{[n/(s-s^2)}$.

If μ (standard deviation) exceeds the desired confidence level, we can conclude that the rate is significantly different from the standard rate (see Table 4-4).

For example, to compute the significance of the birth rate of Liberty County, Georgia:

$$\mu = (r-s)\ \sqrt{[n/(s-s^2)]}$$

Table 4-4 Significance of Observed Standard Deviation

			90%	95%	99%
Standard deviation (σ)	.85	1.28	1.65	1.96	2.33
One-tailed area	.2	.1	.05	.025	.01
Two-tailed area	.4	.2	.1	.05	.025

Source: D. E. Drew and E. Keeler. "Algorithms for Health Planners," *Hypertension* 6 (Prepared for H. R. A. Department of H.E.W., R2215 16-H.E.W. Supp. 1977: Rand Corporation), p. 64.

Observed rate, r = 20.9 per 1,000
Standard rate, s = 16.8 per 1,000
Population (denominator n, on which rate is based) = 16,400

a. (.0168) = .0168 × .0168 = .000282
b. .0168 − .000282 = .016518
c. 16,400/.016518 = 992856.27
d. $\sqrt{992856.27}$ = 996.42173
e. .0209 − .0168 = .0041
f. .0041 × 996.42173 = 4.09 (μ)
(Rounded to nearest tenth)

Since the value 4.09 is greater than 2.33 (Table 4-4), it is significant at the 99 percent level. Thus, there is a significant difference between the birth rate for Liberty County, Georgia, and the state standard.

When rates are very small the actual numbers of events are used instead of rates. Thus, to find if the difference between two small rates is significant, solve for μ in the following formula and find the solution in Table 4-4:[22]

$$\mu = (o - e)/\sqrt{e}$$

where: o = the observed number(s) to be compared
e = the standard number (state, region, nation, etc.)

To calculate this formula:

1. Find the square root of the standard number, e: $\sqrt{e}$.
2. Subtract the standard number, e from the observed number, o: $o - e$.
3. Divide the difference between the observed and standard numbers (Step 2) by the square root of e: $o - e/\sqrt{e}$.

Thus the number significance of infant mortality for a Georgian county may be determined by:

$$\mu = (o - e)/\sqrt{e}$$

Observed rate, o = 20.2 per 1,000 (65 deaths)
Standard rate, e = 17.5 per 1,000 (117 deaths)

a. $\sqrt{117} = 10.81$
b. $65 - 117 = -52$
c. $-52/10.81 = -4.81$

Since the value −4.81 is greater than −1.96, the two rates are significantly different at the 99 percent level.

Why Rates May Show Differences. Differences in rates may result from variations other than statistical differences. Examples of such differences are:[23]

1. Differences in how death certificates are completed by physicians, coroners, and their assistants in different locations.
2. Differences in how health departments' nosologists determine the underlying cause of death and assign a code to it (although this is a highly standardized process done by well-trained and experienced technicians).
3. Differences in the types of coding errors made by data-entry clerks (although this seems unlikely in view of data-processing patterns).
4. Differences resulting from program errors or from choices (such as excluding death records which lack age, sex, and/or county data).
5. Differences among geographical areas in the proportional distribution of residents at each year of age during the time period. Such differences are so great that the U.S. Census count of January 1, 1970, failed to serve equally well in individual areas as an estimate of the population at risk.
6. Differences resulting from the use of the originally published 1970 population counts (before the U.S. Census Bureau discovered that, because of coding errors, all those coded at age 100 or older had been added to the count of those aged 10).
7. Differences in the Census Bureau's undercount percentages among counties and health service areas and between sexes.

Testing for Association Between Variables

When we have two independent and mutually exclusive variables and measurement is on a nominal or binomial scale, the χ^2 test is appropriate in testing for significant differences. In the χ^2 test, we are interested in testing the association between two variables or two proportions. Each must be mutually exclusive and independent, and the expected value in each cell must exceed five. The general format for a 2 × 2 table is:[24]

	Positive	Negative	
Attribute absent	a	b	$a+b$
Attribute present	c	d	$c+d$
Totals	$a+c$	$b+d$	n

The formula for chi square is:[25]

$$\chi^2 = n([ad-bc] - 1/2n)^2/(a+b)(c+d)(a+c)(b+d)$$

where: n = the number of observations
a, b, c, d = the values from the table
$[ad-bc]$ = the absolute value of the difference between ad and bc

For example, suppose we had the following results from a survey of adults in a community health setting in three counties.[26] Of the 200 adults who had not previously exercised, 100 received information on the benefits of exercise and 100 did not receive the information.

	Did Not Exercise	Began Exercising	Total
No exercise information	21	79	100
Exercise information	5	95	100
Total	26	174	200

The formula gives us:

$$\chi^2 = [200\ (|1{,}995 - 395| - 100)^2]/(26)(174)(100)(100) = 9.95$$

From a chi square table for one degree of freedom, we find that the critical value for 95 percent confidence equals 3.841. Since the computed value exceeds the critical value, we conclude that there is an association between the information received about exercising and beginning to exercise.

The chi square test can be extended to a table of dimensions larger than 2 × 2 (referred to as an r x c contingency table). The general form is shown in Figure 4-3.

Figure 4-3 An r x c Contingency Table

Rows \ Columns	1	2	•	•	•	•	c	Total
1	a_1	a_2	•	•	•	•	a_c	t_1
2	b_1	b_2	•	•	•	•	b_c	t_2
↓	↓	↓					↓	↓
r	h_1	h_2					h_c	t_r
Total	n_1	n_2					n_c	N

Source: U.S. DHEW, PHS Center for Disease Control, "Analytical Statistics," *Statistical Methods—Testing for Significance,* p. 3.

In this case, the formula for χ^2 becomes:

$$\chi^2 = \sum (\text{Observed}-\text{Expected})^2/(\text{Expected})$$

The expected value for each cell is calculated by multiplying the raw total *(t)* times the column total *(n),* and dividing by *N*. An example is shown in Table 4-5.[27]

Table 4-5 Immunization Status of Children > 5 Years

Socio-economic Area	Immunization Status			Total
	None	Partial	Full	
Upper	4 (12.7)	7 (12.3)	89 (75.0)	100
Middle	11 (12.4)	13 (12.1)	74 (73.5)	98
Lower	23 (12.9)	17 (12.6)	62 (76.5)	102
Total	38	37	225	300

Source: U.S. DHEW, PHS Center for Disease Control, "Analytical Statistics," *Statistical Methods—Testing for Significance,* p. 4.

The expected value for each cell in Table 4-5 appears in parentheses. Below is an example of computing expected values in cell one (no immunizations and upper socioeconomic area):

$$\text{Expected value} = [(\text{Row total})(\text{Column total})]/N$$
$$= [(100)(38)]/300 = 3{,}800/300 = 12.7$$

The chi square value is:[28]

$$\chi^2 = \sum[(o-e)^2/e$$
$$= (4-12.7)^2/12.7 + (7-12.3)^2/12.3 + (89-75.0)^2/75.0$$
$$+ (11-12.4)^2/12.4 + (13-12.1)^2/12.1 + (74-73.5)^2/73.5$$
$$+ (23-12.9)^2/12.9 + (17-12.6)^2/12.6 + (62-76.5)^2/76.5$$
$$= 5.960 + 2.284 + 2.613 + 0.159 + 0.067 + 0.003$$
$$+ 7.908 + 1.537 + 2.748$$
$$= 23.279$$

From a table of chi square, for four degrees of freedom ($df = (r-1)(c-1) = df\,(3-1)(3-1) = 2 \times 2 = 4$), we find a critical value at the 95 percent level of 9.488, and this value is exceeded. Thus, there is an association between immunization status and socioeconomic area.

Other tests using chi square are available for testing the goodness of fit between an observed and expected or theoretical distribution. An adjusted form for expected values of less than five (Fisher's exact test) is also available.

A Health Planner's Checklist for Statistical Testing

The following checklist is suggested for reviewing procedures in statistical testing.

1. Formulate the problem.
2. State the assumptions. To make use of the statistical tests, confidence intervals, and tests of statistical significance presented in this chapter, the health planner must make certain assumptions about the population(s) and the sampling procedures. (Remember, rates can be assumed to be samples in time and space.) Usually, the assumptions are:
   a. that the data approximate a normal distribution with a population mean (μ) and a population standard deviation (σ),
   b. that S (sample standard deviation) is an unbiased estimate of σ (population standard deviation),
   c. that $\langle X \rangle_{av}$ (sample mean) is an unbiased estimate of μ (population mean), and
   d. that the samples are random and the observations independent.

However, there are methods presented in this chapter for conditions when the rates are not independent.

3. Set the null hypothesis (H_o) in such a way that the planner expects to reject it. In this way, the probability of a Type I error can be calculated and controlled. The null hypothesis usually states that no significant relationship or difference exists.
4. Formulate an alternative (H_1) hypothesis which you will accept upon rejection of the null.
5. Obtain the sampling distribution. Given the assumptions and the characteristics of the data, it is necessary to select the appropriate sampling distribution in which to associate probabilities with outcomes.
6. Select the level of significance (α) or the probability of making a Type I error. Specify n, the sample size or number of observations.
7. Define the critical region. Determine which values of the statistic will cause rejection of the null hypothesis (rejection region) and which values will result in acceptance of the hypothesis. This is done on the basis of the type of sampling distribution at a specified level of significance, whether or not the critical region is to include one or both tails of the sampling distribution.
8. Compute the test statistic. It is the statistic which has the sampling distribution given above. The test statistic is computed from the observed data.
9. Make the decision.
   a. Compare the test statistic for that sampling distribution with the values of the critical region.
   b. Accept or reject the null hypothesis, depending on whether the value obtained is inside or outside the critical region.
   c. Specify the level of significance (confidence) of your decision.
   d. Evaluate the specific problem as formulated in Step 1 above.
10. Review statistical testing procedures (see checklist in statistical testing). Determine whether you are (a) testing for small or large samples and (b) testing means or variances (see Figure 4-4).

Overview of Additional Statistical Techniques

The statistical principles and tests of significance already presented provide a basic foundation for the use of statistics in health. The application of statistics is rapidly growing in both importance and use as practitioners become more proficient, as the demands grow for reliable information collected in a cost efficient manner, and as statistical techniques are developed and applied. In this final section, a brief overview of some

Figure 4-4 Checklist in Statistical Testing

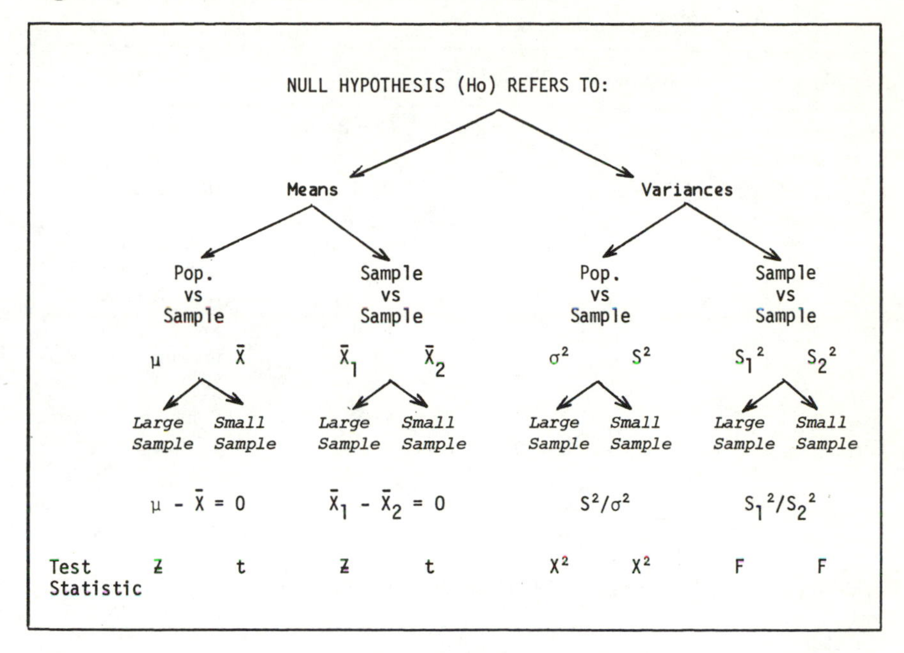

major topics in statistical analysis is presented. The intent is not to be exhaustive or definitive. The number of techniques being applied to health analysis often seems unlimited, frequently with volumes devoted to the theoretical aspects of each technique. A word of caution is in order: the more powerful the technique, the greater the opportunity for misapplication or misunderstanding. Statistical measurements, models, and tests make many assumptions about the nature of relationships within the data set in use, and unknowing violation of these assumptions can result in erroneous conclusions. Before these techniques are applied, competent and experienced advice should be sought. The techniques have much to offer in gaining a greater understanding of relationships within data and an increased ability to produce meaningful information from data, but each should be used with full cognizance of its underlying assumptions.

Correlations

Correlation analysis is a means of examining the degree of association between variables. Correlation techniques are provided for different levels of measurement. The different types of correlation techniques are presented in Table 4-6.

Table 4-6 Appropriate Correlational Techniques for Different Forms of Variables

Technique	Symbol	Variable 1*	Variable 2*	Remarks
Product-moment correlation	r	Continuous	Continuous	The most stable technique
Rank difference correlation	ρ	Ranks	Ranks	Often used instead of product-moment when number of cases is under 30
Kendall's tau	τ	Ranks	Ranks	Preferable to rho for numbers under 10
Biserial correlation	r_{bis}	Artificial dichotomy	Continuous	Sometimes exceeds 1—has a larger standard error than r—commonly used in item analysis
Widespread biserial correlation	r_{wbis}	Widespread artificial dichotomy	Continuous	Used when you are especially interested in persons at the extremes of the dichotomized variable
Point-biserial	r_{pbis}	True dichotomy	Continuous	Yields a lower correlation than r and much lower than r_{bis}
Tetrachoric correlation	r_t	Artificial dichotomy	Artificial dichotomy	Used when both variables can be split at critical points
Phi coefficient	ϕ	True dichotomy	True dichotomy	Used in calculating interitem correlations on multiple choice or two choice items
Contingency coefficient	C	2 or more categories	2 or more categories	Comparable to r_t under certain conditions—closely related to chi square

Table 4-6 continued

*In these columns, a *continuous* variable is one representing an underlying continuum tending to be normally distributed. Examples include such variables as height, weight, and ability or achievement as measured by standardized tests. *Artificial dichotomies* can be constructed by arbitrarily dividing continuous variables into two groups, usually about the center of the data. Examples include such classifications as achiever-nonachiever, above average-below average, pass-fail, and warm-cold on an attitude scale. *True dichotomies* involve relatively clear-cut (though not necessarily absolute) differences, allowing the data to be categorized into two groups. Examples include such dichotomies as male-female, living-dead, teacher-nonteacher, dropout-nondropout, and smoker-nonsmoker. Other variables that can be treated as if they were true dichotomies for the purposes of computing (for example, computing a point-biserial correlation coefficient) include: color blind-noncolor blind, alcoholic-nonalcoholic, and right-wrong responses with respect to a particular test item in item analysis. The distributions underlying true dichotomies, if not absolute differences, tend to be bimodal and/or relatively discontinuous.

Source: S. Isaac. *Handbook in Research and Evaluation* (San Diego: Edits Publishers, 1971), pp. 126–127. Reprinted with permission.

Interpreting correlation coefficients.[29] In its simplest form, a correlation coefficient is a number indicating the degree of relationship between two variables. It measures to what extent variations in one variable go with variations in the other. A perfect positive correlation (1.00) means that changes in one variable are, without exception, accompanied by equivalent changes in the *same* direction in the other variable. No correlation (0.00) means that changes in one variable have no relationship or are randomly related to changes in the other variable. A perfect negative correlation (−1.00) means that changes in one variable are, without exception, accompanied by equivalent changes in the *opposite* direction in the other variable. A correlation coefficient requires two sets of measurements on the same groups of individuals or on matched pairs of individuals. It cannot be computed on one person alone.

Coefficient of determination. The correlation coefficient, r, is a measure of the strength of relationship between two variables. It does not represent a percentage of the determinants they have in common unless it is squared and becomes an estimate of variance called the coefficient of determination (r^2). When the latter is multiplied by 100, it indicates the percentage of variance held in common by the two variables, X and Y, assuming linear regression. It answers the question, How much of the variance in Y is accounted for, associated with, or determined by the variance in X?

Correlation and causation. Our ultimate concern is with identifying cause-and-effect relationships. Since such relationships are always correlated, there is a strong tendency to reverse the process and infer cause-

and-effect status between two or more variables based on an established correlation coefficient. The danger here lies in the fact that correlation does not imply causation; that is, two variables may be correlated with a third variable.

Nonlinear or curvilinear relationships. The standard assumption underlying most correlation coefficients is that the relationship between the two variables is linear. That is, as one variable increases or decreases, so does the other, thus forming a straight line. The simplest procedure for detecting nonlinear trends in correlation data is to construct a scatter diagram and inspect the shape of the plots for bends and curves in the regression line departing from a straight-line function.

Two final precautions. A major weakness of the correlation method is the tendency to adopt a "shotgun" approach to research, utilizing all data in sight indiscriminately. In such cases, the data are extremely difficult to interpret and mostly useless. It should also be noted that the reliability of a correlation coefficient varies directly with the sample size. For problems involving more than two variables—as in partial correlation, multiple correlation, and factor analysis—consult other advanced treatments of correlation methodology.

Regression

Regression is a statistical technique which specifies the relationship between one dependent variable and a set of one or more independent variables. In simple linear regression, we try to estimate a value for Y, the dependent variable, in relation to the value of X, the independent or predictor variable. The estimating equation thus takes the form:

$$Y = a + bX$$

where: a = a constant equal to the Y intercept
b = the estimated regression weight equal to the slope of the regression line

The a and b coefficients both represent estimates of true regression coefficients and thus are measured with error. Like the sample mean, they have a distribution which can be used to develop confidence levels about the regression line, much like a confidence interval on the mean.

The regression coefficients are estimated through solution of a set of normal equations. If more than one set of predictor variables is involved, matrix algebra techniques are used to solve for the regression coefficients.

Regression is one of the most frequently used techniques in the statistical analysis of large data sets where one wants to estimate one value based on a set of other values. Several assumptions are made in a regression analysis. Major violations of these assumptions can cause misleading results. Particular attention must be paid to the error variances of the dependent variable, to intercorrelations within the set of independent variables, and to the functional relationship between dependent and independent variables. Specialized regression techniques have been developed to deal with violations of assumptions.

Statistical Significance and Decision Making

It should be emphasized that statistical significance provides evidence of differences, characteristics, or associations but does not provide proof. This is because statistical significance is based on several underlying assumptions, including those about the properties of the distribution and the sample results. In statistical significance testing, we are concerned with the probability of making an error (or the probability of being correct), given the results obtained. Thus, if we have a 95 percent confidence level (or a 5 percent error level), what we are really saying is that 95 times out of 100 we would get a value that is within two standard errors of the true mean; 5 times out of 100, we would get a value exceeding two standard errors. Thus, if we get a value that exceeds the established critical level and falls outside the range of likely values, two things are possible. Either the true mean is different from the one hypothesized (rejection of the false null hypothesis); or the true mean is not different from the one hypothesized, that is, we have selected a sample value that falls in the 5 percent region only by chance (rejection of a true null hypothesis).

It is also important to realize that statistical significance deals with probabilities based upon repeated sampling from a population. For any one sample, the true probability is either 0.0 or 1.0; that is, either the sample statistic is a reliable estimate of the true population parameter or it is not.

Although the confidence level (often referred to as α) indicates the probability of having a value that exceeds the critical region by chance, it does not indicate the probability that the true statistic is actually different from the hypothesized statistic. The latter is the β probability or the power of the test, dealing with the ability to detect a false null hypothesis. While the computation of the β probability is much more difficult than it is for α, it is important to realize that, once the desired α level and the sample size are set, the β level is fixed. Since this β level value is usually not known and is often very small, we cannot really conclude that it is true, even when we fail to reject a null hypothesis. Rather, we say that the results are inconclusive or, more commonly, that we have failed to reject the null hypothesis. Thus, depending on the results we get from a test of significance, we are likely to make an error—either rejecting a true null hypothesis or failing to reject a false null hypothesis. Any test for significance should consider these probabilities of error, and the decision maker should weigh carefully their consequences.

Practical Significance and Decision Making

While statistical significance is commonly reported in testing hypotheses or making inferences, based upon the theory of sampling distributions and mathematics, serious concern should be shown for its practical significance. By practical significance we mean the real impact or cost of a difference. Practical significance can be assessed only by someone familiar with the hypothesis being tested or with the program being evaluated. It is possible that, though a difference may be statistically significant, it may be so small as to be meaningless in terms of programmatic impact. This is especially true when dealing with large samples or rates based upon large populations. Since statistical significance is a function of both sample size and the variation in the population, it is quite possible that in a large sample any differences will be significant. Thus, consideration must be given to the real impact of a statistically significant difference on the program or population being tested.

A problem for the administrator, then, is the difference between statistical and practical significance. In health services, where we may have data on large populations, indexes such as means or rates may always be significantly different in a statistical sense. The health professional must decide whether the differences are of significant magnitude to justify action, such as revising a program. A common problem in evaluation testing arises when a key index has increased significantly, according to a statistical expert, but the administrator senses that the size of the increase has no programmatic importance. Survey reports on populations often cite differences which are described as "significantly greater" and "significantly longer" but which, even to an untrained analyst, do not seem to matter much.

A final warning about repeated testing for significance: Tests are designed so that the error probability in any one test is small. Yet, if several tests are made, it is quite likely that we may reject true null hypotheses based on chance occurrences. Such repeated testing of a number of related factors is often done when searching for relationships rather than testing specific hypotheses. When statistical significance is found in such cases, the probability is quite high that chance occurrence has caused rejection.

SUMMARY

Statistics provides the tool for health data analysis. Through knowledgeable use of statistical techniques, we can extract the maximum amount of information from a set of data, discover underlying relationships, or predict characteristics based on a set of known characteristics. At the same time, statistics lends itself to misuse. The saying is often heard that one can prove anything with statistics. The fact is that a careful analysis of assumptions and a careful application of statistical techniques can produce useful information that can lead to a better understanding of health data.

NOTES

1. Robert Parsons, *Statistical Analysis: A Decision Making Approach* (New York: Harper & Row, 1974), p. 7.
2. Stephen Isaac, *Handbook in Research and Evaluation* (San Diego: Edits Publishers), pp. 116–148.
3. Isaac, *Handbook,* p. 117.
4. Isaac, *Handbook,* p. 117.
5. Isaac, *Handbook,* p. 117.
6. Joel C. Kleinman, "Mortality," *Statistical Notes for Health Planners,* National Center for Health Statistics (Washington, D.C.: Department of Health, Education, and Welfare, February 1977), p. 16.
7. Paul E. Leaverton, *A Review of Biostatistics* (University of Iowa, 1973), p. 65.
8. Joel C. Kleinman, "Infant Mortality," *Statistical Notes for Health Planners,* National Center for Health Statistics (Washington, D.C.: Department of Health, Education, and Welfare, July 1976), p. 12.
9. Kleinman, "Mortality," p. 6.
10. Kleinman, "Mortality," pp. 13–15.
11. Kleinman, "Mortality," p. 14.
12. Kleinman, "Mortality," p. 14.
13. Kleinman, "Mortality," p. 14.
14. Kleinman, "Mortality," p. 14.
15. Vital and Health Statistics, National Center for Health Statistics, *Synthetic Estimation of State Health Characteristics Based on the Health Interview Survey,* Public Health Service, Series 2, no. 75 (Washington, D.C.: U.S. Government Printing Office, October 1977), p. 22.
16. J. Virgil Peavy and William W. Dyal, *Analytical Statistics: Statistical Methods—Testing for Significance,* Center for Disease Control (Atlanta: Department of Health, Education, and Welfare), p. 1.
17. Peavy and Dyal, *Analytical Statistics,* p. 11.
18. Kleinman, "Infant Mortality," p. 11.
19. Kleinman, "Infant Mortality," p. 11.
20. Kleinman, "Mortality," p. 7.
21. D. E. Drew and E. Keeler, "Algorithms for Health Planners," *Hypertension* 6 (U.S. DHEW, HRA, R-221516, HEW: The Rand Corporation, August 1977), p. 63.

22. Drew and Keeler, "Algorithms," p. 64.
23. Peavy and Dyal, *Analytical Statistics*, p. 1. (I would like to thank the staff at the Center for Disease Control for their permission to quote and reprint much of the material that is used in several sections of this chapter.)
24. William M. Weir, "Confidence Level Estimation to Help Data Users Evaluate Differences in Health Related Rates," The Third Data Use Conference, mimeographed (Phoenix: November 14–16, 1978), pp. III 27–53.
25. Peavy and Dyal, *Analytical Statistics*, p. 1.
26. Peavy and Dyal, *Analytical Statistics*, p. 1. (Data values are used for this example exercise.)
27. Peavy and Dyal, *Analytical Statistics*, p. 4.
28. Peavy and Dyal, *Analytical Statistics*, p. 4.
29. Adapted from Isaac, *Handbook*, pp. 148–151.

Chapter 5
Basic Epidemiological Methods

This chapter presents standard methods for conducting community epidemiological studies. As discussed in Chapter 2, the epidemiological model for health policy analysis considers the nature of health to be holistic, encompassing life style, environment, biology, and the medical care system. The science of epidemiology had its roots in the study and control of infectious diseases. Today, however, emphasis has shifted from infectious diseases to chronic disease epidemiology. The reasons for this change were presented in Chapter 1. Infectious diseases have given way to chronic diseases as the leading causes of death in the modern world. Yet, even with the change in emphasis, many concepts of infectious disease epidemiology continue to be useful in chronic disease epidemiology. This chapter, then, presents some basic methods and concepts that are applicable to epidemiological study and community analysis.

DESCRIPTIVE EPIDEMIOLOGY

Descriptive epidemiology is the "study of the amount and distribution of disease within a population by person, place, and time."[1] It seeks to answer three basic questions regarding disease:[2] (1) Who is affected (person)? (2) Where do the cases occur (place)? (3) When do the cases occur (time)?

While these questions may appear trivial, Friedman[3] points out that descriptive epidemiological studies are of fundamental importance in that they can serve to: (1) indicate what types of persons are most likely to be affected by a disease, where the disease will occur, and when; (2) assist in planning health facilities; (3) provide clues, questions, or hypotheses as to disease etiology for further study; and (4) determine the health status of a population in a geographical area.

Who Is Affected by the Disease?

To answer the first question, we must look at such factors as age, sex, racial or ethnic origin, parental age, birth order, and family size. We must also look at life style, occupation, and socioeconomic group. In community epidemiological studies, we are primarily interested in groups rather than in specific individuals. Thus, rates become a natural tool in the study of the persons whom a disease affects.

Age

Age is the personal attribute most strongly related to disease occurrence.[4] In fact, age is usually included even when studying other personal attributes.

One method of examining the age characteristics of a disease is to graph age-specific death rates. Figure 5-1 shows death rates per 1,000 for white and nonwhite males and females by age. We can see that death rates in all four groups are high at infancy but decline rapidly. The rates increase gradually after age 10 and exponentially after age 40. Chronic diseases, specifically lung cancer, often show a dramatic relationship to age, as in Figure 5-2.

The disease pyramid is an alternate method of examining diseases by age, as well as by sex and race. Constructed in the same manner as a population pyramid, the disease pyramid shows which age groups are affected by diseases. The pyramid provides an immediate visual analysis of disease mortality by age, sex, and race. It can illustrate the dominance of a specific age, sex, or race for the selected disease (see Figure 5-3). Specific target groups may be identified, depending upon the specificity of the age groups utilized. For example, an inverted pyramid indicates a disease that is concentrated in the older ages, whereas a pyramid that bulges to the left of the central axis at midpoint indicates a disease like cirrhosis of the liver which occurs predominantly in males at the middle age group. The pyramid, however, does not give the absolute risk of dying by age, sex, and race because the values are not weighted according to distribution of the population for each age, sex, and race grouping.

Studies by age may be done as current analysis or as cohort analysis. The graphs previously shown are current analysis, showing the relationship between age and, in some instances, sex and race to death or disease at one point in time. In contrast, in a cohort analysis the relationships between successive birth cohorts (persons born during a specified time), age, and death are examined. In Figure 5-4, death rates are plotted using a cohort method. Each line shows the effect of the disease on each cohort as it moves through age groups. Instead of displaying the data cross

Figure 5-1 Death Rates per 1,000 by Age, Color, and Sex, United States, 1968 (semilogarithmic scale)

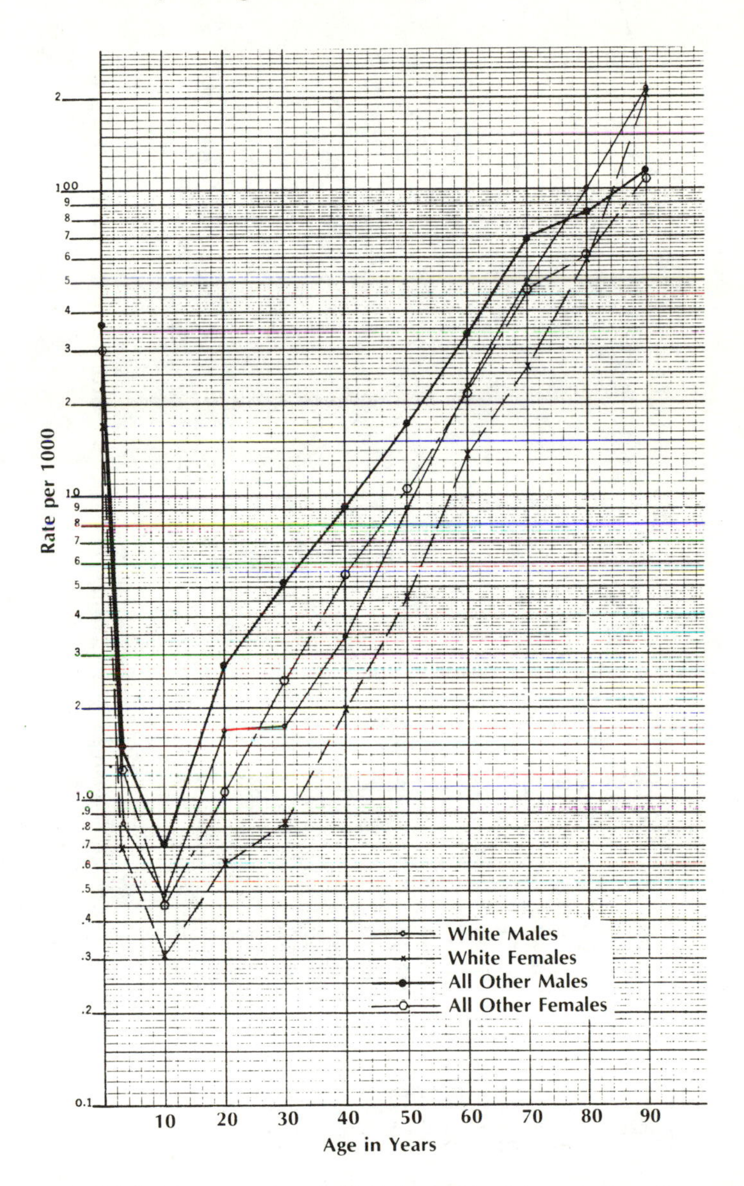

Source: Judith S. Mausner and Antia K. Bahn, *Epidemiology: An Introductory Text,* page 44. Reprinted by permission from W. B. Saunders Co., Philadelphia, Pennsylvania. Copyright 1974. (From National Center for Health Statistics: Vital Statistics of the United States, 1968, Vol. IIA. U.S. Govt. Printing Office, Washington, D.C., 1972.)

Figure 5-2 Age Specific Rates (per 100,000) for Lung Cancer, U.S. Whites

Age	Males	Females
0- 4	0.08	0.06
5- 9	0.03	0.02
10-14	0.04	0.03
15-19	0.08	0.06
20-24	0.22	0.11
25-29	0.51	0.23
30-34	1.95	0.74
35-39	5.67	2.06
40-44	15.04	4.72
45-49	33.43	8.39
50-54	66.66	12.50
55-59	113.21	16.84
60-64	167.49	21.08
65-69	206.52	25.71
70-74	219.25	31.87
75-84	191.28	38.62
85+	120.82	38.74

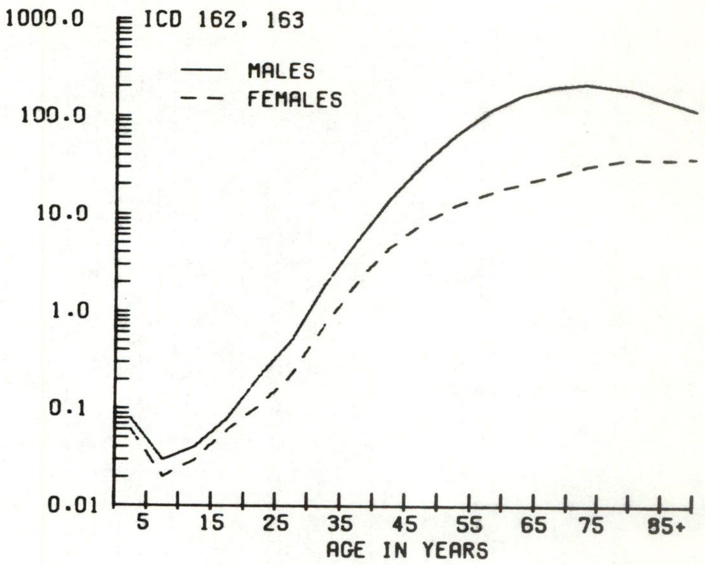

Source: T. J. Mason et al., *Atlas of Cancer Mortality for U.S. Counties, 1950–69,* U.S. DHEW Pub. No. NIH 15-780, p. 81.

Figure 5-3 Disease Pyramids

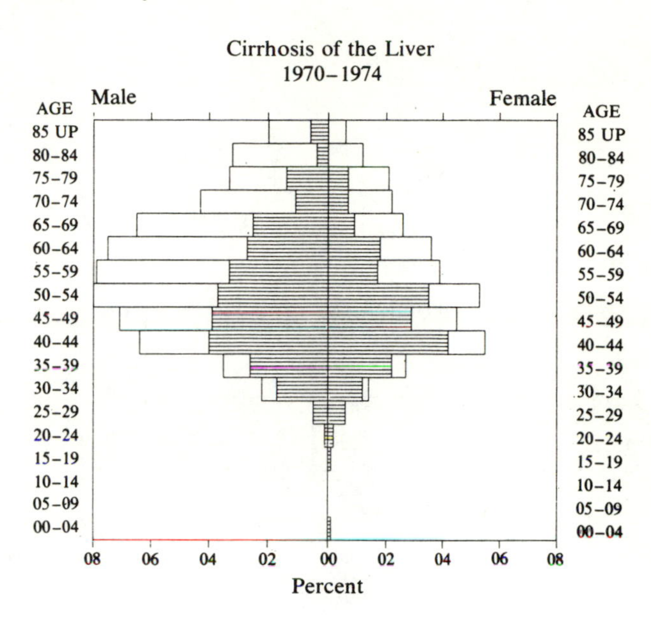

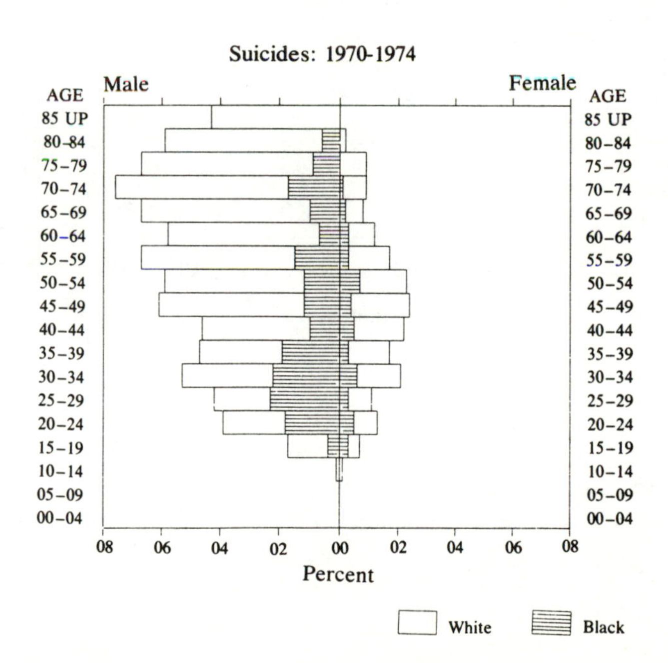

Figure 5-3 continued

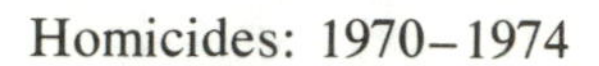

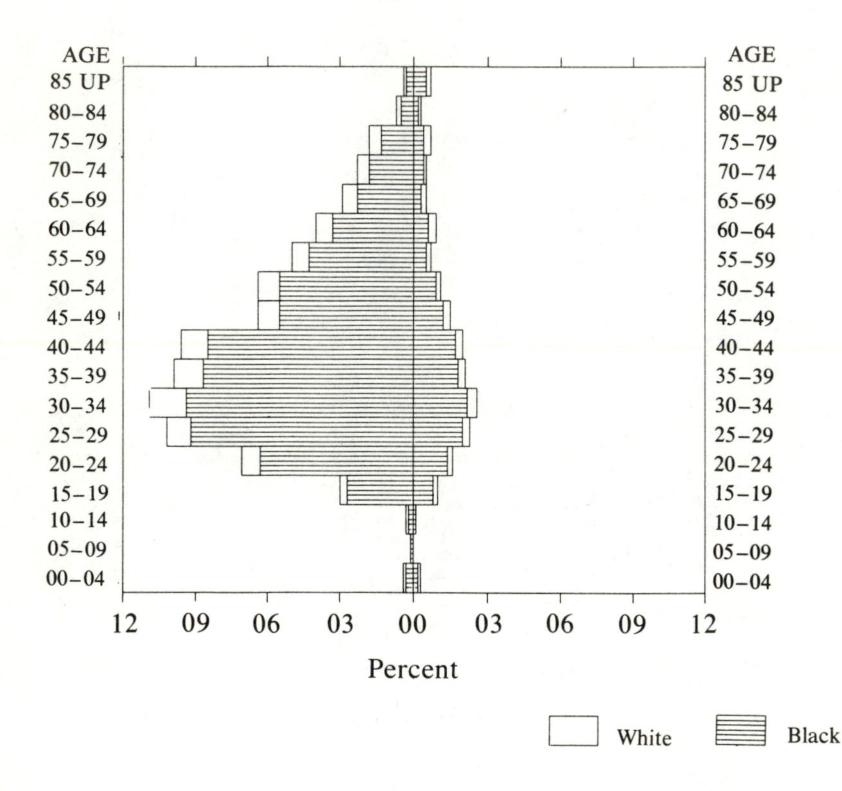

Source: "Disease Patterns of the 70's," *Health Services Research and Statistics,* Division of Physical Health, Georgia Department of Human Resources, August 1976, pp. 116, 121, and 137.

Figure 5-4 Death Rates from Tuberculosis, by Age Group, for Birth Cohorts, United States, 1860–1960

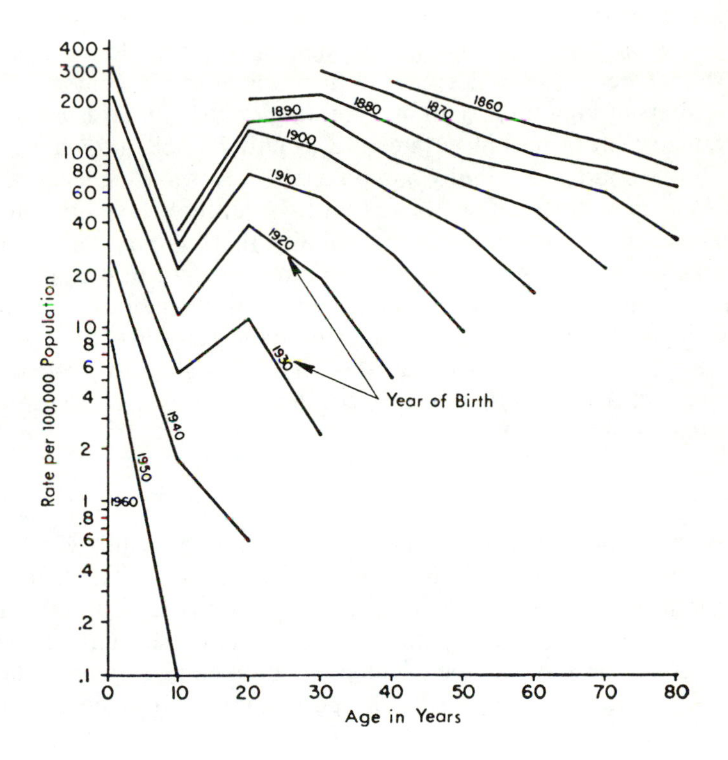

Source: J. S. Mausner and A. K. Bahn, *Epidemiology: An Introductory Text,* p. 84. (Adapted from Doege, T. C.: Tuberculosis mortality in the United States, 1900 to 1960. *J.A.M.A.*, 192:1045, 1965.) Reprinted by permission from W. B. Saunders Co., Philadelphia.

sectionally, cohort analysis shows the relationship between death (or disease) and age through time.

The differential mortality experience of males and females is evident in Figures 5-1 and 5-2. If specific causes were examined, the differences would become even more evident. The ratio of male to female deaths for age-adjusted cancer rates varies from more than three to one to less than one to one.[5] For nearly all forms of cancer, male deaths exceed female deaths. Particularly significant is the fact that the ratio of male deaths to female deaths exceeds three to one for four forms of cancer (larynx, esophagus, tongue, and lung). Lung cancer has been related specifically to the greater incidence of smoking by men. Current evidence suggests, however, that we will see a decrease in this ratio as more women begin to feel the effects of long-term smoking. Although mortality rates are generally higher in males, morbidity rates are usually higher in females.[6] For women, both reported morbidity and physician visits are higher in all age groups. Mausner and Bahn postulate that these differences between men and women may be related to the possibility that women seek medical care at an earlier stage of a disease compared to men or to the possibility that the cited diseases have a less lethal effect on women than on men.[7] As an example of the differences in morbidity and mortality, they point to a study by Silverman[8] which indicates that, though death rates from suicide are higher in men than in women, depression is more common in women than in men.

Race or Ethnic Group

The examination of specific health statistics may be controversial, especially when associated with ethnic or minority groups. Statistical inferences or implications from specialized investigations may justifiably raise more questions than the investigations can answer. While summary health statistics reflect the status of the whole population being examined, health statistics focusing on ethnic or minority populations will reflect the status of that selected population.

Alfred Haynes states that:

> . . . we should insist that adequate statistics be maintained so that health planners do not lose sight of special problems of minority groups. Only by such special focus will minority problems receive due attention. Representing a relatively small percentage of the total population, it is easy for minority problems to be ignored. This must not happen. We must oppose those within minority groups who wish to conceal special problems, and we must oppose those of the majority group who want to ignore these problems.[9]

Adequate health care for all citizens is the goal of the health agency. To reach this goal, the agency must know the disease patterns which may reflect the health status of the population it serves. Ideally, since studies have associated socioeconomic standing with some diseases, the socioeconomic patterns of a state should be most helpful in planning health services. Socioeconomic data, however, are mainly limited to the ten-year census period. For this reason, mortality and, increasingly, morbidity statistics are employed to depict areas of relative need. To plan adequately for the minority population, the health planner should consider racial differences in mortality and morbidity rates.

As shown in Figure 5-1, compared to whites, blacks have a higher death rate at every age group except that of 75 and over. Cause-specific death rates for hypertensive heart disease, cerebrovascular accidents, tuberculosis, syphilis, homicide, and accidental deaths are all higher among blacks.[10] Whites have higher death rates for arteriosclerotic heart disease, suicide, and leukemia. Whites and blacks also have different rates for several forms of cancer; for example, black females have a higher incidence of cervical cancer than white females, while white females have a higher incidence of breast cancer than black females.

Socioeconomic Status

Although, as we have seen, some diseases are related to race or ethnic background, most differences in rates may be accounted for by differences in socioeconomic status and environment. Socioeconomic status may be measured by characteristics such as education, income, occupation, area of residence, and life style. In recent years, the relationship of disease and death with socioeconomic status, particularly occupation and life style, has received particular attention.

In an analysis by socioeconomic class, age-adjusted death rates are usually compared for different classes. Classification may be based on income, occupation, and education, or on some combination of indicators. For example, a study related the ten leading causes of death in Georgia with standardized measures of socioeconomic status, median education, median income, and occupation.[11] The results are shown in Table 5-1. Based on Spearman's rank-order correlation, 7 of the 10 causes of death showed significant inverse relationships to increasing socioeconomic status. Two (ischemic heart disease and cancer of the trachea, bronchus, and lung) showed significant direct relationships, indicating increasing incidence of death from these causes with increasing socioeconomic class.

Table 5-1 Spearman's Rank-Order Correlation Coefficients of Mean Mortality Rates with Combined Socioeconomic Status, Median Education, Median Income, and Occupation, Georgia, 1969–1972

Mortality Categories	Combined Socioeconomic Status		Median Education		Median Income		Occupation	
	"r" Value	Significance	"r" Value	Significance	"r" Value	Significance	"r" Value	Significance
Total Mortality	−.6203	.001	−.5001	.001	−.7233	.001	−.2561	.001
Other Accidents	−.3630	.001	−.3271	.001	−.4515	.001	−.1590	.05
Motor Vehicle Accidents	−.3250	.001	−.3524	.001	−.2936	.001	−.2326	.01
Infant Mortality	−.2762	.001	−.1772	.05	−.3357	.001	−.1611	.05
Ischemic Heart Disease	.2116	.01	.2424	.01	.1376	NS	.1866	.05
Influenza and Pneumonia	−.1885	.05	−.1917	.05	−.2193	.01	−.0498	NS
Cancer of the Trachea, Bronchus, and Lung	.1812	.05	.1657	.05	.0936	NS	.2189	.01
Cerebrovascular Disease	−.1754	.05	−.1116	NS	−.2472	.01	−.0400	NS
Homicide	−.1581	.05	−.0961	NS	−.2350	.01	−.0292	NS
Acute Myocardial Infarction	−.1461	NS	−.1000	NS	−.1482	NS	−.1615	.05
Other Forms of Heart Disease	.0186	NS	.0066	NS	−.0070	NS	−.0457	NS

Note: NS = not significant.

Source: "Socioeconomic Analysis of the Disease Patterns of the 70s," *Health Services Research and Statistics,* Division of Physical Health, Georgia Department of Human Resources, August 1977, p. 10.

The relationship of occupation to disease has been studied frequently in recent years. Occupational exposure to asbestos has been related to mesothelioma and lung and gastrointestinal cancer,[12] free silica exposure to pulmonary fibrosis,[13] and other chemical agents and toxic substances to various forms of morbidity and mortality. Recent studies, like that by Cobb and Rose on air traffic controllers,[14] have focused on stress in the working place, showing increased incidence of hypertension, peptic ulcer, and diabetes associated with certain occupations. A more general study[15] has shown higher rates of mortality from cirrhosis of the liver among higher occupational groups in England and Wales (see Table 5-2). In contrast, a similar study in the United States found a higher mortality rate for cirrhosis of the liver in the semiskilled and laborer classes.[16] Another

Table 5-2 Standardized Mortality Ratios, Cirrhosis of the Liver, Men Ages 20 to 64 Years by Occupational Class, in England and Wales, 1949–1953

Class		Standardized Mortality Ratio
I	Professional occupations	207
II	Intermediate occupations	152
III	Skilled occupations	84
IV	Partly skilled occupations	70
V	Unskilled occupations	96

Source: Milton Terris, "Epidemiology of Cirrhosis of the Liver, National Mortality Data," *AJPH* 47, 1967, pp. 2076–2088.

study has shown that the prevalence of coronary heart disease among workers in agriculture, forestry, and fishing is significantly less than that among workers in other occupational groups.[17]

Other Person-Related Attributes

Although age, sex, and socioeconomic status are the most frequently studied of the person-related attributes of disease and death, other personal attributes should not be overlooked. Studies have shown that religious groups may have different rates, for example, the studies that show that Amish women have a lower rate of cervical cancer morbidity than other groups[18] and the many studies that indicate lower morbidity and mortality rates among Mormons. Marital status also has been shown to have an impact on some causes of death. The unmarried have higher mortality rates; the age-adjusted mortality rate was found to be lower in both married males and females than in single, widowed, or divorced groups.[19] Studies on the birth order and the age of the mother at time of birth have demonstrated considerable variation in stillbirth rates (see Figure 5-5). For instance, no matter what the birth order, mothers over age 40 have high stillbirth rates. It is quite apparent that the 20–24 and 25–29 age groups have the lowest risk of stillbirths. Thus, age of mother and birth order are significant personal characteristics to be investigated in the descriptive phase of a community epidemiological study.

Life Style Characteristics

The relationship of personal characteristics to drinking level is illustrated in Table 5-3. Specifically, consumption of alcohol by persons 18

Figure 5-5 Stillbirth Rates by Birth Order and Age of Mother, Missouri, 1972–74

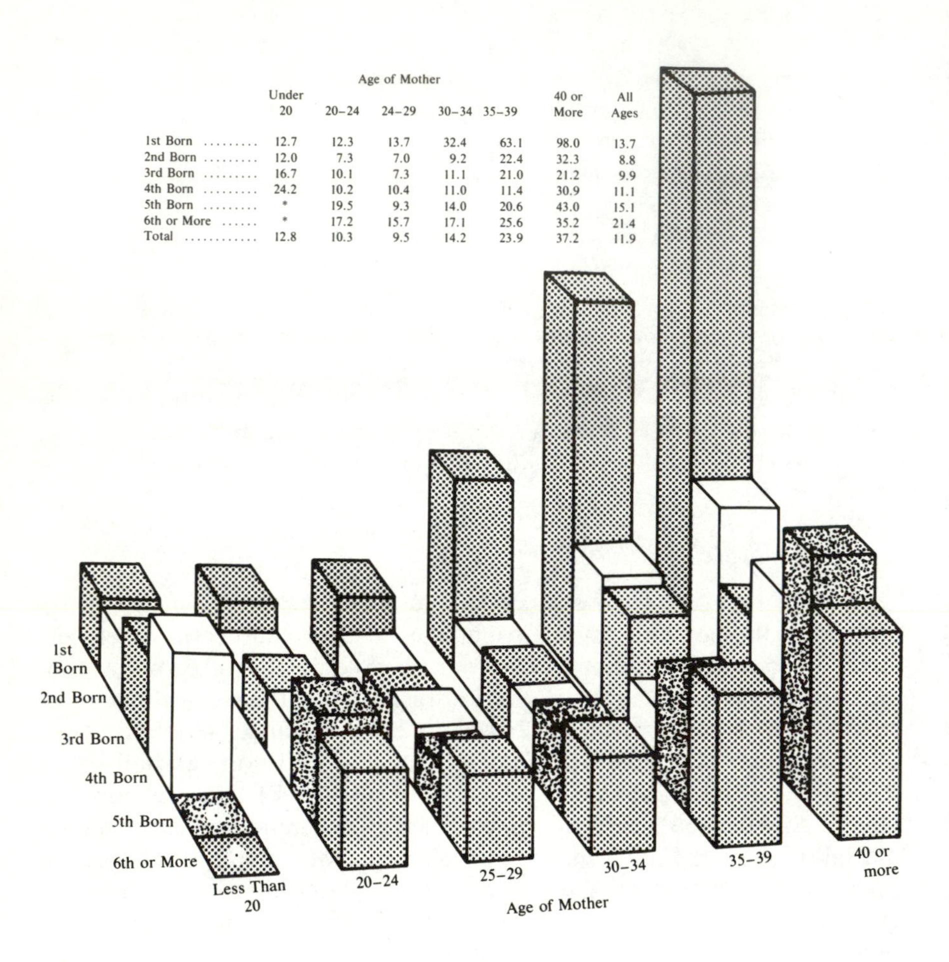

	Age of Mother						
	Under 20	20–24	24–29	30–34	35–39	40 or More	All Ages
1st Born	12.7	12.3	13.7	32.4	63.1	98.0	13.7
2nd Born	12.0	7.3	7.0	9.2	22.4	32.3	8.8
3rd Born	16.7	10.1	7.3	11.1	21.0	21.2	9.9
4th Born	24.2	10.2	10.4	11.0	11.4	30.9	11.1
5th Born	*	19.5	9.3	14.0	20.6	43.0	15.1
6th or More	*	17.2	15.7	17.1	25.6	35.2	21.4
Total	12.8	10.3	9.5	14.2	23.9	37.2	11.9

*Rate not shown because of extremely small numbers in cell.

Source: Missouri Monthly Vital Statistics, Missouri Center for Health Statistics, Dept. of Social Services, Missouri Division of Health, 1975, p. 3.

years of age and over is shown in relation to sex, race, family income, marital status, and education. If we concentrate on the problem area of 0.551 ounces or more of alcohol per day, we can develop a profile. Thus, a heavy drinker may be characterized as a single white male with a family income of $15,000 or more and with either high school or some college education. Such a profile may serve two purposes. First, epidemiological studies could use this information to set up experimental designs. Second, this information provides a market segmentation by which it can be distributed for health education and promotion. Alternatively, major breweries could use such information to market their products. Similar tables from *Health, United States, 1976–77* present other life style characteristics, such as nutritional status, exercise levels, and stress conditions.[20] Many factors related to a disease may go unnoticed if available data on person-related attributes are overlooked. Such life-style data allow us to approach health problems holistically.

Where Does the Disease Occur?

The second major question we seek to answer in descriptive epidemiological studies of a community is, Where does disease occur? As in person-related characteristics, we are again looking for a pattern of disease occurrence, this time in relation to geography. The method of analysis involves mapping disease patterns and making comparisons between geographic areas in tables, graphs, and charts. The objectives are to suggest possible relationships between location and disease for further study and to lay the basis for the planning of specific programs for attacking problem areas.

The most important part of analysis by place is to choose the proper scale. Thus, if information is needed for planning by a health systems agency, the enumeration districts or cities are appropriate levels for analysis. The level of analysis must be specific enough to determine geographic variations of the phenomenon being studied (see Table 7-3). A second aspect of the analysis scale relates to the particular disease being studied. If a disease has a very low incidence, it is often necessary to use a large scale of analysis, for example, a country or a continent, and to plot the location of occurrences. Most community-specific analyses, however, deal with diseases of relatively widespread incidence and prevalence. Consequently, we can make the choice of scale on the basis of need for data.

A classic example of an analysis of epidemiology by place is John Snow's study of cholera in London in 1848–54.[21] Snow mapped the exact

Table 5-3 Consumption of Alcohol by Persons 18 Years of Age and Over, According to Selected Characteristics: United States, January 1975 (Data are Based on Household Interviews of a Sample of the Civilian Noninstitutionalized Population)

		Drinking level					
				Drinkers, average daily consumption of absolute alcohol:			
Characteristic	All levels	Abstainers or less than 1 drink per year	Infrequent drinkers (1–6 drinks per year)	0.100 oz. or less	0.101- 0.200 oz.	0.201- 0.550 oz.	0.551 oz. or more
	Percent distribution						
Total	100	34	10	21	7	11	16
Sex							
Male	100	25	8	18	7	14	25
Female	100	43	11	25	6	8	7
Race							
White	100	33	10	22	7	11	16
Black	100	47	10	19	3	7	9
Family income							
Less than $5,000	100	53	10	16	3	5	11
$5,000–$9,999	100	39	11	15	4	11	16
$10,000–$14,999	100	28	10	25	9	12	15
$15,000 or more	100	16	8	27	10	16	21
Marital status							
Single	100	19	11	22	8	13	28
Married	100	33	9	22	8	11	15
Separated, divorced, or widowed	100	51	11	19	2	6	9
Education							
Less than high school graduate	100	50	9	16	3	6	13
High school graduate	100	27	10	23	8	13	18
Some college	100	22	13	26	8	12	18
College graduate	100	21	6	28	11	16	16

Source: U.S. Department of Health, Education, and Welfare, *Health United States, 1976–77,* Pub. No. (HRA) 77-1232, Table 41, p. 197. Calculated from tables in M. Rappeport, P. Labaw, and J. Williams, *The Public Evaluates the NIAAA Public Education Campaign, A Study for the U.S. Department of Health, Education, and Welfare,* Vols. I and II. Princeton. Opinion Research Corporation, July 1975.

location of cholera deaths occurring during a 10-day period in 1848 (Figure 5-6). Through visual analysis of the distribution of cholera, Snow noted the clustering of deaths around the Broad Street pump, from which residents received their water supply. After removal of the pump handle, no new cholera cases were reported.[22] This fact, coupled with Snow's earlier work, suggested that cholera was transmitted by contaminated water. By determining the relationship between location and disease, many place-related studies attempt to accomplish the same thing Snow accomplished: discovery of the etiological factors of the disease.

Figure 5-6 John Snow's Map of Cholera Deaths in the Soho District of London, 1848

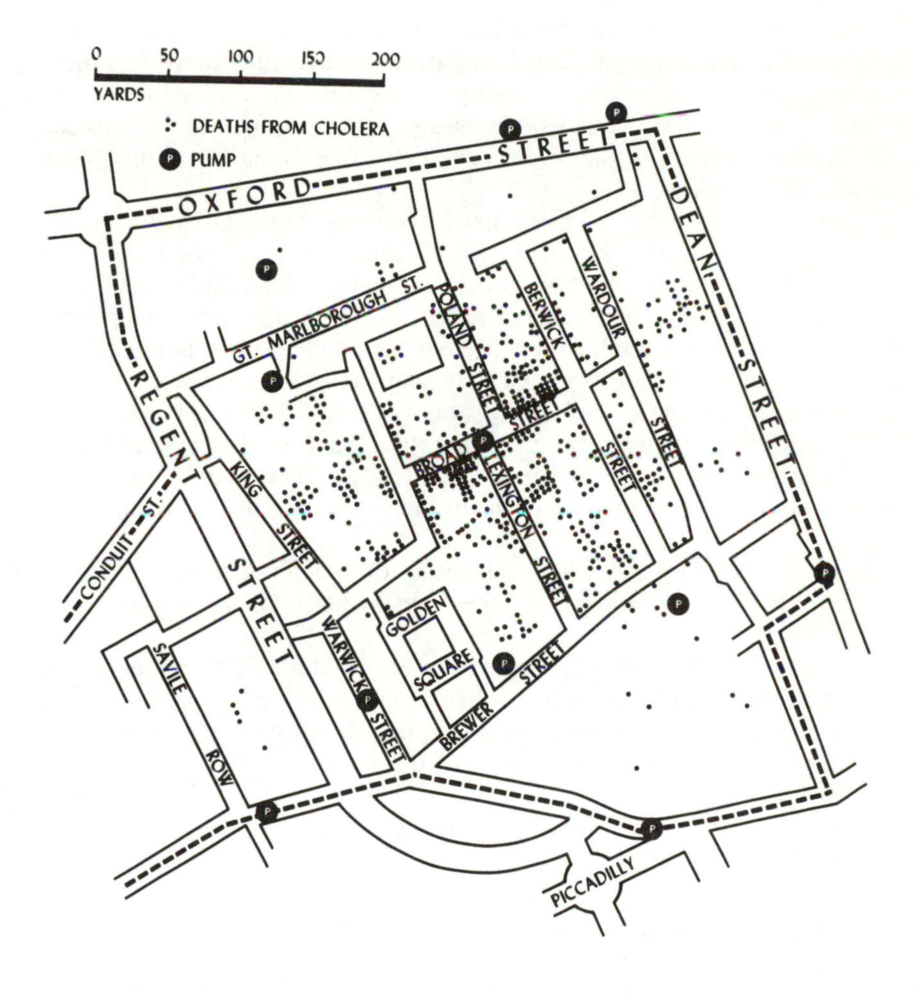

Source: Gary Shannon and G. E. Alan Dever, *Health Care Delivery: Spatial Perspectives* (New York: McGraw-Hill Book Co., 1974), p. 3. From L. D. Stamp, *Some Aspects of Medical Geography* (Oxford University Press, 1964), p. 16.

A second purpose of place-related studies, and probably more common in the field of community health analysis, is the comparison of mortality and morbidity rates of different areas. Age-adjusted rates are compiled and then either plotted or mapped for the areas under consideration. In a study in Georgia, the ten leading causes of death were mapped by county.[23] Figure 5-7 shows one of the maps, which depicts neonatal mortality rates in 1970–74 by county. Similar analyses might be done on the scale of enumeration districts or census tracts, depending upon the purpose of the study.

Probably one of the largest studies of disease occurrence by place was conducted by the National Cancer Institute.[24] This study mapped cancer rates by county and in some cases by state economic area for the entire United States. Several findings may be significant, such as those showing differences in cancer of the digestive system, lung, mouth, and throat by geographic location.

Urban and rural differences in disease patterns may also occur. Table 5-4 shows age-specific death rates for all causes in the United States by urban and rural residence.[25] Note that nonmetropolitan areas had higher death rates for people under age 45 and over age 85 whereas metropolitan areas had higher death rates for those between 45 and 84. Examination of cause-specific death rates showed that lung cancer deaths were higher in urban areas while accidental death rates were higher in rural areas.[26]

The information gained from comparative place studies should be related to differences in environment and life style. The analysis of disease patterns by place can then be used through other graphic techniques to:

1. demonstrate high and low risk areas for specific diseases;
2. provide a "community diagnosis" for further investigation by health officials;
3. provide a basis for determining the health status of the population;
4. provide a tool for planning in health and social programs;
5. provide a reliable method of presenting data to concerned groups;
6. serve as an aid in establishing priorities for allocation of resources; and
7. serve as an aid in developing policy for state, HSA, and community health programs.

When Does the Disease Occur?

The final question to be answered in descriptive epidemiological studies is the relationship of time to disease. The relationship varies with the particular disease under study. Hours are significant when studying an

Figure 5-7 Neonatal Mortality in Georgia, by Health District, 1970–1974

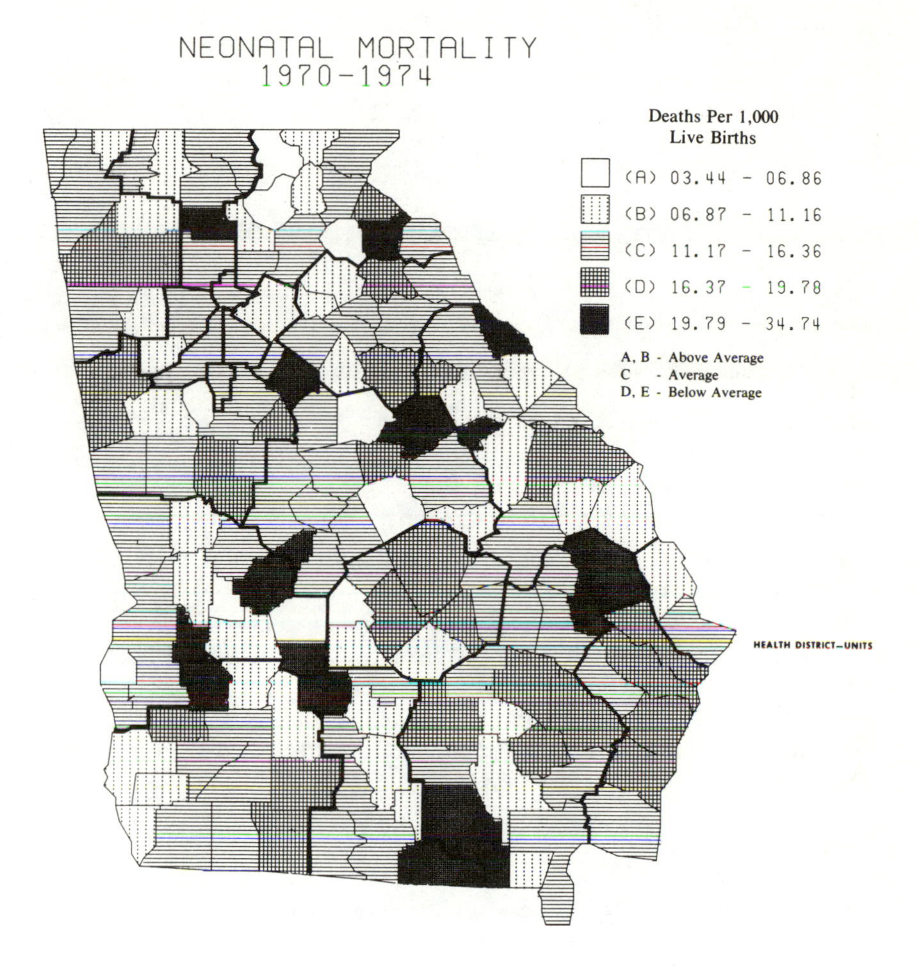

Source: "Disease Patterns of the 70s," *Health Services Research and Statistics*, Division of Physical Health, Georgia Department of Human Resources, August 1976, p. 31.

Table 5-4 Age-Specific Death Rates (All Causes) for Metropolitan and Nonmetropolitan Counties, United States, 1960

Age	Metropolitan Counties	Non-Metropolitan Counties
	u < 1	
	26.0	
	28.7	
1– 4	1.0	1.3
5–14	.4	.5
15–24	.9	1.3
25–34	1.4	1.6
35–44	3.0	3.1
45–54	7.8	7.1
55–64	18.0	16.3
65–74	39.6	36.0
75–84	89.0	85.3
85 +	196.0	200.7
All	9.3	10.0

Source: John P. Fox, Carrie E. Hall, and Lila R. Elveback, *Epidemiology: Man and Disease* (London: Collier MacMillan Ltd., 1970), p. 233.

outbreak of food poisoning. Days may be significant when studying cases of respiratory illness in a boys' camp (Figure 5-8). However, occupational exposure to hazardous substances may not be evident until years or decades later. Indeed, many chronic diseases are characterized by long latency periods and indefinite onset.

In examining diseases, particularly chronic diseases, over time, we commonly look at the changes in mortality rates. Two major kinds of changes may be observed: secular and cyclical trends.

Secular Trends

Secular trends refer to changes which take place over a long period of time, such as years or decades. Figure 5-9 shows the trend of the leading causes of mortality in Georgia in the period from 1956 to 1975. As can be seen, death rates from diseases of the respiratory system and from homicides increased while death rates from birth injuries decreased. Also noteworthy is the fact that about 1969 cancer (all sites) became the second leading cause of death.

Another important application of a line graph showing a secular trend is shown in Figure 5-10. Malaria cases reported in the United States for the period 1933–1977 are highlighted by brief statements citing historical reasons for increases and decreases. For instance, after a long decline of

Figure 5-8 Cases of Respiratory Illness in a Boys' Camp, by Date of Onset, Wisconsin, June 20–July 15, 1978*

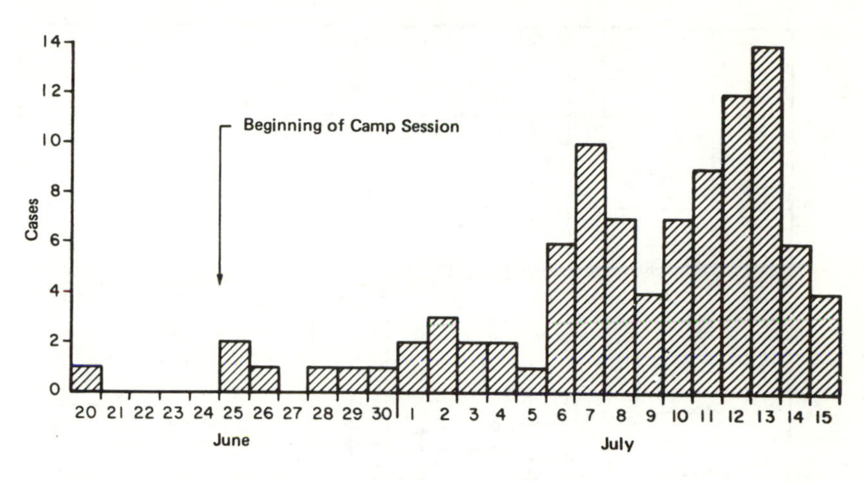

*In 6 cases the date of onset is unknown.
Source: Center for Disease Control, *Morbidity and Mortality Weekly Report,* U.S. Department of Health, Education, and Welfare, Public Health Service, Aug. 4, 1978, Vol. 27, no. 31.

cases, a drastic increase occurred after 1965 as a result of the returning Vietnam veterans. When changes in a line graph can be accounted for in this way, the secular trend approach is highly recommended.

Figure 5-11 shows the seasonally adjusted fertility rate for the period from 1975 through September 1978. The rate reflects births per 1,000 women 15–44 years of age. The graph shows the use of a moving average, which smooths out most random variations occurring within individual time periods (this effect can be seen in a comparison of the line of the moving average with the line showing the monthly data). In some instances, then, the kind of data desired may require the use of a moving average to portray secular trends.

Cyclical Trends

Cyclical trends refer to recurring patterns of disease occurrences over periods of time. In determining cyclical patterns of disease occurrence, we plot rates for a short interval of time, for example, one year. Some of the best known examples of cyclical trends are those depicted in graphs provided by the Center for Disease Control (CDC) on weekly pneumonia and influenza deaths (Figure 5-12). The CDC graphs are used to indicate when epidemic levels are reached.

Figure 5-9 Rates for Leading Causes of Death in Georgia, 1956 to 1975
Death Rates Per 100,000 Population

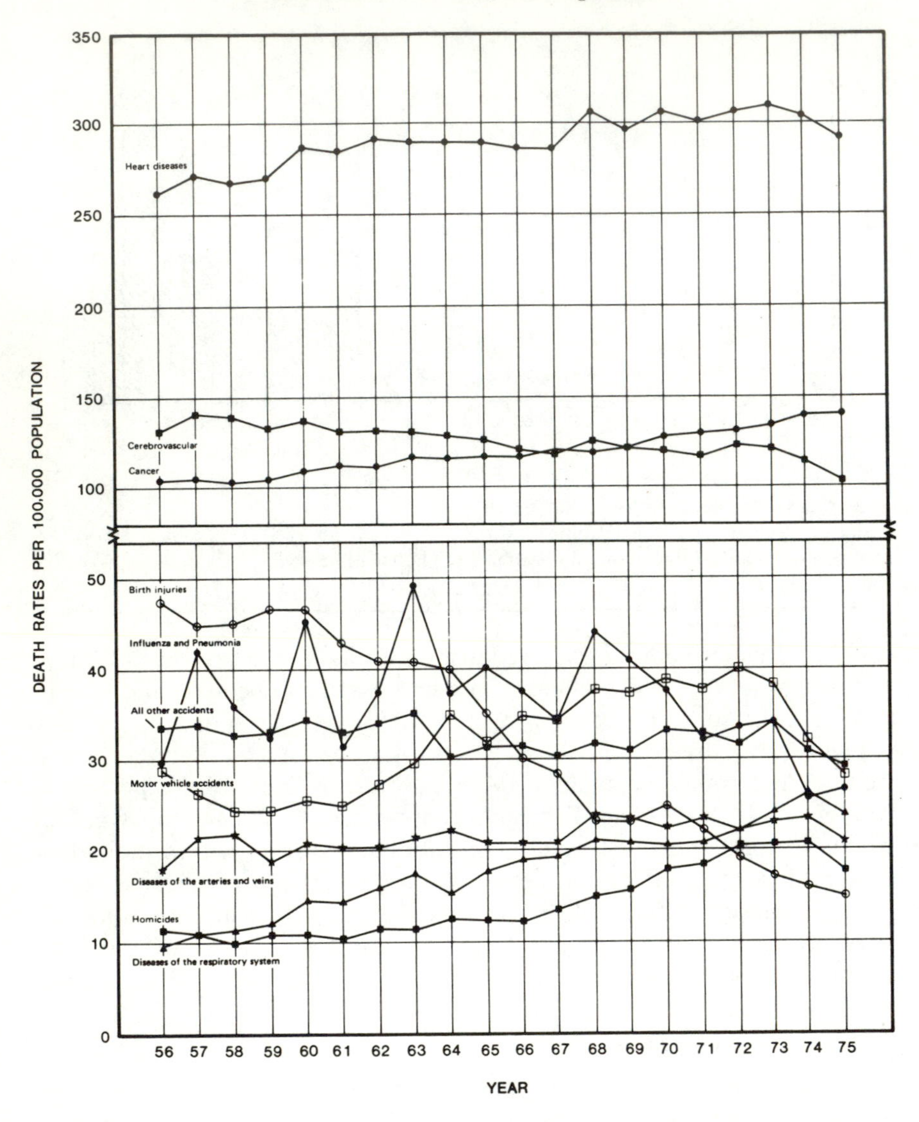

Source: Division of Physical Health, Georgia Dept. of Human Resources, *Georgia Vital and Health Statistics, 1975*, Health Services Research and Statistics, 1977, p. 58.

Figure 5-10 Reported Cases of Malaria by Year, United States, 1933–1977

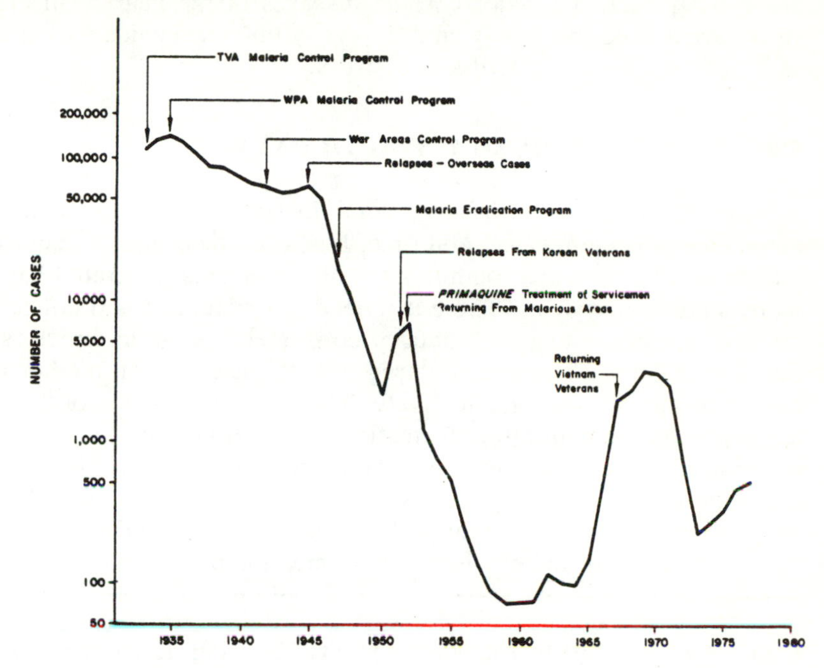

Source: U.S. Department of Health, Education, and Welfare, Public Health Service, *Morbidity and Mortality Weekly Report,* Center for Disease Control, 1978, p. 56.

The concepts of epidemic and endemic are related to both time and place. An epidemic, a short-term fluctuation in a disease cycle, is "the occurrence of a disease in members of a defined population clearly in excess of the number of cases usually or normally expected in that population."[27] Thus, the CDC graphs in Figure 5-12 show for each area the expected number of deaths and an epidemic threshold; when the threshold is exceeded an epidemic is indicated. In contrast, endemic occurrence of a disease is defined as a situation in which the disease is "regularly and continuously present" in a population in a defined place and over a period of time.[28]

Cyclical trends may be observed in deaths or diseases related to seasonal changes: the increase in drownings in summer or some of the infectious diseases transmitted by insects. They may be observed over long periods of time, as in the two-to-three year cycle of influenza Type A epidemics or in the four-to-six year cycle of influenza Type B epidemics, or over short periods, as in the weekly cycle of motor vehicle deaths, peaking on weekends.

Epidemics, it should be emphasized, are not just limited to infectious diseases. In fact, the major chronic diseases of the heart, cancer, and stroke are at epidemic levels, and the really universal epidemics are obesity, poor nutrition, inactivity, and stress.

ORGANIZING COMMUNITY HEALTH DATA

When organizing descriptive epidemiological data to present the characteristics of person, place, and time, health agencies face a major problem in dealing with the voluminous amount of data generated from the many statistical systems. There is a need to understand and utilize basic methods for presenting such data to consumers, program directors, and decision makers. The primary purpose in the use of such methods is to communicate information effectively. Thus, a basic function of the health agency is to communicate information so that informed judgments and decisions may be made about program direction, support, planning, and evaluation. Utilizing the various modes of data presentation (tables, graphs, and charts), the agency's objective should be to provide a product that is an effective and efficient communication device.

Figure 5-11 Seasonally Adjusted Fertility Rate Per 1,000 Women Aged 15–44

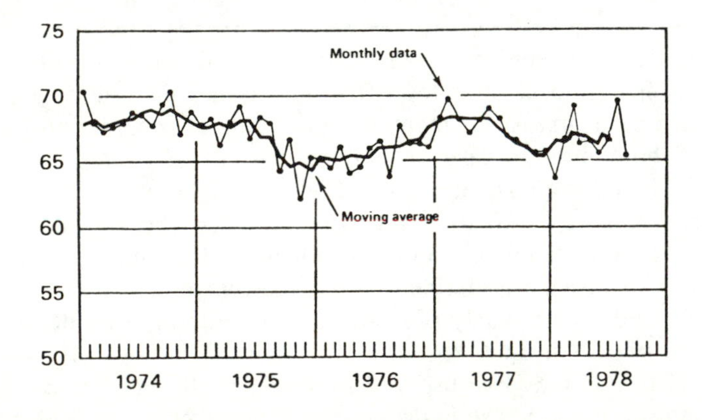

Source: U.S. Department of Health, Education, and Welfare, *Monthly Vital Statistics Report, Provisional Statistics, Birth, Marriage, Divorce, and Death for Sept. 1978.* NCHS Vol. 27, no. 9, Dec. 1978, p. 2.

Figure 5-12 Reported Deaths of Pneumonia and Influenza in 121 Selected U.S. Cities: All Cities by Week, September 1975–June 1978; by Geographic Division by Week, September 1977–June 1978

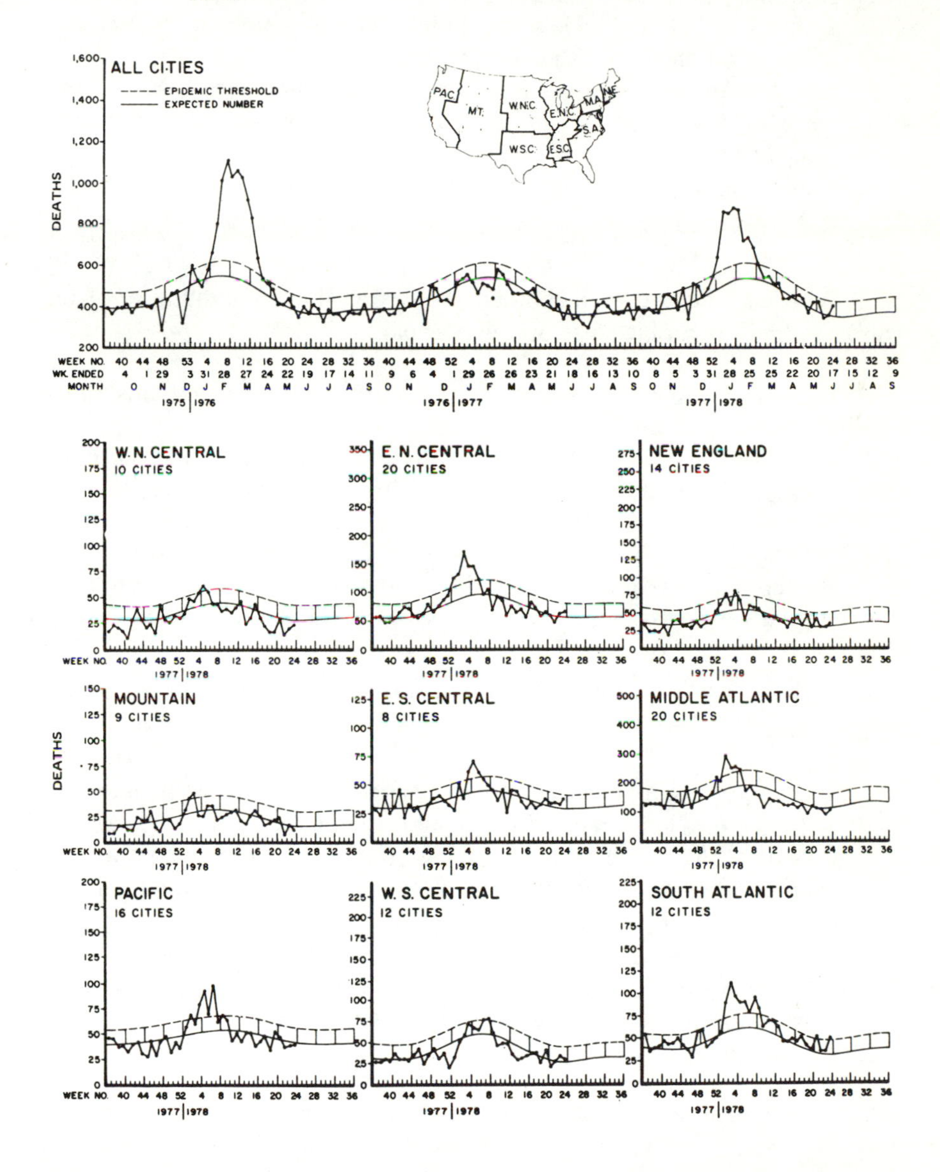

Source: U.S. Department of Health, Education, and Welfare, *Morbidity and Mortality Weekly Report, Annual Summary,* May 1977, Sept. 1978, Vol. 26, no. 53, p. 62.

Organizing data in graphic form has several advantages:

1. Graphic forms make it easy to read data; the lay person as well as the statistician can easily understand graphics.
2. Graphics have popular appeal and can communicate quickly. Readers will often skip lengthy tables or texts; graphics, in contrast, are forceful and attractive as learning devices.
3. Results shown in graphic form are easily remembered. Visual impressions from graphics are more revealing, convincing, and lasting than those from sets of figures or words.
4. Patterns and trends in graphic form are easy to identify and interpret.

As with any method or technique, however, the disadvantages of organizing data in graphic form are also apparent:

1. The use of graphic forms entails a loss of information and thus a loss of precision in the information presented.
2. There is the possibility of oversimplifying information in graphic form. Thus, the input data must be carefully scaled geographically and statistically.
3. In hand-drawn graphics errors and changes can be very costly. (This is becoming less and less of a disadvantage, however, as computer graphics become more and more widespread (see Chapter 9).

Moroney has stated well the need for graphics in organizing community health data:

> Cold figures are uninspiring to most people. Diagrams help us to see the pattern and shape of any complex situation. Just as a map gives us a bird's-eye view of a wide stretch of country, so diagrams help us to visualize the whole meaning of a numerical complex at a single glance. Give me an undigested heap of figures and I cannot see the woods for the trees. Give me a diagram and I am positively encouraged to forget detail until I have a real grasp of the overall picture. Diagrams register a meaningful impression almost before we think.[29]

This is a typical view of health professionals, program managers, policy makers, and directors who are responsible for making timely decisions. Thus, it is imperative that health planners be presented methods for organizing community health data.

Selection of the method for organizing and presenting health data depends on various factors:

1. The purpose of the presentation (oriented toward policymaking, toward management, or toward the consumer).
2. The type of data summary required (by person, place, or time).
3. The type of data message involved (costs, frequencies, rates, ratios, proportions).
4. The type of presentation to be made (slides, transparencies, flip charts).
5. The individual who is to use the data (health planner, epidemiologist, or statistician).

In light of these factors, the basic methods of organizing community health data into tables, graphs, and charts are reviewed below. (Mapping routines, requiring a special type of charting, are reviewed in Chapter 9.)

Tables

Quantitative data are usually organized in tabular form. In many instances, this may be all that is needed. Though valuable, however, tables do have limitations. The basic limitation stems from the fact that interpretation is hindered by the difficulty in determining patterns and trends in the data.

Though no specific rules determine table construction, general standards are more or less accepted:

1. Tables should be as simple as possible and be self-explanatory. Codes, abbreviations, and symbols need explanations in footnotes; titles, rows, columns, and totals should be marked clearly and concisely; and the units of data measurement should be provided.
2. The title should answer the questions, What (person or thing)? When (time)? and Where (place)?
3. The source of reproduced data should be given in a footnote.
4. The layout should be well-spaced, allowing for appropriate vertical and horizontal lines.
5. To enhance reader clarity, not more than three variables should be displayed. Indeed, small tables are often preferred to a single large table (See Table 5-5).

Tabular designs may serve many uses. First, they can display numbers extremely well. Second, the numbers in a tabular design may be expressed in various ways, for example, as absolutes, rates, ratios, per-

Table 5-5 Suicides under Age 35 as a Percent of Total, by Race and Sex, North Carolina Residents, 1977

Race and Sex	Percent
TOTAL	37.3
White male	35.2
White female	34.8
Black male	56.9
Black female	46.7

Source: Modified from North Carolina Department of Human Resources, Divison of Health Services, "Leading Causes of Mortality," *North Carolina Vital Statistics*, 1977, Vol. 2, p. 6.

centages, or correlation coefficients. Third, if absolute numbers are used, the data can be used for allocation of resources. Finally, graphs and charts can be prepared as natural outgrowths of tabular data.

Graphs

One of the oldest forms of graphic presentation, a graph is a method of organizing quantitative data by a coordinate system of x and y points. Examples of graphs are histograms, frequency polygons, and arithmetic, semilogarithmic and logarithmic line graphs.

A line graph has many significant uses. It shows how changes in one quantity are related to changes in another (multiple line graph). The line shows maximum and minimum values and indicates directional change, thereby demonstrating trends. A line graph may project or predict by extrapolating the trend line, representing rates, percentages, or moving averages on a three-, five-, or seven-year basis. Data plotted on a line graph can reflect point or period information. Point data refer to a particular point in time and are seldom used in summarizing health data. Period data, however, refer to a period of time and are frequently used by health planners. Examples of period data are annual mortality rates, average annual occupancy rates, and the annual percentage of the gross national product going to health care.

Following are some general principles outlined in a CDC publication as guidelines for the production of effective line graphs.[30]

1. The simplest graphs are the most effective. The number of lines and symbols in a single graph should be limited to those that the eye can easily follow.

2. Every graph should be self-explanatory.
3. The title may be placed at either the top or the bottom of the graph.
4. When more than one variable is shown on a graph, they should be clearly differentiated by means of legends or keys.
5. Only those coordinate lines that are necessary to guide the eye should be shown.
6. Coordinate lines should be lighter than the lines of the graph itself.
7. Usually, frequency is represented on the vertical scale and method of classification on the horizontal scale.
8. On an arithmetic scale, equal increments must represent equal numerical units.
9. Scale divisions and their units should be clearly indicated.
10. For comparative purposes, the zero point should be shown on the y axis.

Arithmetic Line Graphs

An arithmetic line graph requires arithmetic paper with equal intervals on the vertical (y) axis and the horizontal (x) axis. Some situations, however, may require uneven intervals. For example, a time period displayed on the horizontal axis may be related to infant mortality rates on the vertical axis (see Figure 5-13). Note the scale break in the vertical axis of Figure 5-13 which enables the reader to make the appropriate interpretation. Such a scale break can be used only in an arithmetic line graph. Finally, it should be noted that, on an arithmetic line graph, an arithmetic progression will yield a straight line.

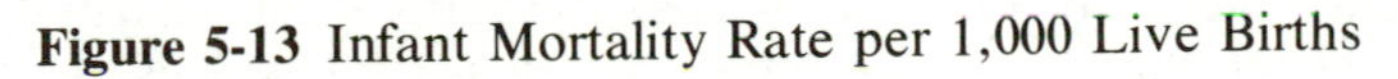

Figure 5-13 Infant Mortality Rate per 1,000 Live Births

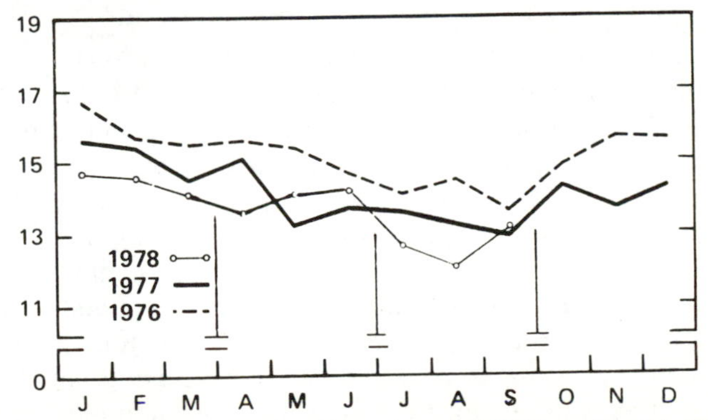

Source: U.S. Department of Health, Education, and Welfare, *Monthly Vital Statistics Provisional Data,* NCHS, Vol. 27, no. 9, Dec. 8, 1978, p. 3.

Semilogarithmic and Logarithmic Line Graphs

On a semilogarithmic line graph, logarithmic units are measured on the vertical axis, and arithmetic units are measured on the horizontal axis. Semilogarithmic and the logarithmic line graphs have specific characteristics. The logarithmic line graph measures logarithmic values on both the vertical and the horizontal axes. The basic reason for using logarithmic scales is to show rates of change. Thus, the choice between arithmetic and logarithmic line graphs depends upon whether the health planner wants to illustrate absolute magnitudes (arithmetic graph) or rates of change (logarithmic graph). Because logarithmic scales can have one or more cycles and do not have to start at zero, the planner can show rates of change. For instance, the scale can begin with 0.1, 1.0, 10.0, 100.0, or 1,000.0, with the larger number always ten times greater than the smaller number (see Figure 5-14). A geometric progression is shown on a logarithmic line graph by a straight line. On a logarithmic line graph, equal increases or decreases represent equal percentage changes, and equal slopes reflect equal rates of change. The basic purposes of semilogarithmic and logarithmic line graphs are to compare proportional rates of change and to illustrate relationships between two or more variables with significant differences (see Figure 5-15).

Histograms and Frequency Polygons

The histogram and the frequency polygon are similar in that they are both special forms of graphics. Each is graphically portrayed on two quantitative scales, a vertical and a horizontal. Data on a variable are usually converted into class intervals on the horizontal axis, and the frequency of the data is plotted on the vertical axis. The vertical and horizontal axes should reflect interval or ratio measurements, for example, the distribution of dentists by age groups.

The *histogram* graphs data as frequency distributions on arithmetic paper. It resembles a bar chart but, unlike the latter, it shows frequencies in both axes. Because the height of each column is being compared, it is not advisable to use a scale break in the histogram. An example of a histogram is shown in Figure 5-16. A histogram must satisfy two conditions: (1) the width of each rectangle must represent the width of the corresponding group, and (2) the area of each rectangle must represent the frequency of the corresponding group. Thus, the area under the histogram (the sum of the area of all rectangles) represents the total frequency.

The *frequency polygon* is constructed from a histogram. It shows a trend line that is constructed by converting the midpoints of the class intervals of the histogram. Because it is able to compare two or more sets

Figure 5-14 Possible Values on a Semilogarithmic Scale

Major Scale Divisions (Semilog Scale)	Possible Values A	B	C	D
1	1000	1.0	100,000	100
9				
8				
7	700	.7		
6	600		60,000	
5				50
4	400	.4		
3	300		30,000	
2	200	.2		20
1	100	0.1	10,000	10
9				
8				
7		.07		
6			6,000	
5	50			5
4				
3		.03	3,000	
2	20			2
1	10	0.01	1,000	1.0
9				
8				
7	7			
6			600	
5		.005		.5
4	4			
3			300	
2				.2
1	1	0.001	100	0.1

Source: U.S. Department of Health, Education, and Welfare, *Methods for Organizing Epidemiological Data,* CDC, Atlanta, Ga., Feb. 1977, p. 15.

of data more concisely and more clearly, the frequency polygon is preferred to the histogram. An example of a frequency polygon is shown in Figure 5-17.

Figure 5-15 Neonatal and Postneonatal Mortality Rates, by Color, United States, 1915–1974

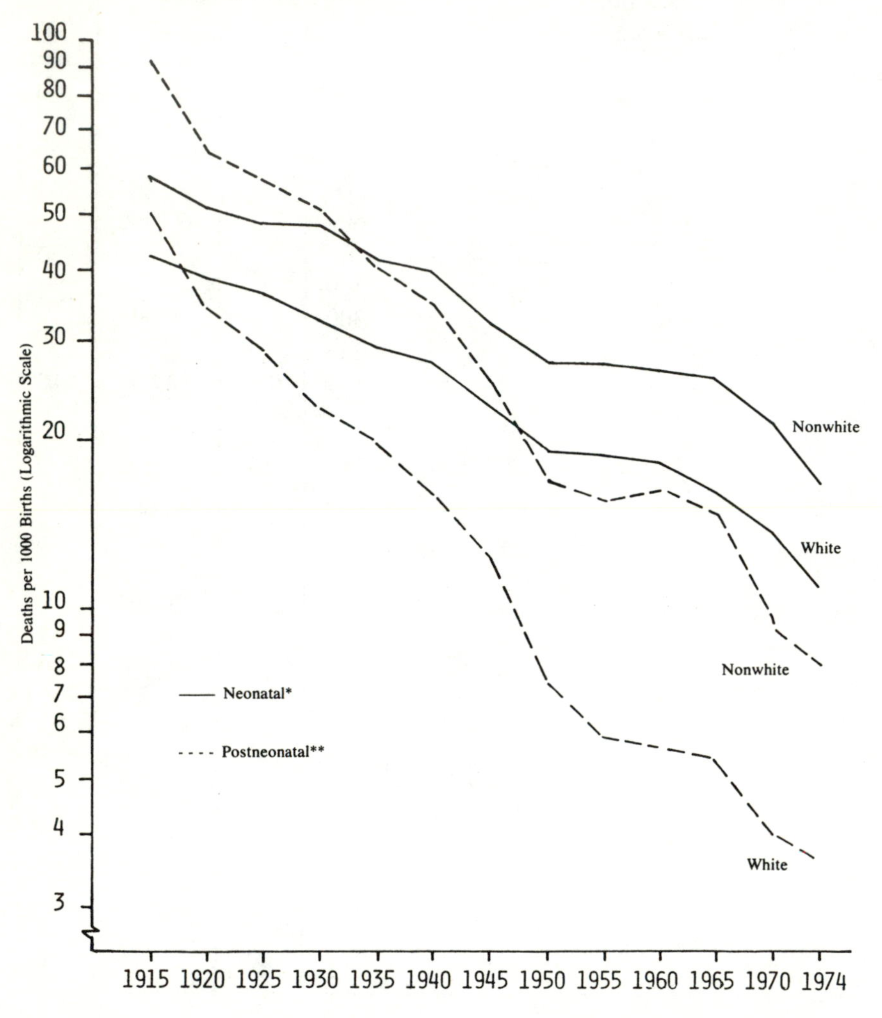

*Neonatal: Deaths under one month per 1,000 live births.

**Postneonatal: Deaths from one month to twelve months per 1,000 live births.

Source: S. I. Axelrod et al., *Medical Care Chart Book,* School of Public Health, Univ. of Michigan, Dept. of Medical Care Organization, 6th ed., rev. Sept. 1976, p. 20.

Figure 5-16 Cases of Rash Illness, Elementary School, Sample City, February 22–March 23, 1970

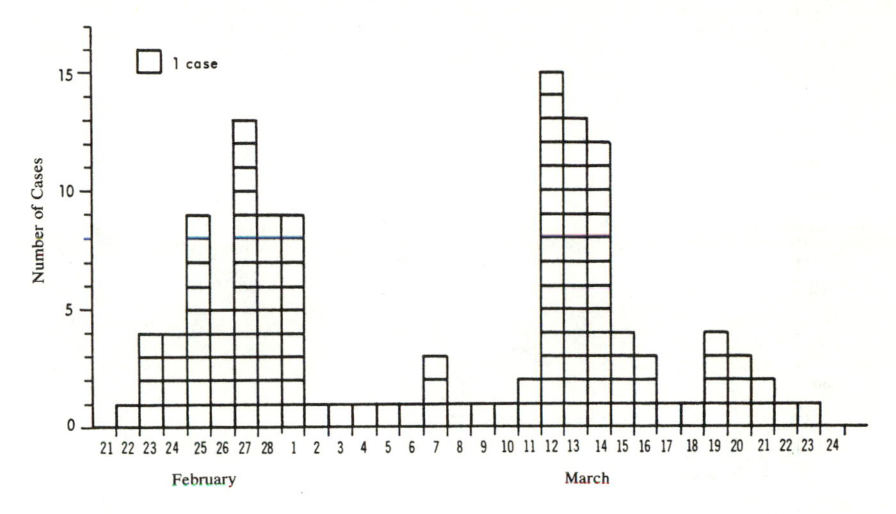

Source: U.S. Department of Health, Education, and Welfare, *Descriptive Statistics: Tables, Graphs, and Charts,* PHS, CDC, Atlanta, Georgia (not dated), p. 8.

Charts

The bar chart is the most widely used of all charts. It is a one-scale chart that portrays data of nominal or ordinal measurement on the vertical axis. No quantitative scale is used on the horizontal axis. The bars may be arranged horizontally or vertically in ascending or descending order. A scale break should never be used on a bar chart. The bars presenting the information should be separated by spaces to avoid the appearance of a histogram. The bar chart can take the form of a two-dimensional bar chart (Figure 5-18), a multiple bar chart (Figure 5-19), a component bar chart (Figure 5-20), or a pie chart (Figure 5-21).

A Guide to Selecting a Method for Organizing Community Epidemiological Health Data

In this section we present a guide for selecting the most appropriate graphic to illustrate community epidemiological data (Table 5-6).[31] Assuming that the health planner has constructed summary tables of com-

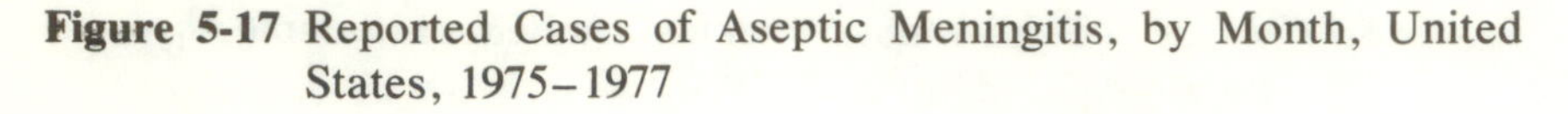

Figure 5-17 Reported Cases of Aseptic Meningitis, by Month, United States, 1975–1977

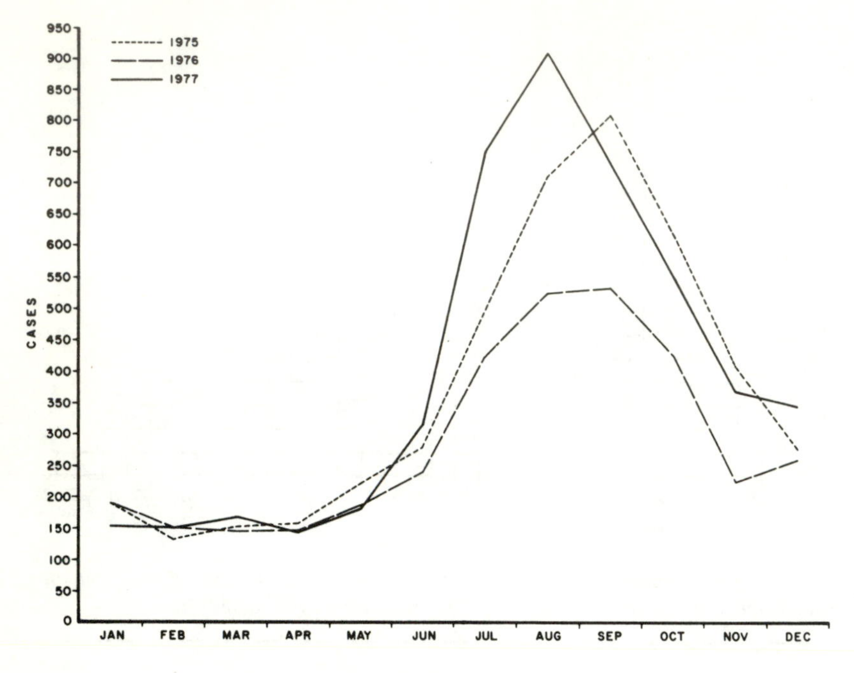

Source: U.S. Department of Health, Education, and Welfare, *Morbidity and Mortality Weekly Report, Reported Morbidity and Mortality in the U.S., Annual Summary, 1977,* CDC, Sept. 1978, Vol. 26, no. 53, p. 50.

munity health data containing important elements that require illustration, the guide will aid in identifying a recommended method for illustrating the data set. Each question in the guide should be answered yes or no. The last column gives appropriate directions either to a follow-up question or to the suggested method.

SUMMARY

By using the basic descriptive epidemiological concepts of person, place, and time presented in this chapter, the health planner should have a better understanding of some of the issues that arise in the analysis of community health data. Both the health planner and the student of health planning and epidemiology should find the material indispensable in the accomplishment of their objectives.

Figure 5-18 Percentage Distribution of Currently Married Women 15–44 Years of Age Using the IUD at Survey Date, by Type of IUD Used: United States, 1976

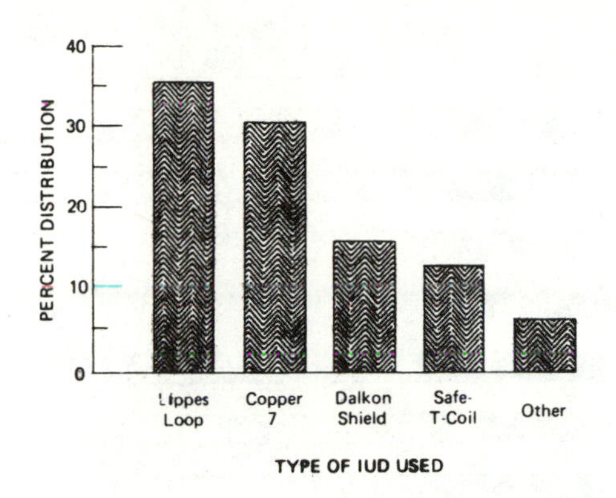

Source: Vital and Health Statistics, "Use of Intrauterine Contraceptive Devices in the U.S.," *Advance Data,* no. 43, Dec. 1978., p. 4.

Figure 5-19 Percentage Change in Population by Race of Selected Age Groups, Georgia, 1970 to 1975

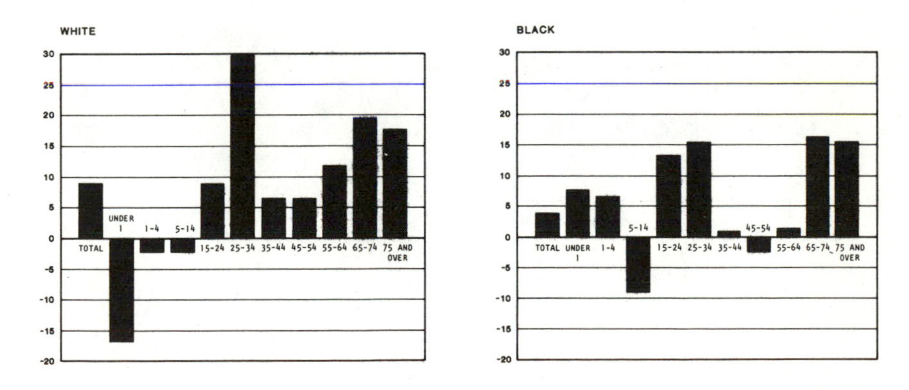

Source: Health Services Research and Statistics, *Georgia Vital and Health Statistics, 1975,* Div. of Physical Health, Georgia Dept. of Human Resources, 1977, p. 18.

Figure 5-20 Physician-Population Ratios by Geographic Area and Selected States, United States, 1973

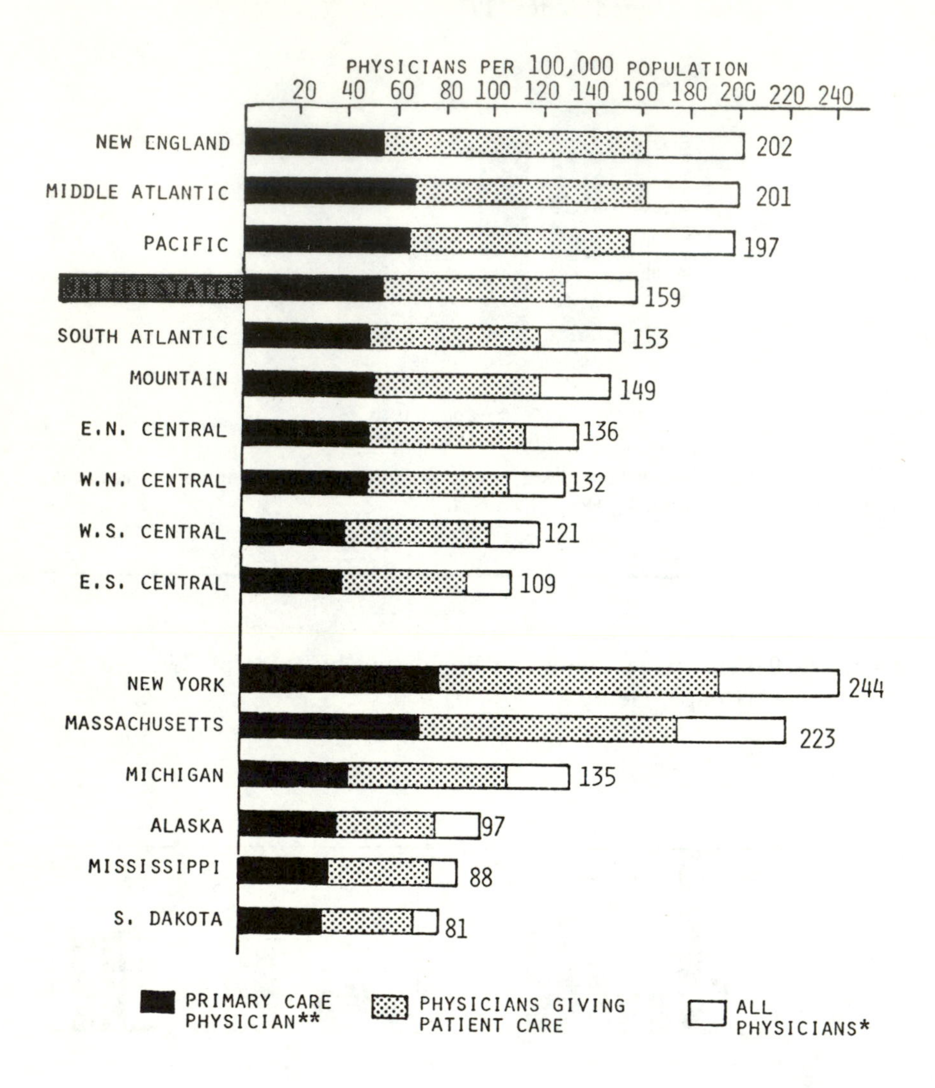

*Excludes physicians working for the federal government and osteopathic physicians.
**Physicians in general practice, internal medicine or pediatrics.
Source: Axelrod et al., *Medical Care Chart Book,* School of Public Health, Univ. of Michigan, Dept. of Medical Care Organization, 6th ed., rev. Sept. 1976, p. 144.

Figure 5-21 Percentage Distribution of National Health Expenditures in Billions of Dollars, by Source of Funds, United States, 1974 (Includes health services and supplies, research and facilities construction)

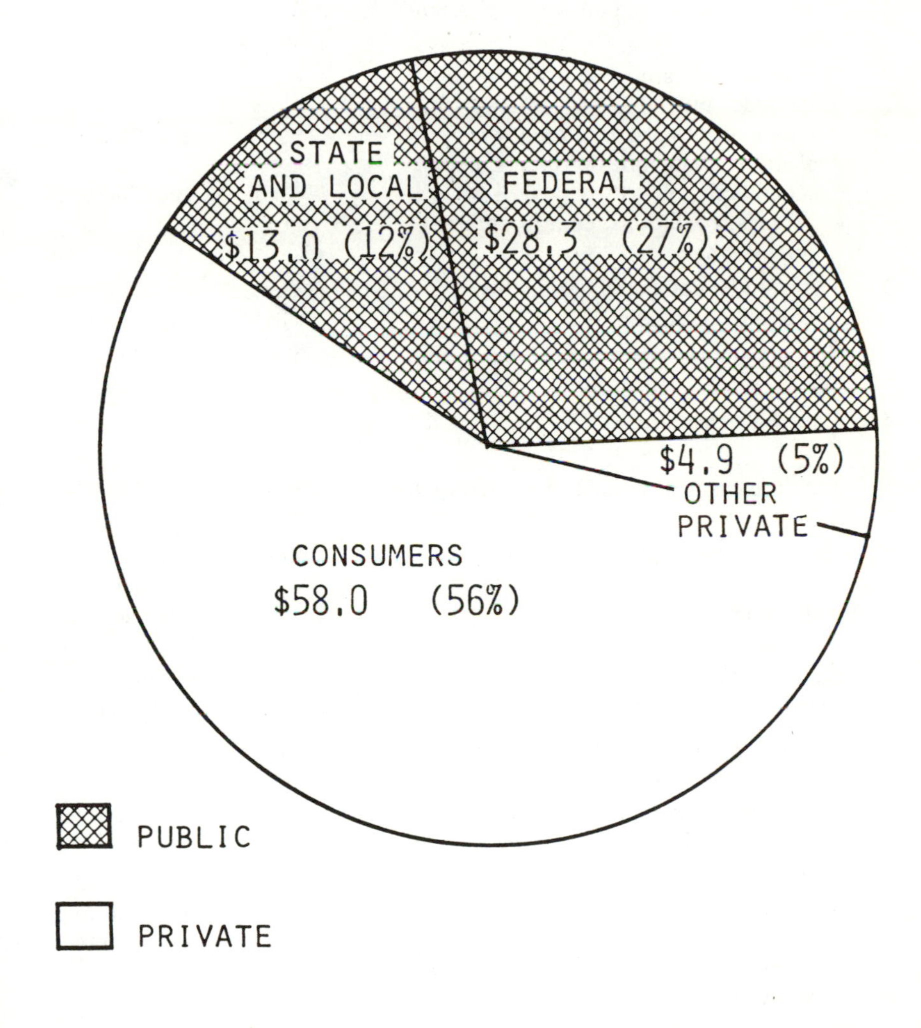

Source: Axelrod et al., *Medical Care Chart Book,* School of Public Health, University of Michigan, Department of Medical Care Organization, 6th ed., rev. September 1976, p. 112.

Table 5-6 Guide for Selecting a Method to Illustrate Community Epidemiological Data

No.	Questions	Answer	Go to Question Indicated or Use Method Shown
1	Data to be illustrated are either continuous or time series	Yes	5
		No	
2	If comparisons are to be made among magnitudes of:		
	a. Component parts of a total, then		Bar Chart
	b. Different categories of things, people, conditions, etc., then		Bar Chart
	c. Things, conditions, etc., in different places, then		3
3	Places to be compared are readily identifiable on a map	Yes	4
		No	Bar Chart
4	Specific site of occurrence is important	Yes	Dot Map
		No	Area Map
5	Data are time series	Yes	6
		No	7
6	Data are cases of disease in an outbreak	Yes	7
		No	9
7	Not more than two sets of data are to be compared (e.g., males and females, cases and deaths)	Yes	Histogram or Frequency Polygon
		No	8
8	More than two sets of data are to be compared		Frequency Polygon
9	Intent is to show *variation* in frequency of one or more items	Yes	10
		No	11
10	Range from minimum to maximum values to be illustrated does not exceed two orders of magnitude	Yes	Arithmetic Line Graph
		No	11
11	Either the intent is to show rates of change in one or more items, or the range of values to be illustrated exceeds two orders of magnitude		Semilogarithmic Line Graph

Source: Modified from "Methods for Organizing Epidemiological Data," DHEW, PHS, Center for Disease Control, Atlanta, Georgia, February 1977, pp. 33–36.

NOTES

1. Judith S. Mausner and Anita K. Bahn, *Epidemiology: An Introductory Text* (Philadelphia: W. B. Saunders Co., 1974), p. 43.
2. Ibid.
3. Gary D. Friedman, *Primer of Epidemiology* (New York: McGraw-Hill, 1974), pp. 52–53.
4. Abraham M. Lilienfeld, *Foundations of Epidemiology* (New York: Oxford University Press, 1976), p. 190.
5. Lilienfeld, *Foundations of Epidemiology*, p. 96.
6. Mausner and Bahn, *Epidemiology*, p. 47.
7. Mausner and Bahn, *Epidemiology*, pp. 48–49.
8. C. Silverman, *Epidemiology of Depression* (Baltimore: Johns Hopkins University Press, 1968).
9. Alfred M. Haynes, *Urban Health* (Minorities and Health Statistics, June 1975), p. 14.
10. Mausner and Bahn, *Epidemiology*, p. 44.
11. Health Services Research and Statistics, Division of Physical Health, *Socioeconomic Analysis of the Disease Patterns of the '70s* (Atlanta: Georgia Department of Human Resources, August 1977), p. 51.
12. I. J. Selikoff et al., "Asbestos Exposure, Smoking, and Neoplasia," *Journal of the American Medical Association* 204, 1968.
13. V. M. Trasko, "Silicosis, A Continuing Problem," *Public Health Reports* 73, 1958.
14. S. Cobb and R. M. Rose, "Hypertension, Peptic Ulcer, and Diabetes in Air Traffic Controllers," *Journal of the American Medical Association* 224, 1973.
15. Milton Terris, "Epidemiology of Cirrhosis of the Liver, National Mortality Data," *American Journal of Public Health*, 47, 1967.
16. John P. Fox, Carrie E. Hall, and Lila R. Elveback, *Epidemiology: Man and Disease* (London: Collier MacMillan 1970), p. 339.
17. Fox, Hall, and Elveback, *Epidemiology*.
18. H. E. Cross, E. F. Kennel, and A. M. Lilienfeld, "Cancer of the Cervix in the Amish Population," *Cancer* 21, 1968.
19. Fox, Hall, and Elveback, *Epidemiology*, p. 202.
20. U.S. Department of Health, Education, and Welfare, *Health, United States, 1976–77*, Pub. No. (HRA) 77-1232, 1977, pp. 133–217.
21. Gary Shannon and G. E. Alan Dever, *Health Care Delivery: Spatial Perspectives* (New York: McGraw-Hill, 1974), p. 141.
22. L. D. Stamp, *Some Aspects of Medical Geography* (New York: Oxford University Press, 1964), p. 103.
23. Health Services Research and Statistics, Division of Physical Health, *Disease Patterns of the '70s*, Georgia Dept. of Human Resources, 1976), p. 167.
24. T. J. Mason et al., *Atlas of Cancer Mortality for U.S. Counties, 1950–1969*, U.S. DHEW Pub. No. NIH 15-780, 1975, p. 103.
25. Fox, Hall, and Elveback, *Epidemiology*, p. 233.
26. William Haenszel and Michael B. Shimkin, "Smoking Patterns and Epidemiology of Lung Cancer in the United States: Are They Compatible?" *Journal of the National Cancer Institute* 16, 1956.
27. Friedman, *Primer of Epidemiology*, p. 67.
28. Fox, Hall, and Elveback, *Epidemiology*, p. 240.
29. M. J. Moroney, *Facts from Figures* (Baltimore: Penguin Books, 1963), p. 20.
30. Center for Disease Control, *Methods for Organizing Epidemiological Data*, U.S. Department of Health, Education, and Welfare, Public Health Service, Atlanta, Georgia, Feb.

1977, p. 9.

31. Adapted from the CDC publication, DHEW, PHS, *Methods for Organizing Epidemiological Data*, Atlanta, Georgia, February 1977, pp. 33–36.

Chapter 6

Community Health Surveys

The basic objective of planning and conducting community health surveys is to determine the occurrence and distribution of selected environmental, socioeconomic, and behavioral conditions important to disease control and wellness promotion. Surveys become essential as a basis for analysis when data sources are lacking. Because data on health and other characteristics are seldom available locally, surveys play an extremely important role in analyzing community health. Though the national, regional, state, and county levels may provide vital data for health analysis, surveys are often the only way to obtain information specific to a community. Surveys serve as an important means of reducing gaps in our knowledge of ways to promote competent and intelligent health planning.

CONDUCTING THE COMMUNITY HEALTH SURVEY

Community health surveys are conducted to determine immunization levels, the incidence and prevalence of diseases, health care utilization patterns, population demographic characteristics, housing characteristics, attitudes, health practices and beliefs, and many other things. Health surveys conducted by the National Center for Health Statistics and sometimes replicated at the community level, include the Health Interview Survey, the Health Examination Survey, and the Ambulatory Care Survey.

Steps in Designing and Completing a Survey

Before embarking on a health survey, planners should be particularly aware of approaches to survey design. Weiss and Hatry have outlined basic steps in designing and completing a survey:[1]

1. Determine the objectives. Why is information needed? In rough terms at least, what degree of accuracy is needed?

2. Define the population groups to be studied. Are they tenants or homeowners, or both? Are they workers or residents? Are their ages to be 21 and over or 18 and over?
3. Determine the specific data to be collected and the methods of measurement. Should behavior, values, or opinions be reported? Should information on health be obtained by asking people or by examining clinical records? Can data already developed in other studies be used or modified for present purposes?
4. Choose the sampling unit. Should it be the individual, the household, or the city block? What size sample is needed? What should be done about nonresponses? Which sampling method is most appropriate and feasible?
5. Determine the method of contacting individuals. Should this be done with personal interviews, mailed questionnaires, or telephone calls?[2] Should interviews be conducted in certain facilities, such as health clinics or schools, or in homes?
6. Construct the questionnaire to obtain the desired information.
7. Organize and carry out the interviews. This includes hiring interviewers and supervisors, training interviewers, fieldtesting the questionnaire and adjusting it as necessary, assigning interviews, collecting and editing interview schedules, checking on the completion and quality of work, and dealing with nonresponses and refusals.
8. Process and analyze the data. This includes coding, keypunching, tabulating, constructing indexes, running cross tabulations, and using appropriate statistical methods to specify relationships and significance.
9. Report the results. These should include implications and recommendations for actions.

Because an adequate design will increase the likelihood of getting required results, survey design is the most important part of the survey. The lack of an adequate survey design guarantees failure. The step-by-step approach outlined above is one way to design a survey. Even though some of the steps may seem trivial or appear to be foregone conclusions, each should be carefully considered.

Size and Accuracy of Sample

In designing a health survey, three major points to consider are (1) the size of the sample needed, (2) the level of accuracy required, and (3) the type of sample.

Size of the Sample

The sample size needed depends on the characteristic being measured and the desired level of accuracy. It has little relationship to the size of the total population, except that as the sample size increases, so does the accuracy of the results. But increases in sample size also raise survey costs, which diminishes the advantages of sampling. Still, very high degrees of accuracy can often be obtained with relatively small samples. The degree of accuracy required is an administrative, not a statistical, decision. The administrator or the person requesting a survey must determine how accurate the estimates derived from the survey must be to meet decision-making requirements. Once this decision is made, the health planner can then determine the size of sample necessary to meet the desired accuracy.

Level of Accuracy

Figure 6-1 shows the relationship between sample size and accuracy.[3] It is interesting to note that accuracy declines with increasingly larger samples. Thus, little is gained by enlarging sample size beyond a certain point. For example, as seen in Figure 6-1, if a survey shows that 50 percent of the population have some characteristic, at the 95 percent confidence level a sample size of 100 has an accuracy of ± 9.8 percent, whereas a sample of 1,000 has an accuracy of ± 3.1 percent. Thus, increasing the sample size ten times reduces the error potential by about one-third. Yet if a sample size increased ten times means a cost is also increased ten times, that one-third increase in accuracy becomes very costly indeed.

Figure 6-1 also shows the relationship between confidence level and accuracy. As the level of confidence increases, the range of accuracy decreases. As with accuracy, the desired level of confidence is an administrative decision. The statistician or health planner should provide the administrator with an estimate of the cost to achieve stipulated levels of accuracy and confidence and let the administrator determine the required levels.

As noted, the sample size required depends upon the characteristic being measured as well as upon the desired level of accuracy. This means that, because the sample size increases with the increase in the variation of the characteristic being measured, a previous estimate of the variance of the characteristic is needed. When sampling for proportions, the sample size reaches a maximum at a level of 50 percent; but when sampling to estimate a mean, the sample-size formulas have no maximum but depend

Figure 6-1 Relation Between Sample Size and Precision in a Simple Random Sample (95 Percent Confidence Intervals)

If the percent giving the same answer to a question is . . .	And the sample size is: 50	100	200	400	500	1000
	Then there is a *95 out of 100* chance that the percent of the *total* population that would respond the same way would fall between these ranges:*					
2	0- 5.9	0- 4.7	0.1- 3.9	0.6- 3.4	0.8- 3.2	1.1- 2.9
5	0-11.1	0.7- 9.3	1.9- 8.1	2.8- 7.2	3.1- 6.9	3.6- 6.4
10	1.8-18.2	4.1-15.9	5.9-14.1	7.1-12.9	7.5-12.5	8.1-11.9
20	8.8-31.2	12.2-27.8	14.5-25.5	16.1-23.9	16.5-23.5	17.5-22.5
50	36.1-63.9	40.2-59.8	43.1-56.9	45.1-54.9	45.7-54.3	46.9-53.1

*More precisely, if an infinite number of samples of indicated size were taken, 95 percent of them would contain the true value of the total population in the given confidence ranges.

Notes: The above ranges apply if simple random sampling is used. If cluster sampling is used, the errors will be greater. Also, the ranges apply only if the total population from which the sample is drawn is large relative to the sample size. If not, the accuracy of the sample estimate should be greater and therefore the ranges narrower than given in this table. Nonsampling errors are not included.

Source: Carol H. Weiss and Harry P. Hatry, *An Introduction to Sample Surveys for Government Managers* (Washington, D.C.: The Urban Institute, March 1971), p. 27. Based on *Supplemental Courses for Case Studies in Surveys and Censuses: Sampling Lectures*, U.S. Bureau of the Census, Washington, D.C., 1968, p. 20.

upon the expected variation. Though it may be argued that we are sampling to determine this variation and that no estimate is available, a general estimate of the degree of variation will be available from surveys of similar characteristics in other areas. Even when an estimate is not available from any other source, it is possible to conduct a small survey to get an initial estimate for completing the survey.

Sample-size formulas, based on the particular survey to be conducted, are quite numerous. An excellent guide to determining sample size is found in a United Nations' publication, *A Short Manual on Sampling*.[4] (Details of a method for selecting the sample size are presented in the following section.)

Type of Sample

The third question to be addressed in survey design is, What type of sample is required? There are two major types of sampling: nonprobability and probability. Nonprobability sampling means that the probability of drawing a respondent is unknown. It often takes the form of judgment samples, in which respondents are drawn on the basis of known, preconceived characteristics, or of convenience samples, in which respondents are drawn on the basis of convenience or availability. Nonprobability samples are often helpful in gathering certain types of information. It is impossible, however, to make any statements from nonprobability samples about sampling error or population estimates. Conversely, probability samples imply that every individual in a population has a known probability of being selected. Based on this knowledge, it is possible to assess the degree of accuracy in making population estimates. Following are some major types of probability sampling:[5]

- "Simple random sampling [which] involves drawing units at random from the whole population. A table of random numbers (which is readily available) is traditionally used.
- "Stratified random sampling [which] involves drawing samples separately from subgroups of the universe (white males, white females, black males, black females).
- "Cluster sampling [which] can reduce costs because batches of people who live near each other are selected, thus reducing travel time. However, for a given sample size, there is somewhat less confidence in the findings."

Other types of sampling include (1) systematic sampling, in which units are drawn from an existing list or distribution in a regular manner (as in every fifth unit), and (2) multistage samples, in which the population is divided into smaller groups, the groups sampled, and further sampling done within the groups. For example, if a sample of households were taken from a community and the residents within the households sampled, we would have a two-stage sample design.

Each method has certain advantages and disadvantages. Frequently, a simple random sample will be sufficient to meet the needs of an agency. Certain gains can be made, however, using other techniques. Since each technique was developed to meet certain requirements, the design that is most appropriate and cost efficient for the characteristic being measured should be used.

A SAMPLE SURVEY DESIGN FOR A COMMUNITY PROGRAM IN DIETARY COUNSELING

To determine if a program of dietary counseling is effective in altering dietary habits and producing positive changes in health, a sample survey of the population (1249 people) which has received dietary counseling services is required.

Requirements for Sampling

For a sample to be valid, several important requirements must be met. First, the sample must be truly representative of the population to be surveyed. This usually requires random sampling. Second, the size of the sample must be large enough to ensure that any measures obtained from the survey will apply to the population as a whole with a specific degree of precision. Two measures of precision are the error limit and the confidence level. Basically, the error limit is the amount of variation permitted between the sample measure and the actual population measure. The confidence level is the degree of certainty that the sample measure is within the desired error limits. A generally accepted error limit is 5 percent with a confidence level of 95 percent.

Selection of the Sample

The selection of the sample is based on a specific formula for estimating sample size. Inputs for the formula include the size of the population to be sampled, the error limit, the confidence level, and the proportion of the population having the characteristic being sampled. Since we do not know this proportion, the sample size is maximized by making this proportion equal to 50 percent; that is, one-half the population has the desired characteristic.

The selection of the sample then becomes a step-by-step procedure:

1. Select the desired error limit.
2. Select the desired confidence level.
3. Determine the proportion of the population having the characteristic being sampled. If this is not known, and we do not wish to estimate the population, a value of 50 percent can be used. This says, in effect, that one-half the population has the characteristic and the other half does not. The result is a maximum sample to attain the desired degree of precision.
4. Compute the sample size for a very large population, using the following formula:

$$n_0 = t^2 pq/d^2$$

where: n_o = first estimate of sample size, given large population
t^2 = the number of standard errors in which lie the desired limits of reliability (confidence interval)
p = proportion of the population having 1 characteristic
q = proportion of the population having the second characteristic (not having characteristic 1) equal to (1-p)
d^2 = the error limit which will be acceptable

5. If the population is not very large, an adjustment of the initial sample size estimate is made, using the following formula:

$$n = n_o/\{1+[(n_o-1)/N]\}$$

where: n = adjusted sample size
n_o = initial estimate of the sample size from Formula 1, above
N = number in the total population to be sampled

In our survey on dietary counseling, with a sample population of 1,249 people, the results are as follows:

1. The error limit is 5 percent.
2. The confidence level is 95 percent.
3. Since we do not know the proportion having the characteristics of improved or unimproved dietary habits, we maximize the sample by setting the proportion to 50 percent.
4. Solving the formula for the initial estimate of sample size:

$n_o = (1.96)^2(.50)(.50)/.05^2$

$n_o = (3.8400)(.2500)/.0025$

$n_o = .9604/.0025$

$n_o = 384.16$

5. Rounded to a whole number, the initial estimate is a sample size of 384 people. Since we are dealing with a small population, we apply the appropriate correction factor:

$n = 384/\{1+[384-1/1{,}249]$

$n = 384.00/1.31$

$n = 293.88$

Rounded to a whole number, this becomes 294, the sample size required to attain the stated degree of precision.

Method of Sampling

In this case, the best sampling method would be either a personal interview with each of the 294 people in the sample, a personal phone call to each, or a combination of the two methods. Personal contact ensures a high degree of response, in contrast to the mail-out method which often produces a response of only 10 to 20 percent. A mail survey would require sending questionnaires to all 1,249 people in the population. Even then, the desired degree of precision might not be attained.

Two procedures are required to ensure a representative sample: First, the sample must be proportioned according to the population in each county. Table 6-1 shows the number to be sampled in our dietary counseling survey in each county.[6] Second, the individuals to be sampled from each county must be randomly selected. This is done most easily by use of a random-number table and a numbered list of the people who originally received dietary counseling. A starting point is chosen from a page of random numbers by looking away from the page while touching it with the point of a pencil. The random starting point is the digit closest to where the pencil touched the page. Let us assume that this procedure led to a random starting point of 137. The 137th person in the list from Baldwin County is therefore selected as the first person in our sample. The random number is recorded so that we do not reselect this person, and the process is continued until we have selected a sample of the required size. In the case of Baldwin County, this is 44 people. The same method is applied to the remaining four counties; in each the appropriate number of people to be surveyed is selected. Those selected are then interviewed, and the results of the survey are tabulated. Assuming that these procedures have been followed, the results may be assumed to represent, within the stated degree of precision, the total population receiving the dietary counseling.

COMMUNITY STRATIFICATION

Community stratification is "the delineation of a community into graded geographic areas (strata), each of which is highly homogeneous internally with respect to certain preselected behavioral or socioeconomic characteristics, such as housing conditions, income, and education."[7] The purpose of stratification is to facilitate comparison of health statuses within a community across different strata and between communities for comparable strata. The basic reason for stratification within a community

Table 6-1 Sample Size for Dietary Counseling Survey

County	Number Receiving Original Dietary Counseling	Proportion and Percent of Total Receiving Dietary Counseling		Multiplication to Obtain Sample Size		Size of Sample Needed to Attain Degree of Precision
		Proportion	Percent			
Baldwin	187	.1497	14.97	.1497 × 294	=	44
DeKalb	530	.4243	42.43	.4243 × 294	=	125
Dougherty	324	.2594	25.94	.2594 × 294	=	76
Laurens	27	.0216	2.16	.0216 × 294	=	6
Muscogee	181	.1449	14.49	.1449 × 294	=	43
Total	1,249	1.00	100.00	—		294

Source: G. E. Alan Dever and Charles Plunkett, *A Sample Design Demonstration: A Sample Design for a Program of Dietary Counseling,* Division of Physical Health, Georgia Department of Human Resources, Health Services Research and Statistics, Atlanta, Georgia, 1975, p. 5.

is that members of each stratum are similar with respect to the characteristics of stratification and thus present a base for comparison with known characteristics.

Between differing communities, stratification makes it possible to compare groups that are similar with respect to the stratification variables. For example, if we compared the health statuses of two communities on an overall basis, we might find that one status is significantly below the other. With stratification, however, we could compare similar groups of people within each community. Thus, we might find that the community with the lower health status has a higher proportion of lower income people but that the latter's health status is actually higher than that of the low income group in the community with the higher health status. Thus, stratification makes it possible to compare similar groups.

Two principal methods of community stratification are (1) the analysis of residential structures and (2) the use of census data.

Stratification by Residential Structures

This method is based on a community block survey of residential structure conditions within a community. Guidelines for conducting such a survey can be found in the CDC publication *Community Block Surveys*.[8] (For a discussion of the method for selecting the sample, see Weiss and Hatry.[9]) The procedure consists of surveying a community's residential structures and, on the basis of housing conditions, classifying them by socioeconomic class, such as upper, middle, and lower. Any given area within the community may have all types of socioeconomic groups, but stratification is based on the predominant group. The characteristics to be considered include housing conditions and types, nature of vacant land, solid waste disposal, animal types, mosquito breeding areas, sewage disposal, water supply, and possibly other environmental conditions. In a total survey for the purpose of community stratification, each block in the community is visited to assess housing and environmental conditions and is then assigned a score based on its conditions. The most common method of scoring is to color-code a community block map based on the characteristics. After the entire community has been surveyed, the blocks are grouped to form more general community strata. This technique results in the type of distribution of housing conditions and strata shown in Table 6-2.[10]

Stratification by Census Data

The chief advantage of this second method of developing strata within a community is that actual social characteristics are used for classifying strata. Since census information is available only at ten-year intervals, however, actual conditions may change significantly. In general, stratification by census data is valid if the data are used within a relatively short

Table 6-2 Characteristic Range of Housing Conditions in Each Stratum of a Community

Stratum	Range of Housing Conditions
Upper	90% or more good housing and less than 2% poor housing
Middle	Less than 90% good housing and less than 10% poor housing
Lower	More than 10% poor housing; or more than 7% poor, if 20% or more of structures are fair

Source: Wayne G. Brown and Virgil Peavy, *Community Stratification: Techniques of Community Health Analysis*, U.S. DHEW, CDC, Atlanta, Ga., 1973, p. 6.

period of time after the census is taken and if the community has been relatively stable since the time of the census.

Suggested variables from the census for use in stratification include:[11]

1. Median school years completed for persons 25 years of age and older
2. Percent of unskilled workers (employed persons 16 years old and over)
3. Median income of families
4. Percent of housing units with 1.01 or more persons per room

The census tracts within a community are assigned scores based on levels of these characteristics, and score values are added. Tables 6-3, 6-4, 6-5, and 6-6 show the recommended guidelines.[12] When the point values are added, we can classify the community into strata (Table 6-7).[13] Each census tract is placed in a socioeconomic stratum, based on its total score.

Table 6-3 Median School Years Completed

Range of Median School Years	Point Value
12.6 and above	4
11.6–12.5	3
10.6–11.5	2
9.1–10.5	1
0.0– 9.0	0

Source: Wayne G. Brown and V. Peavy, *Community Stratification: Techniques of Community Health Analysis,* U.S. DHEW, CDC, Atlanta, Georgia, 1973, p. 5.

Table 6-4 Percentage of Unskilled Workers

Range of Unskilled Workers	Point Value
0%– 8.0%	4
8.1%–16.0%	3
16.1%–24.0%	2
24.1%–32.0%	1
32.1% and above	0

Source: Wayne G. Brown and V. Peavy, *Community Stratification: Techniques of Community Health Analysis,* U.S. DHEW, CDC, Atlanta, Georgia, 1973, p. 5.

Table 6-5 Median Income Families

Range of Median Income	Point Value
$13,000 and above	4
$ 9,290 – $12,999	3
$ 6,300 – $ 9,289	2
$ 3,290 – $ 6,299	1
$ 0 – $ 3,289	0

Source: Wayne G. Brown and V. Peavy, *Community Stratification: Techniques of Community Health Analysis,* U.S. DHEW, CDC, Atlanta, Georgia, 1973, p. 6.

Table 6-6 Percentage of Housing Units With 1.01 or More Persons Per Room

Range of Crowded Housing Units	Point Value
0% – 4.9%	4
5.0% – 9.9%	3
10.0% – 14.9%	2
15.0% – 19.9%	1
20.0% and above	0

Source: Wayne G. Brown and V. Peavy, *Community Stratification: Techniques of Community Health Analysis,* U.S. DHEW, CDC, Atlanta, Georgia, 1973, p. 6.

Table 6-7 Socioeconomic Strata

Socioeconomic Strata	Total Point Value
Upper	13–16
Middle	7–12
Lower	0– 6

Source: Wayne G. Brown and V. Peavy, *Community Stratification: Techniques of Community Health Analysis,* U.S. DHEW, CDC, Atlanta, Georgia, 1973, p. 7.

Stratification by Residential Structures and Census Data– An Example

The use of both community block survey and census data for stratification is shown in a sample design for a survey on lead poisoning.[14] In this example, a community block survey was conducted on the basis of housing conditions, and each block in the city was classified as having good, moderate, or deteriorating residential structures. Next, since lead poisoning is found primarily in children under age six, stratification from census data was required to determine where children under age six might be living. Census tapes showed the number of children under age six by enumeration district within the city. Thus, two measures were available for stratification: the percentage of housing classified as moderate, good, or deteriorating, and the percentage of children under age six. Next, three strata were identified as a basis for conducting blood-lead tests of the children. Table 6-8 shows how the enumeration districts were stratified. Housing units were then selected in a sample procedure, with first priority being given to Stratum 1. (Appendix 6A outlines the entire stratification procedure for this project.)

The survey results pointed up one of the problems in using census data. The data were five years old at the time of the survey, and, although birth records and local observations indicated that the population under age six in Brunswick was not changing rapidly, surveyors in Stratum 1 found very few children in deteriorating housing. Although the census data indicated a high proportion of children in the stratum, they had apparently either moved out of the area or, more likely, had not been replaced with younger brothers and sisters.

SUMMARY

Community health surveys lead to the identification of target groups for the development of a full health service program. Of course, community health surveys are not without problems. Although the basic concern is cost, secondary concerns are the survey design, type of sampling method, sample size, and precision of results. Housing and census surveys are of considerable importance when data are not available to determine program target areas and to conduct subsequent evaluation.

Community health surveys are essential to community health analysis[15] but must be dovetailed with the other methods and techniques to develop successful holistic health programs.

Table 6-8 Determination of Strata in a Lead Screening Project

Enumeration District	Number of Children Age 0-5	Percent of Total Population (A)	Estimated Number of Housing Units in Moderate or Deteriorating Condition	Percent of All Housing Units (B)	Sum of A&B (C)	Rank of C	Stratum
25	125	14.3	42	17.5	31.8	10	2
26	156	9.8	0	0	9.8	19	3
27	179	11.6	99	20.0	31.6	11	2
28	137	10.8	21	4.9	15.7	17	3
29	107	10.8	35	10.8	21.6	16	3
30	136	11.1	112	30.2	41.3	8	2
31	143	12.5	147	39.7	52.2	6	1
32	46	8.7	24	13.7	22.4	14	3
33	103	10.1	141	40.3	50.4	7	2
34	181	14.4	212	64.4	78.8	2	1
35	71	9.1	4	1.5	10.6	18	3
36	117	11.1	153	43.1	54.2	5	1
37	78	9.4	160	50.2	59.6	4	1
38	80	7.9	78	21.7	29.6	12	2
39	70	10.9	130	50.0	60.9	3	1
40	107	11.8	109	27.4	39.2	9	2
41	84	10.3	233	70.0	80.3	1	1
42	102	10.0	52	13.2	23.2	13	2
43	92	8.6	45	12.3	20.9	15	3

*U.S. Census Tapes, Georgia, U.S. Bureau of the Census, 1970.
Source: Charles Plunkett and G. E. Alan Dever, *Brunswick Lead Screening, A Sample Survey,* monograph, *Health Services Research and Statistics,* Division of Physical Health, Georgia Dept. of Human Resources, 1975, p. 20.

APPENDIX 6A
COMMUNITY STRATIFICATION FOR A LEAD SCREENING PROJECT

In order to reduce the statistical variance of the sample results for the entire city and to allow estimates of high, medium, and low risk areas within the city, the city of Brunswick was divided into three sampling strata.[16] The three strata were based on the addition of the percentage of the population under age six and the percentage of housing units in a moderate or deteriorating condition (see Table 6-8). The enumeration districts were ranked according to this sum and divided into three strata, each containing approximately one-third of the enumeration districts. Table 6A-1 shows the breakdown for these values by strata and the total sample size of each stratum. The sample size was based on the total number of housing units within each stratum. These sample sizes will allow us to estimate the incidence of lead poisoning with an accuracy level of 5.0 percent at the 95 percent confidence level within strata and at an accuracy level of 3.1 percent at the 95 percent confidence level within the city.

Within each stratum the sample is divided among the enumeration districts according to the proportion of the population under age six and the proportion of dwelling units within the stratum which are in moderate or deteriorating condition. Tables 6A-2, 6A-3, and 6A-4 show the proportion of each enumeration district's sample size for each of the three strata. The procedure for selecting the sample size is displayed in Tables 6A-5, 6A-6, and 6A-7.

Table 6A-1 Determination of Sample Size

	Stratum 1	Stratum 2	Stratum 3	Total
Total Housing Units*	1966	2610	2052	6628
Total Moderate And Deteriorating Housing Units	1035	814	129	1978
Percent of Total	52.6	31.2	6.3	29.8
Population Age 0–5*	673	832	609	2114
Percent of Total	11.7	10.9	9.8	10.8
Sample Size	277	287	279	843

*U.S. Census Tapes, Georgia, U.S. Bureau of the Census, 1970.
Source: Charles Plunkett and G. E. Alan Dever, *Brunswick Lead Screening, A Sample Survey,* monograph, Health Services Research and Statistics, Division of Physical Health, Georgia Department of Human Resources, 1975, p. 7.

Table 6A-2 Sample Size by Enumeration District, Stratum 1

Enumeration District	Percent of Stratum's Population Age 0–5*	Percent of Stratum's Housing Units in Moderate Or Deteriorating Condition	Total Housing Units*	Sample Size
31	21	14	370	48
34	27	21	329	67
36	17	15	355	44
37	12	15	319	38
39	10	13	260	32
41	13	22	333	48
Stratum Total	100%	100%	1966	277

*U.S. Census Tapes, U.S. Bureau of the Census, 1970.
Source: Charles Plunkett and G. E. Alan Dever, *Brunswick Lead Screening, A Sample Survey,* monograph, Health Services Research and Statistics, Division of Physical Health, Georgia Department of Human Resources, 1975, p. 9.

The actual selection of the sample is a systematic procedure based on the sample size and the resulting sample fraction. The sample fraction is the ratio of the number of sample units to the total number of dwelling units. Thus, for Enumeration District (ED) 31, with a sampling fraction of one-eighth, we are sampling one of every eight dwelling units. A further breakdown is necessary, since a complete enumeration of housing units is unavailable. The sampling fraction is divided in such a way that we draw just a sample of blocks and then sample a portion of those blocks chosen. Thus, for ED 31, the sampling fraction is divided into one-fourth and one-half. We first draw a sample of blocks based on a ratio of one in four.

Table 6A-3 Sample Size by Enumeration District, Stratum 2

Enumeration District	Percent of Stratum's Population Age 0–5*	Percent of Stratum's Housing Units in Moderate or Deteriorating Condition	Total Housing Units*	Sample Size
25	15	5	240	28
27	22	12	496	49
30	16	14	371	43
33	12	17	350	42
38	10	10	360	29
40	13	13	398	37
42	12	29	395	59
Stratum Total	100%	100%	2610	287

*U.S. Census Tapes, U.S. Bureau of the Census, 1970.

Source: Charles Plunkett and G. E. Alan Dever, *Brunswick Lead Screening, A Sample Survey,* monograph, Health Services Research and Statistics, Division of Physical Health, Georgia Department of Human Resources, 1975, p. 10.

Table 6A-4 Sample Size by Enumeration District, Stratum 3

Enumeration District	Percent of Stratum's Population Age 0–5*	Percent of Stratum's Housing Units in Moderate or Deteriorating Condition	Total Housing Units*	Sample Size
26	25	0	496	36
28	22	16	431	53
29	18	27	323	62
32	8	19	175	38
35	12	3	260	20
43	15	35	367	70
Stratum Total	100%	100%	2052	279

*U.S. Census Tapes, U.S. Bureau of the Census, 1970.

Source: Charles Plunkett and G. E. Alan Dever, *Brunswick Lead Screening, A Sample Survey,* monograph, Health Services Research and Statistics, Division of Physical Health, Georgia Department of Human Resources, 1975, p. 11.

Table 6A-5 Sample Size Determination, Stratum 1

Enumeration District	Population Age 0–5*	Population Age 0–5 as a Proportion of Stratum Total	Proportion of Total Sample (A)	Estimate of Moderate and Deteriorated Housing Units	Proportion of These Units to Stratum Total	Proportion of Total Sample (B)	ED Sample Size Average of A and B (C)	Total Housing Units*	Sample Fraction C/D	Sample Frac-tion Among Blocks	Sample Frac-tion Within Blocks
31	143	.21	59	147.0	.14	38	48	370	1/8	1/4	1/2
34	181	.27	75	212.1	.21	58	67	329	1/5	1/3	1/2
36	117	.17	47	153.0	.15	41	44	355	1/8	1/4	1/2
37	78	.12	34	159.6	.15	41	38	319	1/8	1/4	1/2
39	70	.10	28	129.8	.13	36	32	260	1/8	1/4	1/2
41	84	.12	34	233.1	.23	63	48	333	1/7	1/4	1/2
Total	673	1.00	277	1034.6	1.00	277	277	1966	1/7		

*U.S. Census Tapes, U.S. Bureau of the Census, 1970.

Source: Charles Plunkett and G. E. Alan Dever, *Brunswick Lead Screening, A Sample Survey,* monograph, Health Services Research and Statistics, Division of Physical Health, Georgia Department of Human Resources, 1975, p. 21.

Table 6A-6 Sample Size Determination, Stratum 2

Enumeration District	Population Age 0–5*	Population Age 0–5 as a Proportion of Stratum Total	Proportion of Total Sample (A)	Estimate of Moderate and Deteriorated Housing Units	Proportion of These Units to Stratum Total	Proportion of Total Sample (B)	ED Sample Size Average of A and B (C)	Total Housing Units*	Sample Fraction C/D	Sample Fraction Among Blocks	Sample Fraction Within Blocks
25	125	.15	43	42.3	.05	14	28	240	1/9	1/5	1/2
27	179	.22	63	99.0	.12	35	49	496	1/10	1/5	1/2
30	136	.16	46	111.6	.14	40	43	371	1/9	1/5	1/2
33	103	.12	34	141.2	.17	49	42	350	1/8	1/4	1/2
38	80	.10	29	78.0	.10	29	29	360	1/12	1/4	1/3
40	107	.13	37	108.6	.13	37	37	398	1/11	1/4	1/3
42	102	.12	35	233.1	.29	83	59	395	1/7	1/4	1/2
Total	832	1.00	287	813.8	1.00	287	287	2610	1/9		

*U.S. Census Tapes, U.S. Bureau of the Census, 1970.

Source: Charles Plunkett and G. E. Alan Dever, *Brunswick Lead Screening, A Sample Survey,* monograph, Health Services Research and Statistics, Division of Physical Health, Georgia Department of Human Resources, 1975, p. 21.

Table 6A-7 Sample Size Determination, Stratum 3

Enumeration District	Population Age 0–5*	Population Age 0–5 as a Proportion of Stratum Total	Proportion of Total Sample (A)	Estimate of Moderate and Deteriorated Housing Units	Proportion of These Units to Stratum Total	Proportion of Total Sample (B)	ED Sample Size Average of A and B (C)	Total Housing Units*	Sample Fraction C/D	Sample Fraction Among Blocks	Sample Fraction Within Blocks
26	156	.26	72	0	0	0	36	496	1/14	1/7	1/2
28	137	.22	61	21.0	.16	45	53	431	1/8	1/4	1/2
29	107	.18	50	35.0	.27	75	62	323	1/5	1/3	1/2
32	46	.08	22	23.9	.19	53	38	175	1/5	1/3	1/2
35	71	.12	33	4.5	.03	8	20	260	1/13	1/7	1/2
43	92	.15	41	44.6	.35	98	70	367	1/5	1/3	1/2
Total	609	1.00	279	129.0	1.00	279	279	2052	1/7		

*U.S. Census Tapes, U.S. Bureau of the Census, 1970.

Source: Charles Plunkett and G. E. Alan Dever, *Brunswick Lead Screening, A Sample Survey*, monograph, Health Services Research and Statistics, Division of Physical Health, Georgia Department of Human Resources, 1975, p. 23.

Table 6A-8 Sample Units by Selected Enumeration District

Enumeration District	Block Number To Be Sampled	First House Sampled	Sample Every __ House
25	1	2	2
	6	1	2
	11	2	2
	16	1	2
26	6	2	2
	13	2	2
	20	2	2
27	5	1	2
	10	1	2
	15	1	2
	20	2	2
	25	1	2
	30	1	2
	35	1	2
	40	1	2
	45	2	2
	50	1	2
28	1	2	2
	5	1	2
	9	2	2
	13	1	2
	17	2	2
	21	2	2
	25	2	2
	29	2	2
	33	2	2
	37	1	2

Source: Charles Plunkett and G. E. Alan Dever, *Brunswick Lead Screening, A Sample Survey,* monograph, Health Services Research and Statistics, Division of Physical Health, Georgia Department of Human Resources, 1975, p. 24.

This is done by drawing a random number between one and four, using this as the first block to sample, and taking every fourth block after the first. Each selected block is then sampled by selecting a random starting point of one or two and sampling every second house thereafter. This involves a process of screening all children within the selected dwelling units.

The results will be roughly equivalent to a stratified random sample without replacement of all dwelling units. By selecting many blocks within each enumeration district and sampling a portion of each, we avoid the possible bias which would result in sampling fewer blocks with complete enumeration. Table 6A-8 contains the selected blocks to be sampled for each enumeration district.

NOTES

1. Carol H. Weiss and Harry P. Hatry, *An Introduction to Sample Surveys for Governmental Managers* (Washington, D.C.: The Urban Institute, 1971), pp. 13–14.
2. Harry T. Phillips and Angell G. Beza, "The Use of Health Surveys in Health System Agency Planning," *American Journal of Public Health*, 1979, Vol. 69, no. 3, pp. 221–222. See also Jack Diemiatycki, "A Comparison of Mail, Telephone, and Home Interviews: Strategies for Household Health Surveys," Ibid. pp. 238–245. Diemiatycki notes that a telephone survey, if followed up by household interviews, can lead to a high response at a comparatively low cost.
3. Weiss and Hatry, *An Introduction to Sample Surveys*, p. 20.
4. Vol. I, Elements of Sample Survey Theory, United Nations, Series F, No. 1, Rev. 1, 1972, p. 325.
5. Weiss and Hatry, *An Introduction to Sample Surveys*, p. 19.
6. G. E. Alan Dever and Charles Plunkett, *A Sample Design Demonstration: A Sample Design for a Program of Dietary Counseling*, Health Services Research and Statistics, Ga. Dept. of Human Resources, Sept. 1975, p. 16.
7. Wayne G. Brown and Virgil Peavy, *Community Stratification: Techniques of Community Health Analysis*, U.S. DHEW, CDC, Atlanta, 1973, p. 1.
8. Wayne G. Brown, *Community Block Surveys: Techniques of Community Health Analysis*, U.S. DHEW, CDC, Atlanta, 1972, p. 29.
9. Weiss and Hatry, *An Introduction to Sample Surveys*, p. 20.
10. Brown and Peavy, *Community Stratification*, p. 6.
11. Brown and Peavy, *Community Stratification*, p. 4.
12. Brown and Peavy, *Community Stratification*, pp. 5, 6.
13. Brown and Peavy, *Community Stratification*, modified from p. 7.
14. Charles Plunkett and G. E. Alan Dever, *Brunswick Lead Screening, A Sample Survey*, Health Services Research and Statistics, Div. of Physical Health (Ga. Dept. of Human Resources, 1975), p. 20.
15. U.S. DHEW *Health Survey Research Methods*. NCHSR, DHEW Pub. No. (PHS) 79-3207, 1979, p. 96.
16. Modified from Plunkett and Dever, *Brunswick Lead Screening*, p. 28.

Chapter 7

Health-Status Indicators and Indexes

Building on previous approaches to health and our belief systems and to an epidemiological model for community health policy analysis, the present chapter deals with the development of community health-status indicators and indexes as they relate to holistic and wellness issues impacting on community health status. The development of health-status goals and objectives is essential to the construction of meaningful indicators and indexes. In addition, criteria and data requirements must be determined to develop the various types of community health-status indicators and indexes.

The development of health policy through the epidemiological model is a prerequisite to the formulation of health-status goals and objectives. The epidemiological model outlines policy direction and analysis for the organization. The most beneficial aspect of this model is that it may be applied on a disease-by-disease basis to provide information for program management and policy analysis. In essence, the model provides a comprehensive needs assessment of the health status of a population (disease specific). The detailed application of this model is the subject of a subsequent chapter.

HEALTH-STATUS GOALS AND OBJECTIVES

Operational Definitions

One cannot develop responsible and realistic objectives unless one analyzes the community's health and its health system. This involves analyzing the statuses of several geographical areas and population groups and of the health services presently available to them. The major purpose of a community needs assessment by a health organization, therefore, is to determine: (1) the characteristics and health status of the area's population; (2) the characteristics of existing health systems; (3) which areas have the greatest potential for positive change; and (4) which health services require priority in the health plan, assuming that other functions (e.g., review functions) will be based on the plan.[1]

The needs assessment and the policy analysis of the epidemiological model are necessary in order to offer in the health plan explicit statements of goals and objectives. Such an approach, embodying a new health outlook of holism and wellness, must guide the selection of health-status indicators and indexes (Figure 7-1).

Figure 7-1 A Model Showing the Relationship of the Health-Field Concept to Health Status

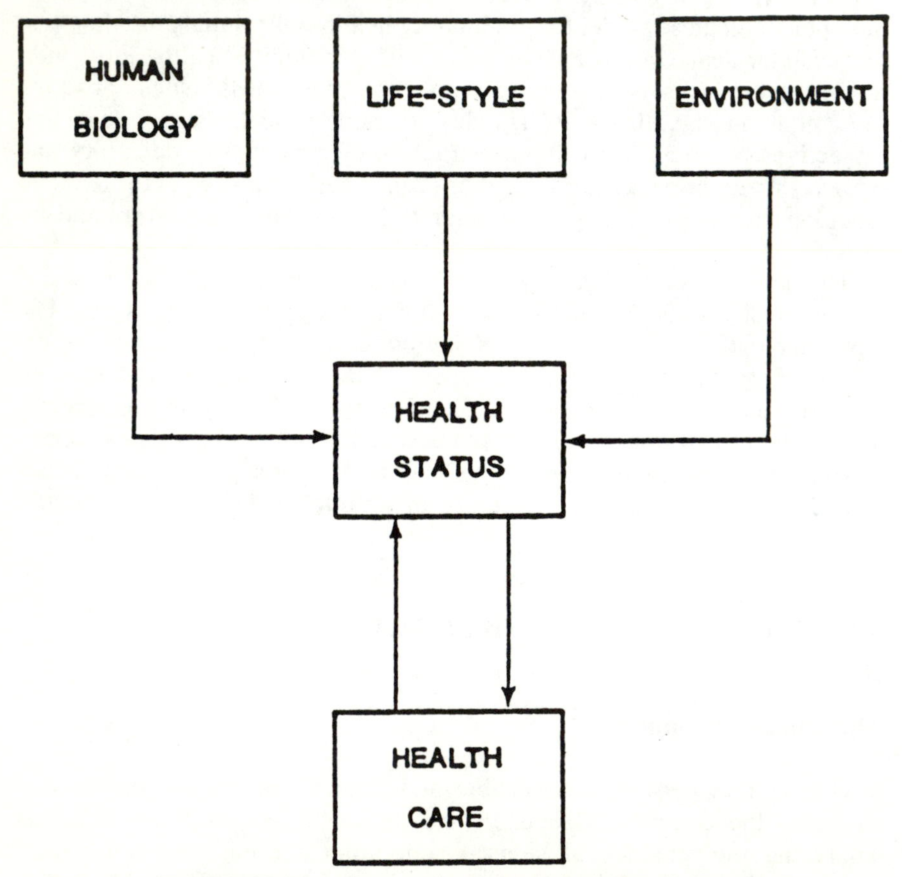

Source: G. B. Hill and J. M. Romeder. "Health Statistics in Canada" (Paper presented at the Society for Epidemiological Research, Toronto, Ontario, June 18, 1976), p. 11.

In an approach of this type, the association of health-status statistics with life style, environment, and biology, will be useful in assessing the effect of the health services (health-system goals) on the health and well-being (health-status goals) of the population. The achievement of such an association is not easy. The health planner or the data coordinator must, nevertheless, understand that an integrated statistical system is required. Though the data and the statistical system needed for their collection are generally lacking or inadequately developed, the methods for such a system are available.

Definitions

Questions of considerable concern during the process of formulating policy are, What is a "goal" and what is an "objective?" These two terms have different meanings, cause indecisive debates, and involve time-consuming procedures. Program plans have been delayed six months or more because of the inability to reach consensus on a set of definitions for these terms. Clarification of the terms is thus essential to the process of establishing meaningful health-status measures.

- "*Goals* are expressions of desired conditions of health status and health systems expressed as quantifiable, timeless aspirations. Goals should be both technically and financially achievable and responsive to community ideals."[2]
- "*Objectives* should be prepared for goals which have been identified as high priority. Objectives generated from the goals contained in the health plan should express particular levels of expected achievements in health status or health system by a specific year."[3]

Examples of a health-status goal and objective would be the following: A quantifiable goal would be to keep the mortality rate from motor vehicle accidents to less than 15 per 100,000 population per year. The objective related to this goal would be to reduce the mortality rate from motor vehicle accidents to 12 per 100,000 population by 1980. Table 7-1 shows the results of an analysis of 149 statements examined for specificity and clarity in terms of time, direction, magnitude, definition of measure, and the measure of the characteristic to be changed.[4]

The actual process of establishing health-status goals and objectives involves several facets, depending on the current level of operations. Presumably, the goals and objectives will be stated as comprehensively as necessary. Blum has suggested that the analytic steps in qualitative goal analysis should be a function of whether the planning body decided (1) to set a qualitative goal for all (broadened to reflect the holistic model, that is, wellness and not just medical care) or (2) to study the present delivery system in terms of the community problem that warrants priority.[5] These

Table 7-1 Analyzing Statements for Clarity

Goals and Standards	Elements of Clarity				
	Time	Direction	Magnitude	Measure	Definition of Measure
Health Status (N = 15)					
Specified	9	13	8	12	8
Not Specified	6	2	7	3	7
Health Promotion & Protection (N = 44)					
Specified	5	41	1	35	7
Not Specified	39	3	43	9	37
Health Care Services (N = 41)					
Specified	13	33	12	31	10
Not Specified	33	13	34	15	36
Health Data Systems (N = 15)					
Specified	6	18	0	18	1
Not Specified	12	0	18	0	17
Health Innovation (N = 13)					
Specified	3	10	0	11	3
Not Specified	10	3	13	2	10
Health Care Financing (N = 13)					
Specified	3	11	1	8	4
Not Specified	10	2	12	5	9
Total					
Specified	39	126	22	115	33
Not Specified	110	23	127	34	116

Source: U.S. DHEW. "The Conditions of Health and Health Care: Context for Goals and Standards," in *Baselines for Setting Health Goals and Standards,* HRA 77–640, January 1977, pp. 47–51.

two approaches should be dovetailed. Use of the holistic model would entail the definition of quantitative goals related to the qualitative goals of good care and wellness. With such an approach, one could analyze each problem to develop prevention and intervention measures to attack the causes and consequences of a disease.

Quantitative Goals and Objectives

How do we determine a realistic level of attainment of goals and objectives? The level of attainment may be determined on the basis of realistic assumptions or value-derived standards of expectations, that is, committee or professional opinion as to what the level of attainment should be; or it may be determined quantitatively by applying general, promulgated standards, for example, the use of the national average as the standard for infant mortality.

The use of generally promulgated standards to establish goal and objective levels has several advantages:[6]

1. Such standards serve as a quick reference to what is regarded as adequate.
2. By matching standards to local conditions, local areas (HSAs) that fall significantly short of desired levels can demonstrate health gaps.
3. By comparing multiple health gaps (revealed by standards), a community can see gaps that are proportionately worse and that may deserve higher priority.
4. Though local standards are not well accepted, national standards are capable of demonstrating meaningful comparisons of what "is" versus what "could be" or "should be."
5. Community comparisons of national standards can provide impetus to the measurement of health status.

It is imperative that trends or standards be determined for specified health-status measures. Professional and committee opinion, a review of past trends, and promulgated standards may all reveal appropriate targets or standards for attainment of objectives. As noted earlier, for example, the reduction of infant mortality by 20 percent within the next year may be a totally unrealistic objective in view of the fact that it has been reduced by only 3 percent per year over the last ten years, to a level that is already below the national rate.

When setting objectives, it should be kept in mind that a rate may change within probability limits based on the standard deviation or variation of the variables over time. For example, the use of an absolute value of 3.0 percent for a specific variable would be misleading when a ± 1.00 standard deviation for the data set of observations is 1.5 percent. In this case, a more valid objective would be a range of 1.5 to 4.5 percent instead of 3.0 percent. In setting realistic objectives, it is important to account for such a variation in the data set. Readjustment of objectives in the light of unforeseen issues which surface and impact on the program is always feasible.

Kinds of Goals and Objectives

The goals and objectives selected for inclusion in the plan reflect several considerations. First, such goals and objectives are direct consequences of the adopted health policy (wellness and holistic) as shown in Table 7-2. If the health policy is comprehensive—including elements of the environment, human biology, life style, and system of medical care organization—the goals and objectives should reflect such a policy. In the near future, however, the health agency must concentrate on more nontraditional goals and objectives, such as life style and environmental measures, which have a decisive impact on changing disease patterns. Second, national priorities dictate to a health-systems agency the types of goals and objectives to be included in the health-system plan. Third, it is necessary to do a needs assessment which identifies disease and social patterns (specific problems) for each health service or geographic area. This is an obvious need but one which is not always satisfied. Thus, the kinds of goals and objectives included in the plan are a function of the health agency's policy, national priorities, and a needs assessment—all of which form a very dynamic process.

Numbers of Goals and Objectives

Another major concern is the number of goals and objectives to be included in the plan. No magic formula can determine how many goals and objectives should be listed. One rational approach would be to determine the extent to which disease morbidity and mortality and social problems are crippling and killing the selected population. Proportional Mortality Ratios (PMRs) or specific death rates by cause, age, sex, race, etc., are health indicators that might enable one to set priorities and thereby limit the number of health status goals and objectives within the plan. Other considerations, however, will affect the number of health-status goals and objectives to include in the plan. After determining PMRs and specific death rates, for example, one must take into account how much a community can accomplish.

The plan includes both priority health-status goals and objectives that must be developed with recommended actions and resource requirements and nonpriority ones that do not need to be developed. For health-status goals with high priority, one would develop selected health-system goals and objectives, depending on the plan format in some cases and on recommended actions in all cases. So, in setting goal priorities, criteria such as the extent of the problem, agency resources, and feasibility of impacting on the problem must be considered.

Table 7-2 The "Honor Roll" of Wellness—Involved HSAs

Name of HSA	Location	A Clear Definition of Wellness/ Health Promotion	B Conceptual Framework Articulated	C Inventory of Community Wellness Resources
Health Planning Council, Inc. (HPC)	Madison, WI	X	X	X
Oklahoma Health Systems Agency (OHSA)	Oklahoma City, OK	X	X	
Northern Alaska Health Resource Association, Inc.	Fairbanks, AK	X	X	
Southern New Jersey Health Systems Agency, Inc.	Bellmawr, NJ			
Central Maryland Health Systems Agency, Inc.	Baltimore, MD	X	X	
Comprehensive Health Planning in Southern Illinois, Inc. (CHPSI)	Carbondale, IL	X	X	
PEE DEE Regional Health Systems Agency, Inc.	Florence, SC			
Northwest Oregon Health Systems Agency, Inc.	Portland, OR	X	X	
Western Oregon Health Systems Agency, Inc.	Eugene, OR	X	X	
West Michigan Health Systems Agency, Inc.	Grand Rapids, MI		X	
Central Arizona Health Systems Agency, Inc.	Phoenix, AZ	X	X	
Health Planning Council for Greater Boston	Brighton, MA		X	
Eastern Washington Health Systems Agency, Inc.	Spokane, WA	X	X	
Southeastern Colorado Health System Agency, Inc.	Colorado Springs, CO	X	X	
South Central Health Planning and Development, Inc.	Anchorage, AK	X	X	X
TRI-Region Health Systems Agency, Inc.	Abilene, TX	X	X	X
Birmingham Regional Health Systems Agency, Inc.	Birmingham, AL	X	X	
Panhandle Regional Planning Commission Health Systems Agency, Inc.	Amarillo, TX	X	X	
HSA of Northeastern New York	Albany, NY		X	
HSA of Southwestern Pennsylvania	Pittsburgh, PA			

(Columns D through L continued on page 176)

Table 7-2 continued

D Sponsor Wellness Publications & Seminars etc.	E Wellness Presented As Part of Cost Containment	F Efforts to Influence Public Policy Toward Wellness	G Wellness Programs for Employees	H Wellness Programs for Hospitals	I Wellness Programs for Health Providers	J Wellness Programs for Schools	K Insurance-Directed Wellness Initiatives	L Other (See Text)
X	X	X	X	X	X	X	X	X
	X	X	X					
X								
X	X	X		X	X	X		X
	X							
X	X							X
X	X	X		X	X	X		X
X				X	X	X	X	X
	X							X
					X	X		X
X	X	X	X	X	X		X	X
X	X	X				X	X	
X				X	X	X	X	
X					X	X	X	
X	X				X	X		
X				X		X	X	
X			X		X	X	X	
X						X		X
		X			X	X		
X		X				X		

Source: Donald B. Ardell. "High Level Wellness and the HSAs: A Health Planning Success Story," *American Journal of Health Planning,* vol. 3, no. 3, July 1978, pp. 1–18.

Summary

In short, the health agency should be aware of the following considerations when establishing health-status goals and objectives.

1. Appropriate operational definitions of goals and objectives are related to the planning process.
2. Quantitative goals and objectives, that is, attainment levels, result from community and professional inputs as well as from data analysis.
3. The kinds of goals and objectives included in the plan are a reflection of health agency policies, national priorities, and needs assessment.
4. The number of goals and objectives to be included in the plan can vary. By using such aids as PMRs and specific death rates, however, one can set priorities, thereby limiting the number of goals and objectives. In any event, their number and priority must be weighted in accordance with the extent of the problem, the feasibility of impacting on the problem, and agency resources.

DEVELOPMENT OF HEALTH-STATUS INDICATORS AND INDEXES

To measure the extent of achievement in terms of stated health-status goals and objectives, it is necessary to develop indicators and, if possible, an index relating to health status. Several criteria for a health-status indicator or index should be considered, however, before using a specific type.

The difference between a health indicator and a health index can be seen in the following definitions:

- A health-status indicator is a single measure which is obtained from a single component (variable) and which purports to reflect the health status of an individual or defined group; for example, infant mortality, Proportional Mortality Ratio.
- A health-status index is a composite measure which summarizes data from two or more components (variables) and which, like an indicator, also purports to reflect the health status of an individual or defined group;[7] for example, a Z-Score Model or Regression Correlation Model.

Criteria for Selection

Because of inappropriate data and imperfect measures of health status, the health agency must utilize what data, indicators, or indexes are currently available. Consequently, the agency should concentrate on using basic health indicators or simplified applications of a health index. Whichever approach is followed, it is important to note basic criteria for selecting appropriate health indicators or an index to reflect the status of the population being investigated.

The following criteria should serve as a guide for the agency health planner in determining the requirements for a health-status indicator or index:

Data Availability

The mere existence of data does not mean they are ready for incorporation in the health plan. The manipulation required may be as simple as collapsing categories or as complex as abstracting subset categories. Generally, the data should be available without conducting detailed, complex investigations. To meet this requirement, Miller suggests the following possibilities:[8]

1. Data from published reports and monographs may be available from public health agencies. Considering the value of the data and the

importance of the research questions, special analysis may require additional funding.
2. Current data collection systems can be utilized with slight modifications, though such data analysis may require expenditures.
3. The collection and analysis of data by special surveys can expedite results.

Data may also be gleaned from *Examples of Data Used in Diverse Settings for a Variety of Planning Purposes* (produced by the Bureau of Health Planning and Resources Development, Division of Planning Methods and Technology, June 1977).

Level of Analysis

The unit of investigation or level of analysis must be specific enough to determine geographic variations of the phenomenon being studied. Levels of analysis may be summarized as in Table 7-3. Thus, if the universe to be investigated is a particular health service area, then the level of analysis for investigation should be the township, enumeration district, other subcounty geographic area, or city.

Levels of Measurement

Four levels of measurement may characterize a set of data: nominal, ordinal, interval, and ratio.[9] The levels are important in the use of a health indicator or in providing summary statements which are usually of more practical value than the complete distribution. The four levels of measurement are described as follows:

Nominal. In nominal data one data element is distinguished from another but no direction is implied. Examples include male and female; health service areas A, B, or C; and religion categories, like Baptist, Lutheran, and Mormon. Nominal data may be displayed using bar charts and pie charts. Appropriate statistics are the mode and frequency counts.

Ordinal. In ordinal data the data items are ranked. The level shows that one value is more or less than another value but does not indicate by how much. For example, we may rank health service areas by socioeconomic status, such as high, medium, or low. Appropriate statistics include the median, percentile, Spearman r_s, and Kendall τ.

Interval. In interval data the data items are characterized by identical distance between adjacent points on a scale. Interval scales reflect direction and number of points between two values. Appropriate statistics would be the mean, standard deviation, Pearson product-moment correlation, multiple correlation, and tests such as t and F.

Ratio. The ratio is represented by a true zero. Thus, a value of 20 can be conceived as being twice the value of 10. Because ratio measurement is the highest level of measurement, any statistical test is usable. Appropriate statistics requiring knowledge of true zero are the geometric mean and the coefficient of variation.

Data Quality

The data should not represent varying time periods or different geographical areas. If they do, it could have a substantial effect on the health-status indicator or the health-status index. Every effort should be made to ensure comparability in time and space of the data, and the planner should carefully examine the data for gaps that may be detrimental to their utility.

Table 7-3 Levels of Analysis in Rank Order for Identifying Health Needs and Resources

Universe	Levels of Analysis for Investigation
World	Continents
Continent	Countries
Country	States
State	Counties Health Service Areas
County	Townships
Health Service Area	Enumeration Districts Cities
City	Neighborhoods
Neighborhood	Census Tracts
Census Tract	Blocks
Block	Households
Household	Families
Family	Individuals

Comprehensiveness

This applies only to the health-status index. The index could cover a broad range of diseases and conditions which have a decided impact on the health levels of a population or which focus on a specific disease and all risk factors associated with that disease. A Q Index would be an example of the former, and a regression model would be an example of the latter. It should be clear, however, that such an index indicates only a general level of well-being, and its application to program evaluation, resource allocation, and the setting of goals and objectives is limited.

Specificity

This also applies only to the health-status index. The health index should be as disease-specific as possible.[10] An index relating to a specific population subgroup is recommended. An example would be an infant health status index. The more specific the index, the more useful it will be in program analysis and resource allocation.

Indicator or Index Calculation

The indicator or index should be calculated by the simplest method feasible. It should not be expensive in terms of resources required. In a subsequent section, the various methods of calculation will be detailed.

Utility

For an indicator or index to have maximum utility, it should gain wide acceptance and be easy to reproduce. Above all, it must have practical applicability.

The purpose of providing the above criteria is to encourage the planning agency to follow a standardized procedure for selecting a health indicator or index. Failure to do so will result in invalid comparisons or differences in results and, potentially, erroneous conclusions. If these criteria are followed, problems of comparability should occur less frequently. This should become more apparent in the discussion of types of health-status indicators and indexes in a subsequent section.

Data Requirements for Health-Status Measurement

Data must be collected to reflect potential solutions to problems posed by the health-status objectives, goals, and policies of the agency. Often data are collected without reference to the problems they are supposed to answer. Adoption of the wellness or holistic approach to planning for health will make it necessary to begin thinking about the use of nontraditional as well as traditional data for health-status measurement. Consequently, traditional and nontraditional data must reflect broad categories like community health status, the health system, the life style, human biology, the environment, and social indicators.[11]

Within these categories there is also a need for specific data sets. For example:

1. Community health-status data. These are data related to the status of community health which provide a community health diagnosis. Appropriate measures include mortality rates, disability rates (workday loss), incidence and prevalence of specific diseases, and morbidity rates. These measures are obvious traditional health-status indicators of disease processes. Though they reflect deeply entrenched belief systems, the measures are important for developing indicators for acceptable goals and objectives.

2. Health-system data. Figure 7-1 indicated the relationship of health-system data to health status. It is evident that changes in life style, biology, and the environment will impact on health status and, in turn, on the health system. The health system will also have a limited impact on health status. Selected specific categories of health-system data are presented below:

    a. Health service utilization data
        (1) Hospital admissions
        (2) Discharges
        (3) Visits for ambulatory care
        (4) Patient-origin data
        (5) Residential data
        (6) Measurements accessibility in terms of geographic, economic, and cultural factors, or distance to facilities in terms of time, mileage, social aspects, and cost
    b. Facility and management data (availability)
        (1) Institutional resources like hospital beds, nursing homes, health access stations (primary care), and county health departments
        (2) Human resources like physicians, nurses, dentists, and other essential personnel
    c. Cost data
        (1) Diagnosis and care costs
        (2) Indirect costs of lost wages and lost productivity

(3) Indirect costs attributed to investment in individuals, that is, premature illness or death
(4) Government subsidies, such as Medicare and Medicaid

3. Life style data. Life style or health-behavior data will probably have to be (although not always) collected by a survey instrument. Examples are:
   a. Reasons for seeking health care
   b. Barriers to health care
   c. Spatial restrictions
   d. Life style components like drugs, nutrition, carelessness (alcohol, driving behavior), and risktaking (smoking, obesity, level of exercise)
   e. Marriage
   f. Divorce
4. Human biology data. These data are necessary to identify target groups at risk of a disease or to provide health information via promotional and awareness programs. Examples are:
   a. Demographic characteristics like age, sex, race, and ethnic group
   b. Genetic risks
   c. Intelligence
5. Environmental data
   a. Air, water, and soil conditions
   b. General climatic conditions
   c. Prevalence of rats and other pests presenting disease risks
   d. General environmental quality
   e. Housing data to reflect the quality and type of housing:
      (1) Crowding
      (2) Plumbing facilities
      (3) Social restrictions due to inadequate planning
      (4) Psychological needs and satisfactions
      (5) Neighborhood quality
   f. Occupational health
6. Social-indicators data
   a. Income, wealth, employment status, and income supplements
   b. The living environment, including housing, the neighborhood, and the physical environment
   c. Physical and mental health
   d. Education in terms of achievement, duration, and quality
   e. Social order (or disorganization) indicated by personal pathologies, family breakdown, crime and delinquency, and public order and safety
   f. Social belonging (alienation and participation) reflected in demo-

cratic participation, criminal justice, and segregation/ desegregation

g. Recreation and leisure in terms of recreational facilities, culture and the arts, and leisure available[12]

The health agency should use the above list of data requirements as a guide to present and future data needs. Since some of the data categories mentioned will not be available for some time, the agency should concentrate in the meantime on the more traditional categories.

Types of Health Status Indicators

Many indicators have been developed to measure the health status of a population. Some are simple and easily applied, while others are quite advanced and require skills of considerable sophistication. By applying the definition of a health-status indicator cited earlier to a review of the types of indicators available, a health agency can choose an indicator with relevance to the agency's skills and abilities. Following are some selected examples of the health indicators.

Age-Specific Death Rates

These may be expanded to include rates specific to sex, race, occupation, cause, and so forth. Differences in the magnitude of the rates in time and place suggest "poor" and "good" areas of health status. This type of rate approximates the risk of death from a specific condition and is perhaps the most important epidemiologic indicator available.

This type of rate may also be expanded to include adjusted or standardized rates. The crude rate and the adjusted rate can be compared to the state rates for a particular disease category. If the crude rate of a county or a community has been stable over the past few years, a community diagnosis can be determined by comparing it with the adjusted rate (Table 7-4).

An example of age-sex specific rates for cancer in Utah in 1976 is shown in Table 7-5. The two basic requirements are data on population and deaths, distributed by age and sex groups. To provide adjusted rates the same procedure noted in the age-sex specific rate example is followed to obtain the specific rate. The age-specific rate, however, is multiplied by a factor which is the proportion of population of each group in a standard million. The standard chosen should closely resemble the population being investigated. The multiplication of the factor by the age-specific rate gives expected death, and the sum of all expected deaths provides the age-adjusted death rate. This is the direct method of computation. Table

7-6 shows the procedure applied to determine expected deaths from cancer in Utah in the period 1972–76. The resulting state rates are those which would be expected; any differences found in the adjusted rates must be due to differences in age-specific rates. Table 7-7 shows the advantages and disadvantages of crude, specific, and adjusted rates when used as health-status indicators. Well-presented documents showing how to calculate these rates, standard errors, and confidence intervals may be found in Kleinman's material;[13] this subject is also discussed in Chapter 4.

The Proportional Mortality Ratio

The proportional mortality ratio (PMR) is not a rate, since it refers to total deaths and not to the population at risk. The ratio indicates what proportion of deaths is attributable to a specific disease. It is useful because it permits estimation of the proportion of lives to be saved by reducing a given cause of death. The PMR may be calculated as the number of deaths from a given cause in a specified period, divided by the

Table 7-4 Community Health Diagnosis Using Crude and Adjusted Rates

Relative Crude Rate	Status of Adjusted Rate	Community Diagnosis
Low	Low	Low mortality is not due to age, race, and sex factors; other mortality conditions are favorable.
Low	High	Low mortality is due to favorable age, race, and sex factors; other mortality conditions are unfavorable.
High	Low	High mortality is due to unfavorable age, race, and sex factors; other mortality conditions are favorable.
High	High	High mortality is not due to age, race, and sex factors; other mortality conditions are unfavorable.

Source: North Carolina Vital Statistics, Leading Causes of Mortality, Vol. 2, 1977, p. 8.

total number of deaths in the same time period, times 100. See Table 2-1 for an application of this health-status indicator. In community health, the PMR is quite useful because one can estimate the proportion of lives saved by reducing or eradicating a particular cause of death.

Indicator of Unnecessary Deaths

Using mortality data, it is possible to calculate an indicator showing a value for unnecessary deaths (UD).[14] This indicator is useful as a means of demonstrating variations in death rates in any given population compared to another population. The indicator is simply the difference be-

Table 7-5 Age-Sex Specific Rates for Cancer (ICDA Codes 140–209), Utah, 1976

Age Group	Population		Number of Deaths		Age-Sex Specific Rate	
	Male	Female	Male	Female	Male*	Female*
	(1)	(2)	(3)	(4)	(5)	(6)
≤4	67,645	64,814	4	3	5.91	4.63
5– 9	59,265	56,418	2	3	3.37	5.32
10–14	61,513	59,786	4	1	6.50	1.67
15–19	65,263	62,742	3	5	4.60	7.97
20–24	60,114	60,601	5	4	8.32	6.60
25–29	47,572	53,500	10	2	21.02	3.74
30–34	36,998	37,364	6	10	16.22	26.76
35–39	29,425	30,052	5	10	16.99	33.28
40–44	26,889	28,007	9	12	33.47	47.85
45–49	27,328	27,763	25	30	91.48	108.06
50–54	25,845	27,141	0	0	.00	.00
55–59	23,416	24,879	0	0	.00	.00
60–64	19,395	20,809	2	1	10.31	4.81
65–69	15,303	17,521	254	198	1,659.81	1,130.07
70–74	10,510	13,511	132	118	1,255.95	873.36
75–79	7,195	10,141	85	57	1,181.38	562.07
80–84	4,017	6,305	80	66	1,991.54	1,046.79
85+	2,325	3,871	54	46	2,322.58	1,188.32

*(5) = (3)/(1) • 100,000 = Age-Sex Specific Rate.
(6) = (4)/(2) • 100,000 = Age-Sex Specific Rate.

tween an expected death rate and the actual death rate of the population under study. Thus:

$$UD = DR_A - DR_E$$

where: UD = Unnecessary deaths
DR_A = Actual death rate
DR_E = Expected death rate

Table 7-6 Age-Adjusted Table for Cancer (ICDA Codes 140–209) Utah, 1972–1976

Age Group	Average Deaths	Age-Group Population	Age-Specific Rate*	Proportion of Population in a Standard Million	Expected Deaths*
	(1)	(2)	(3)	(4)	(5)
≤4	6.2	132,459	4.6807	.08536088	.3995
5– 9	7.2	115,683	6.2239	.09931664	.6181
10–14	5.0	121,299	4.1220	.10346954	.4265
15–19	8.8	128,005	6.8747	.09350754	.6428
20–24	8.8	120,715	7.2899	.07600068	.5540
25–29	12.8	101,072	12.6642	.06569550	.8320
30–34	11.4	74,362	15.3304	.05593244	.8575
35–39	14.2	59,477	23.8748	.05436577	1.2980
40–44	24.6	54,896	44.8120	.05922990	2.6542
45–49	49.0	55,091	88.9437	.06011021	5.3464
50–54	79.2	52,986	149.4734	.05517646	8.2474
55–59	105.8	48,295	219.0703	.04961604	10.8694
60–64	132.6	40,204	329.8179	.04288187	14.1432
65–69	168.4	32,824	513.0392	.03479489	17.8511
70–74	158.4	24,021	659.4230	.02709088	17.8643
75–79	144.2	17,336	831.7951	.01907850	15.8694
80–84	118.0	10,322	1,142.1893	.01136951	12.9975
85+	83.6	6,196	1,349.2576	.00700275	9.4485
			State Age-Adjusted Death Rate		120.9201 (6)*

*(3) = (1)/(2) • 100,000 = Age-Specific Rate; (5) = (4) • (3) = Expected Deaths; (6) = sum of all values of (5) = Age-Adjusted Death Rate.

In the case of infant mortality in a county where the state is selected as a standard:

$$UD_{County} = DR_A \text{ (county)} - DR_E \text{ (state)}$$
$$UD_{County} = 15.3 - 10.1$$
$$UD_{County} = 5.2$$

To make statistically valid comparisons, the death rates should be specific, although crude rates may be used if one is reasonably assured that the age and sex structures of the population under investigation are similar. The expected death rate could be the rate for the national, regional, or state populations or it could be another calculated rate. This rate may be

Table 7-7 Advantages and Disadvantages of Using Crude, Specific, and Adjusted Rates for Health Status Indicators

Health Status Indicators	Advantages	Disadvantages
Crude Rates	Easy to calculate. Summary rates. Widely used for international comparisons (despite limitations).	Because population groups vary in age, sex, race, etc., the differences in crude rates are not directly interpretable.
Specific Rates	Applied to homogeneous subgroups. The detailed rates are useful for epidemiological and public health purposes.	Comparisons can be cumbersome, if many subgroups are calculated for two or more populations.
Adjusted Rates	Represents a summary rate. Differences in composition of groups reviewed allowing unbiased comparison.	Not true rates (fictional). Magnitude of rates is dependent upon the standard million population chosen. Trends in subgroups can be masked.

Source: Modified from J. S. Mausner and A. K. Bahn, *Epidemiology: An Introductory Text* (Philadelphia, Pa.: W. B. Saunders Co., 1974), p. 138.

quite useful to the health agency in setting objectives to reduce the value and in determining the success of its achievements. Because of its relatively clear expression of the frequency of deaths, it should be useful for community education and may also serve to support resource-allocation decisions. The indicator may also be used as a community-rating scale when various counties are compared to determine overall health statuses.

Years-of-Life Lost

The years-of-life lost or YLL indicator allows the health planner to use deaths at different ages from a specific cause to calculate estimated total years of life lost. The example in Table 7-8 shows estimated years of life lost for various age groups and gives a total number of years of life lost for acute myocardial infarction. This indicator may be applied to disability statistics to denote productive workday loss. The health agency may also use this type of analysis to set priorities in terms of specific ages and particular diseases. Goals and objectives may be determined in terms of clear quantitative statements. Because the requisite data are usually readily available to the agency, this indicator should be easy to use.

Other Health-Status Indicators

Other measures traditionally used as health-status indicators are shown

Table 7-8 Estimated Years of Life Lost from Acute Myocardial Infarction

Age Group	Deaths 1976		Average Years of Life Lost*	Estimated Total Years of Life Lost
35–39	81	×	30	2,430
40–44	201	×	25	5,025
45–49	433	×	20	8,660
50–54	692	×	15	10,380
55–59	1,101	×	10	11,010
60–64	1,426	×	5	7,130
Total	3,934			44,635

*Based on a life expectancy of 69 years.

in Table 7-9. The general format for these indicators is a numerator over a denominator multiplied by a constant; thus:

$$(x/y)(k)$$

where: x, y, and k are defined as in Table 7-9.

Table 7-9 Health-Status Indicators Most Frequently Used for Describing Natality, Morbidity, and Mortality

No.	Description of Indicator	Numerator (x)	Denominator (y)	Expressed per Number at Risk (k)
	NATALITY			
1	Birth Rate			
	Crude; specific for age of mother, sex of child, socioeconomic status, etc.	Number of live births reported during a given time interval	Estimated mid-interval population	1,000
2	Fertility Rate			
	Crude; specific for age of mother, race, socio-economic status, etc.	Number of live births reported during a given time interval	Estimated number of women in age group 15–44 years at mid-interval	1,000
3	Low Birth Weight Ratio			
	Crude; specific for age of mother, race, socio-economic area, etc.	Number of live births under 2,500 grams (or 5½ lbs.) during a given time interval	Number of live births reported during the same time interval	100
	MORBIDITY			
1	Incidence Rate			
	Crude by cause; specific for age, race, sex, socioeconomic area, state of disease, etc.	Number of new cases of a specified disease reported during a given time period	Estimated mid-interval population	Variable: 10^x where $x = 2, 3, 4, 5, 6$
2	Attack Rate			
	Crude by cause; specific for age, race, socio-economic area, etc.	Number of new cases of a specified disease reported during a specific time interval	Total population at risk during the same time interval	Variable: 10^x where $x = 2, 3, 4, 5, 6$
3	Point Prevalence Rate (Ratio)			
	Crude by cause; specific for age, race, sex, socioeconomic area, stage of disease, etc.	Number of current cases, new and old, of a specified disease existing at a given point in time	Estimated population at the same point in time	Variable: 10^x where $x = 2, 3, 4, 5, 6$

Table 7-9 continued

No.	Description of Indicator	Numerator (x)	Denominator (y)	Expressed per Number at Risk (k)
4	Period (Case Load) Prevalence Rate (Ratio) Crude by cause; specific for age, race, sex, socioeconomic area, stage of disease, etc.	Number of current cases, new and old, of a specified disease occurring during a given time interval	Estimated mid-interval population	Variable: 10^x where x = 2, 3, 4, 5, 6
	MORTALITY			
1	Crude Death Rate Crude; specific for age, race, sex, socioeconomic area, etc.	Total number of deaths reported during a given time interval	Estimated mid-interval population	1,000
2	Cause-Specific Death Rate Crude by cause; specific for age, race, sex, socioeconomic area, etc.	Number of deaths assigned to a specific cause during a given time interval	Estimated mid-interval population	100,000
3	Proportional Mortality Ratio Crude by cause; specific for age, race, sex, socioeconomic area, etc.	Number of deaths assigned to a specific cause during a given time interval	Total number of deaths from all causes reported during the same interval	100 (percentage)
4	Case Fatality Rate (Ratio) Crude; specific for age, race, sex, socioeconomic area, etc.	Number of deaths assigned to a specific disease during a given time interval	Number of new cases of that disease reported during the same time interval	100
5	(a) Fetal Death Rate I Crude; specific for age of mother, race, socioeconomic area, etc.	Number of fetal deaths of 28 weeks or more gestation reported during a given time interval	Number of fetal deaths of 28 weeks or more gestation reported during the same time interval plus the number of live births occurring during the same time interval	1,000

Table 7-9 continued

No.	Description of Indicator	Numerator (x)	Denominator (y)	Expressed per Number at Risk (k)
	(b) Fetal Death Rate II			
	Crude; specific for age of mother, race, socioeconomic area, etc.	Number of fetal deaths of 20 weeks or more gestation reported during a given time interval	Number of fetal deaths of 20 weeks or more gestation reported during the same time interval plus the number of live births occurring during the same time interval	1,000
6	(a) Fetal Death Ratio I			
	Crude; specific for age of mother, race, socioeconomic area, etc.	Number of fetal deaths of 28 weeks or more gestation reported during a given time interval	Number of live births reported during the same time interval	1,000
	(b) Fetal Death Ratio II			
	Crude; specific for age of mother, race, socioeconomic area, etc.	Number of fetal deaths of 20 weeks or more gestation reported during a given time interval	Number of live births reported during the same time interval	1,000
7	(a) Perinatal Mortality Rate I			
	Crude; specific for age of mother, race etc.	Number of fetal deaths of 28 weeks or more gestation reported during a given time interval plus the reported number of infant deaths under 7 days of life during the same time interval	Number of fetal deaths of 28 weeks or more gestation reported during the same time interval plus the number of live births occurring during the same time interval	1,000
	(b) Perinatal Mortality Rate II			
	Crude; specific for age of mother, sex, socioeconomic area, etc.	Number of fetal deaths of 20 weeks or more gestation reported during a given time interval plus the reported number of infant deaths under 28 days of life during the same time interval	Number of fetal deaths of 20 weeks or more gestation reported during the same time interval plus the number of live births reported during the same time interval	1,000

Table 7-9 continued

No.	Description of Indicator	Numerator (x)	Denominator (y)	Expressed per Number at Risk (k)
8	Infant Mortality Rate Crude; specific for race, sex, socioeconomic area, birth weight, cause of death, etc.	Number of deaths under one year of age reported during a given time interval	Number of live births reported during the same time interval	1,000
9	Neonatal Mortality Rate Crude; specific for race, sex, socioeconomic area, birth weight, cause of death, etc.	Number of deaths under 28 days of age reported during a given time interval	Number of live births reported during the same time interval	1,000
10	Postneonatal Mortality Rate Crude; specific for race, sex, socioeconomic area, cause of death, etc.	Number of deaths from 28 days of age up to, but not including, one year of age, reported during a given time interval	Number of live births reported during the same time interval	1,000
11	Maternal Mortality Rate Crude; specific for age of mother, race, socioeconomic area, etc.	Number of deaths assigned to causes related to pregnancy during a given time interval	Number of live births reported during the same time interval	10,000

Source: Descriptive Statistics, Rates, Ratios, Proportions, and Indices, U.S. DHEW, PHS, Center for Disease Control, Atlanta, Georgia, pp. 3–8.

Types of Health-Status Indexes

The construction and use of a health index can require very elaborate statistical techniques and methodologies. It is recommended that the health agency use health indicators where possible and develop health indexes to provide a composite description of health status. Table 7-10 shows the various uses of health-status indexes for community and individual diagnosis.

Health-status indexes may be used to demonstrate community health status on a community rating scale. An example of this is the index derived from regression analysis. A health index may also be used as a baseline or benchmark measure if the methodology is standardized so that future comparisons will be valid.

To be useful, an index must satisfy certain practical requirements. It must be simple in construction, use, and application. It should be acceptable to both respondents and users. It should be economical and make use of available data or data that are readily gathered.

Clearly, under the definition of health index given earlier, many forms of indexes can be constructed. For any index, four points should be considered:

1. What is the purpose of the index?
2. What are the exact components of the index?
3. What is the form of interpretation?
4. What are the limitations of the index?

As noted in the annotated guide to the papers of the 1976 Health Status Indexes Conference (*Health Services Research,* Winter 1976, p. 340):

> The general impression of the state of the art in the development of health status indexes is one of ferment. Some work is methodologically sophisticated, some is naive. Certain approaches offer early programmatic uses, others appear purely theoretical. In some cases in which the work is both advanced and sophisticated, there is a danger that it is too complex or conceptually confused to be used readily in policy analysis and planning. One lesson is clear: solid results require competent methodological input, and much current work is deficient in that respect.

Following are some selected examples of health indexes. The first two are more nontraditional; the remainder are more traditional measures for use when certain types of data and information are available. It is recommended that agencies use the most appropriate index in light of their needs and resources.

Wellness Appraisal Index

The data from a wellness index developed for individuals may be aggregated to reflect populations at a small-area analysis level. The wellness index centers on the four main components of self-responsibility, nutri-

Table 7-10 Uses of Health-Status Indexes

Use	Community	Individual
Comparison	Social indicators	Clinical status indicators
Evaluation	Program trials	Clinical trials, peer review
Allocation	Program planning	Patient management
Baseline measurement	Program planning	Patient management

Source: Modified and reproduced with permission from *Health Services Research* Vol. 8, No. 2, Summer 1973, p. 154. Copyright 1973 by the Hospital Research and Educational Trust, 840 N. Lake Shore Drive, Chicago, Illinois 60611.

tion, stress control, and physical awareness.[15] From several detailed questionnaires on these four components, a summary of 16 wellness-index questions were selected (see Table 7-11). The reader may easily answer the 16 selected questions and determine a personal level of wellness without referring to the full-scale questionnaires. It is recommended, however, that if greater detail is needed, the *Wellness Workbook* be consulted.

The responses of "rarely," "sometimes," or "very often" in Table 7-11 may be portrayed graphically to illustrate a picture of wellness. Figure 7-2 shows a blank pie chart, divided into quarters representing the four dimensions of wellness. The inner broken circle corresponds to "rarely," the middle broken circle to "sometimes," and the outer broken circle to "very often." After answering the questions in Table 7-11, fill in the appropriate area of the Figure 7-2 graphic. That is, if your response to question one is "sometimes," color in area one of the graph, up to the second broken circle (b). Complete this for each question. The resulting shape of the index will provide a self-evaluation of your level of wellness.

This approach may be modified by inserting percentages to broaden the categories beyond "rarely," "sometimes," and "very often." The result would be a numerical index which, through minor statistical analysis, would reflect levels of wellness for population groups. For example, a health agency could apply this wellness evaluation to their employees, by section or unit, to determine the overall level of wellness in the organization. The results would enable the director to provide the employees with appropriate solutions as designated by the wellness evaluation. Further, simple telephone or newspaper surveys utilizing this approach could provide results or measures on a community basis. This health status index on wellness is in obvious correspondence with the epidemiological model on health policy outlined in a previous chapter.

Table 7-11 Wellness Appraisal Index: Questions and Evaluation Criteria

Area of	Question No.	Wellness Evaluation Questions	Categories	Evaluation Criteria	Survey Instrument	Response
Nutrition	1	I am conscious of the food ingredients I eat and their effect on me.	R, S, VO	Conscious about nutrition	Eating Habits Survey (64 questions)	VO
	2	I avoid overeating and abusing alcohol, caffeine, nicotine, and other drugs.	R, S, VO	Awareness of overuse of substances	Eating Habits Survey	VO
	3	I minimize my intake of refined carbohydrates and fats.	R, S, VO	Reduced carbohydrate and fat intake	Computerized Nutrition Survey	VO
	4	My diet contains adequate amounts of vitamins, minerals, and fiber.	R, S, VO	Adequacy of vitamins, minerals, fiber	Computerized Nutrition Survey	S
Physical Awareness	5	I am free from physical symptoms.	R = > 10 S = 5–10 VO = < 5	Absence of physical symptoms	Symptom Checklist	VO
	6	I get aerobic cardiovascular exercise.	R, S, VO = 12–20 min. 5 times/wk.	Aerobic exercise level (running, swimming, bicycling)	Wellness Inventory	VO
	7	I practice yoga or some other form of limbering/stretching exercise.	R, S, VO	Body flexibility and training	Wellness Inventory	S
	8	I nurture myself. (Nurturing means pleasuring and taking care of oneself; e.g., massages, long walks, buying presents for oneself, sleeping late without feeling guilty.)	R, S, VO	Awareness of self-nurturing	Wellness Resource Book (Part 3) Survey Questions	R

Table 7-11 continued

Area of	Question No.	Wellness Evaluation Questions	Categories	Evaluation Criteria	Survey Instrument	Response
Stress Control	9	I pay attention to changes occurring in my life and am aware of them as stress factors. (A score of 300 from the Life Change Index is considered very stressful.)	R, S, VO	In control of life changes	Life Change Index	S
	10	I practice relaxation regularly. (20 minutes a day, "centering" or "letting go" of thoughts, worries, etc.)	R, S, VO	Regular relaxation needs	—	R
	11	I am without excess muscle tension.	R, S, VO	Levels of muscle tension, stress	Body Stress Assessment	S
	12	My hands are warm and dry.	R, S, VO	Tense, uptight	Body Stress Assessment	VO
Self-Responsibility	13	I am both productive and happy.	R, S, VO	Productivity and aliveness	Wellness Resource Book (Part 1)	VO
	14	I constructively express my emotions and creativity.	R, S, VO	Enlightenment and happiness	Wellness Resource Book (Part 6)	VO
	15	I feel a sense of purpose in life, and my life has meaning and direction.	R, S, VO	Purpose in life directed and clear	Purpose in Life Test	VO
	16	I believe I am fully responsible for my wellness or illness.	R, S, VO	Locus of control internal versus external	Wellness Work Book (Part 4) Summary Questions	VO

Table 7-11 continued

R = Rarely, S = Sometimes, VO = Very Often.

Source: This table is a modification of p. 20 in the *Wellness Workbook*. Questions and full-length questionnaires are available from the *Wellness Workbook*, Wellness Resource Center, 42 Miller Avenue, Mill Valley, California 94941. Reprinted with permission from the *Wellness Workbook for Health Professionals*, Copyright 1977, John W. Travis, M.D. Published by the Wellness Resource Center, 42 Miller Avenue, Mill Valley, CA 94941.

Health Hazard Appraisal Index

In line with the basic premise of this book, the health hazard appraisal (HHA) index is based on wellness and holistic principles. Many types of appraisals are equally useful in developing a risk profile based on wellness and holistic practices. Examples include Risk Analysis Detection and Reduction (RADAR), Life Style Profile, and Risk (the Heart Association of Greater Miami).[16]

The basic aim of the HHA is to obtain information from individuals concerning their personal life styles. In each case, the chronological age is compared with the appraisal age, and an attainable age is calculated based on responses to the questions. To reach the attainable age, recommendations may include more exercise, cessation of smoking, and the loss of weight, with benefits measured in years. If known, certain medical facts, such as those pertaining to blood pressure, cholesterol, and triglyceride levels, are also weighted in the final recommendations. Exhibit 7-1 shows a sample output from the HHA index, and Table 7-12 indicates what each category means in the sample output.

In a community survey, the HHA index might be administered on a random-sample basis in a health-service area encompassing several counties. The results from each county could be tabulated and an index constructed. The HHA index could include questions like What is the average risk reduction by county? What is the average benefit in years from an exercise program? or, What is the average patient risk by county for comparable age and sex groups? Essentially, this procedure would apply an individual clinical questionnaire to a community population. The health agency would certainly benefit in many respects from such an application.

The HHA index provides: (1) a community diagnosis, (2) baseline measurements, (3) an excellent educational and awareness program, and (4) an evaluation of health status for the health plan. The only potential drawback to this approach might be the dollar resources needed to complete the HHA. A complete analysis by computer, however, costs from three to five dollars. The HHA index is indeed nontraditional and can address very effectively the holistic and wellness epidemiological policies of life style, environment, human biology, and medical care system.

Exhibit 7-1 Sample Health Hazard Appraisal

RISK ANALYSIS DETECTION AND REDUCTION- -
A SERVICE OF THE FULTON COUNTY
HEALTH DEPARTMENT, ATLANTA, GA.

1PATIENT NAME#DOE JOHN
2PATIENT NO# 32 BIRTHDATE#121525
3PROV/PHYS# FULTON COUNTY HEALTH DEPARTMENT

7TOTAL REDUCIBLE RISK 7 YRS

4CHRONOLOGIC AGE 42
5APPRAISAL AGE 47
6ACHIEVABLE AGE 40

8CAUSE OF DEATH	9 AVERAGE	10 APPRAISED	11 ACHIEVABLE
ARTERIOSCLEROTIC HEART DISEASE	2278.	5467.	1990.
CANCER OF THE LUNG	436.	130.	87.
CIRRHOSIS	382.	764.	76.
MOTOR VEHICLE ACCIDENT	314.	722.	282.
SUICIDE	263.	263.	263.
STROKE	257.	642.	347.
CANCER OF THE INTESTINES,RECTUM	112.	336.	112.
PNEUMONIA	102.	102.	102.
HOMOCIDE	100.	100.	100.
RHEUMATIC HEART DISEASE	77.	0.	0.
ACCIDENTS MACH. NON-MOTOR VEH.	64.	64.	64.
ALCOHOLISM	50.	50.	50.
OTHER (NOT GRAPHED)	15 2117.	2117.	2117.
TOTAL	16 6552.	17 10757.	18 5590.

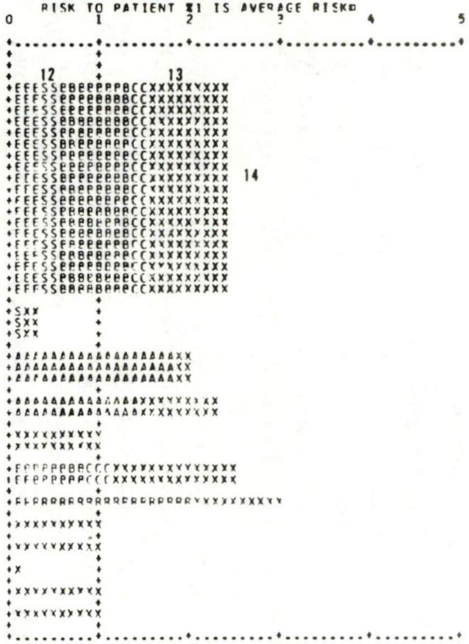

COMPUTATIONS BASED ON 1971 DATA; CHANCES OF DYING PER 100,000

RISK TO PATIENT (1 IS AVERAGE RISK): 0 1 2 3 4 5 (markers 12, 13, 14 on graph)

19LEGEND AND REDUCIBLE RISK IN YEARS

X#IRREDUC.											
E#EXERCISE	1.0	S# SMOKING	0.6	B# BP SYST	2.5	A# ALCOHOL	1.5	F#	0.0	L#	0.0
W# WEIGHT	0.0	D# DIABETES	0.0	N# NEG/PAP	0.0	V# SEATBELT	0.0	P# PROCTO	0.0	C# CHOLESTR	0.7
R#RECTAL BLOOD	0.3	G#	0.0	T#	0.0	H# DEPRESS	0.0	J# RH FEVER	0.0		

20FOR HEIGHT 68 INCHES AND MEDIUM FRAME, 172 LBS. IS APPROXIMATELY 15 PERCENT OVERWEIGHT DESIRABLE WEIGHT IS 149 LBS.

- - - ACHIEVABLE - - -

21YOUR HEALTH RISKS WILL BE REDUCED BY MAKING ANY OR ALL OF THE FOLLOWING CHANGES IN YOUR BEHAVIOR---

EXERCISE	FROM	LOW MODERATE	TO	EXERCISE PROGRAM
SMOKING	FROM	PIPE NOT INHALED	TO	STOPPED SMOKING
BP SYST	FROM	180 MM.	TO	146 MM.
BP DIAS	FROM	94 MM.	TO	90 MM.
ALCOHOL	FROM	7-24/WEEK	TO	1-2/WK NONE B4 DRVNG
WEIGHT	FROM	172 LBS.	TO	149 LBS.
CHOLESTR	FROM	220 MGS. PERCENT	TO	196 MGS. PERCENT
RCTBLEED	FROM	BLOOD IN STOOL	TO	BLOOD IN STOOL&DIAG.

****
* * * DETAIL * * *

FILE NO 13

22 CAUSE OF DEATH	23 PRECURSORS	24 APPRAISAL YOUR CURRENT CHARACTERISTIC	25 RISK FACTOR	26 COMP R-FAC	27 ACHIEVABLE YOUR POTENTIAL CHARACTERISTIC	28 RISK FACTOR	29 COMP R-FAC
ARTERIOSCLEROTIC HEART DISEASE	BL.PRESS	PH 0/ 0 180/ 94	2.2/1.3		146/ 90	1.5/1.1	
	CHOLESTR	220	1.00		196	0.70	
	DIABETES	NOT DIABETIC	1.00		NOT DIABETIC	1.00	
	WEIGHT	172	1.00		149	1.00	
	EXERCISE	LOW MODERATE	1.00		EXERCISE PROGRAM	0.50	
	SMOKING	PIPE NOT INHALED	1.00		STOPPED SMOKING	0.70	
	FAM/HIST	NO	0.90	2.40	NO	0.90	0.87
CANCER OF THE LUNG	SMOKING	PIPE NOT INHALED	0.30	0.30	STOPPED SMOKING	0.20	0.20
CIRRHOSIS	ALCOHOL	7-24/WEEK	2.00	2.00	1-2/WK NONE B4 DRVNG	0.20	0.20
MOTOR VEHICLE ACCIDENT	ALCOHOL	7-24/WEEK	2.00		1-2/WK NONE B4 DRVNG	0.50	
	MIL/YEAR	15000	1.50		15000	1.50	
	SEATBELT	75-100 PERCENT	0.80		75-100 PERCENT	0.80	
	DRUG/MED	NONE BEFORE DRIVING	1.00	2.30	NONE BEFORE DRIVING	1.00	0.90
SUICIDE	DEPRESS	SELDOM OR NEVER	1.00		SELDOM OR NEVER	1.00	
	FAM/HIST	NO	1.00	1.00	NO	1.00	1.00
STROKE	BL.PRESS	PH 0/ 0 180/ 94	2.2/1.3		146/ 90	1.5/1.1	
	CHOLESTR	220	1.00		196	0.70	
	DIABETES	NOT DIABETIC	1.00		NOT DIABETIC	1.00	
	SMOKING	PIPE NOT INHALED	1.00	2.50	STOPPED SMOKING	1.00	1.35
CANCER OF THE INTESTINES,RECTUM	POLYP	HAS NOT HAD	1.00		HAS NOT HAD	1.00	
	PROCTO	NOT HAD IN PAST YEAR	1.00		NOT HAD IN PAST YEAR	1.00	
	RCTBLEED	BLOOD IN STOOL	3.00		BLOOD IN STOOL&DIAG.	1.00	
	ULCERCOL	HAS NO SYMPTOMS	1.00	3.00	HAS NO SYMPTOMS	1.00	1.00
PNEUMONIA	ALCOHOL	7-24/WEEK	1.00		1-2/WK NONE B4 DRVNG	1.00	
	BACTPNEU	HAS NOT HAD	1.00		HAS NOT HAD	1.00	
	SMOKING	PIPE NOT INHALED	1.00		STOPPED SMOKING	1.00	
	EMPHYSEM	DOES NOT HAVE	1.00	1.00	DOES NOT HAVE	1.00	1.00
HOMICIDE	ARRESTS	NO ARRESTS	1.00		NO ARRESTS	1.00	
	WEAPONS	DOES NOT CARRY	1.00	1.00	DOES NOT CARRY	1.00	1.00
RHEUMATIC HEART DISEASE	RH FEVER	NO R.F. + NO MURMUR	0.10		NO R.F. + NO MURMUR	0.10	
	RH S/C/S	NO SYMPTOMS	0.10	0.01	NO SYMPTOMS	0.10	0.01

* RISK FACTORS ADAPTED FROM HOW TO PRACTICE PROSPECTIVE MEDICINE , DRS. ROBBINS AND HALL, METHODIST HOSPITAL OF INDIANA.
* ACKNOWLEDGEMENT TO H.N. COLBURN, MD-MPH HEALTH AND WELFARE CANADA AND J.W. TRAVIS,MD-MPH U.S. P.H. SERVICE BALTIMORE,MD

Source: Reprinted with permission from the *Wellness Workbook for Health Professionals,* Copyright 1977, John W. Travis, M.D., published by the Wellness Resource Center, 42 Miller Ave., Mill Valley, CA 94941.

Figure 7-2 Wellness Appraisal Index Graphs

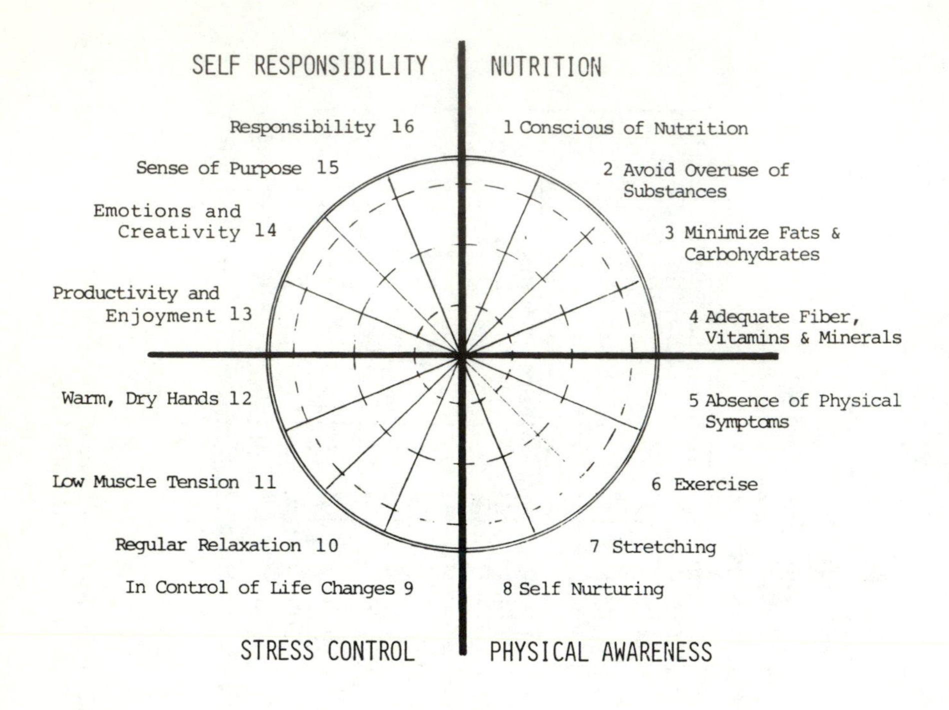

Completed Wellness Appraisal Index Graph

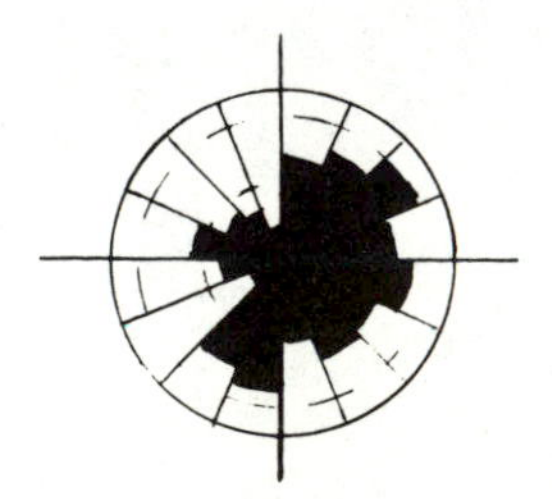

a = rarely
b = sometimes
c = very often

Source: Reprinted with permission from the *Wellness Workbook for Health Professionals*, Copyright 1977, John W. Travis, M.D., published by the Wellness Resource Center, 42 Miller Avenue, Mill Valley, CA 94941, p. 21.

Table 7-12 RADAR (Risk Analysis Detection and Reduction) Report—Key to Understanding Your Health Hazard Appraisal

---

Your computerized risk analysis is basically a statistical comparison of three different risk situations. In each case, risk refers to the number of deaths expected from specified diseases or accidents in the next ten years. These three risks are stated in the usual numerical fashion of the expected or projected number of deaths per 100,000 in the population group. The three situations are:

1. Average—this is the average risk for all persons of your age, race and sex;
2. Appraised—this is an estimate of your particular risk as calculated from data supplied in your questionnaire;
3. Achievable—this is a minimum risk situation for you if you make all the suggested changes in your life style.

In order to make these risks most meaningful, appraisal and achievable *ages* are also shown. See items 5 & 6.

An illustrated example report is attached. Each item is numbered according to the following explanations.

1. *CLIENT NAME - DOE, JOHN*—Name of individual having Health Risk Appraisal.
2. *CLIENT NUMBER, 32 - BIRTHDATE, 12/15/35*—Identification number assigned to individual. Name and number are entered separately for confidentiality. Birthdate - individual's date of birth.
3. *PROV/PHYS - FULTON COUNTY HEALTH DEPARTMENT*—The provider's or physician's office where individual had his or her appraisal done. If done through a company or organization, this would be indicated here.
4. *CHRONOLOGICAL AGE - 42*—John Doe's present age.
5. *APPRAISAL AGE - 47*—The age John Doe is in terms of his risks. He stands the same chance of dying in the next 10 years as a person 47 years old. It does not say he will die 6 years earlier but his chances of dying are that of a person 6 years older than John Doe.
6. *ACHIEVABLE AGE - 40*—The age John Doe might have if he made all the recommended behavioral changes. He then stands the same chance of dying in the next 10 years as a person 40 years old.
7. *TOTAL REDUCIBLE RISK - 7 YEARS*—This is the difference between the appraised and achievable age, and is the sum of the different behavior changes recommendation (see No. 19).

Table 7-12 continued

8. *CAUSE OF DEATH*—This column lists in rank order John Doe's 12 leading causes of death in the next 10 years.
9. *AVERAGE DEATHS/100,000*—These are the number of expected deaths associated with each disease. The data are taken from the National Center for Health Statistics and reflect the 1971 United States Mortality experience. This shows that 2,278 deaths from arteriosclerotic heart disease can be expected for 100,000 white males 42 years old in the next 10 years. Similarly, 436 deaths from lung cancer, etc.
10. *APPRAISED DEATHS/100,000*—This column shows the adjusted mortality figures for John Doe. This shows John Doe's risk of heart attack as compared to the average is 2.4 times the average; 2.4 is the risk multiplier for arteriosclerotic heart disease for John Doe and is shown in two components below (Items 12 and 13).
11. *ACHIEVABLE DEATHS/100,000*—This column reflects the expected deaths per 100,000 for John Doe assuming modification of *all* risk reducing behavioral changes are made.
12. *EEESSBBBBBBBCC*—This is the reducible risk broken down from the codes at the bottom of Figure 1 (No. 19).
13. *XXXXXXXXX*—This is the irreducible component of the risk multiplier. The combined irreducible and reducible risk made up the total risk multiplier for arteriosclerotic heart disease and is read as 2.4 from the horizontal scale.
14. The height of the bar graph reflects the relative significance of each cause of death in terms of its contribution to the total number of expected deaths for an average 42-year-old white male.
15. *OTHER*—All other causes of death are lumped together. None account for more than 1 percent of the total deaths.
16. *TOTAL 6552*—The sum of this column shows that the average risk for 42-year-old white males is 6552 deaths per 100,000 individuals over the next 10 years.
17. *TOTAL 10,757*—The sum of this column shows that John Doe's specific risks place him in a group which would have 10,757 deaths per 100,000 individuals, giving him an appraisal age of 47 years.
18. *TOTAL 5590*—The sum of this column shows that by complying with recommendations made (No. 19) John Doe can reduce his risk to 5,590 deaths per 100,000 individuals, giving him an achievable risk of 40 years.

Table 7-12 continued

19. *LEGEND AND REDUCIBLE RISKS IN YEARS*—This is the legend for the letters used in the bar graph. Each is followed by an expression (in years) of its contribution to the total reducible risk.

    *If you stop smoking, your risk of dying from heart disease, lung cancer, emphysema, pneumonia, and stroke will be reduced .6 years.

    *If you adhere to a prescribed exercise program your risk of dying from heart disease will be reduced 1 year.

    *If you stop drinking alcohol, or limit your consumption of it and do not drink before driving, your risk of dying from motor vehicle accidents, cirrhosis of the liver, and pneumonia will be reduced 1.5 years.

    *If you reduce your cholesterol, your risk of dying from heart disease and stroke will be reduced .7 years.

    *If you have a rectal examination to diagnose blood in stool, your risk of dying from cancer of the intestines and rectum will be reduced .3 years.

    *If you lower your blood pressure to 146/90, your risk of dying of heart disease and stroke will be reduced 2.9 years.

By complying with these recommendations, you can reduce your risk to 5,590 deaths per 100,000 for an achievable risk age of 39 years.

20. This describes John Doe's frame, weight, and height taken with shoes and indoor clothing. This shows he is 15 percent overweight (based on Metropolitan Life Insurance Company, New York's desirable weight tables for adult males) and his desirable weight is 149 pounds. A 42-year-old white male, *15 percent* overweight is at average risk; as this percent increases, so does the risk.
21. The suggestions in this section cover the most important behavior changes John Doe should make in order to achieve the same risk of dying in 10 years as a person 39 years old.
22. *CAUSE OF DEATH*—This column lists John Doe's 12 leading causes of death (same as No. 8, Figure 1).
23. *PRECURSORS*—For each cause of death the contributing factors or precursors are listed, i.e., for *arteriosclerotic heart disease,* blood pressure, cholesterol, diabetes, weight, exercise, smoking, family history: *cancer of the lung,* smoking, etc.
24. APPRAISAL - YOUR CURRENT CHARACTERISTIC—This section provides corresponding patient data. For arteriosclerotic heart

Table 7-12 continued

disease, the patient's blood pressure is 180/94, and his cholesterol is 220 Mgs. He is not diabetic, his exercise level is low moderate. He has no family history of heart disease. He smokes 20 plus cigarettes a day and is 15 percent overweight.

25. *RISK FACTOR*—This column lists the risk factors for each precursor. The risk factor answers the question, "To what degree does the individual with this precursor deviate from average?" For example, this patient's blood pressure is 180/94 which corresponds with the risk factor 2.2/1.3. His cholesterol being 220 is average or 1.0, while his smoking behavior gives him a risk factor of 1.0 or average risk, but is still reducible.
26. *COMPOSITE RISK FACTOR*—Each composite represents a combination of all the single risk factors in a particular disease category. If a disease category has only one precursor, this risk factor is used as the composite.
27. *ACHIEVABLE - YOUR POTENTIAL CHARACTERISTIC*—This column indicates recommended behavioral changes for all the precursors found in Nos. 23 and 24.
28. *RISK FACTOR*—This column lists the risk factors for each precursor assuming the recommended behavioral changes have been made. By decreasing blood pressure from 180/94 to 146/90, John Doe has reduced his risk from 2.2/1.3 to 1.5/1.1.
29. *COMPOSITE RISK FACTOR*—Indicates combination of all the single *new risk* factors after recommended behaviors have been modified. The total of this column indicates the individual's achievable age.

Source: Reprinted with permission from the *Wellness Workbook for Health Professionals,* Copyright 1977, John W. Travis, M.D., published by the Wellness Resource Center, 42 Miller Ave., Mill Valley, CA 94941.

Standard Scores (Z-Score Additive Model)

An important score used in statistical analysis is a Z-score or standard score. It is defined as:

$$Z_j = X_j - \langle X \rangle_{av}/S$$

where: Z_j = the standard score for county j

X_j = the original value for county j. This could be an infant mortality rate, a hypertension death rate, or another specific mortality, morbidity, natality, fertility, or disability rate.

$\langle X \rangle_{av}$ = the average or mean of the death rate(s) for the nation, state, or health agency

S = the standard deviation of the death rate(s) for the nation, state, or health agency

To translate a set of *n* measures into standard scores, first express each value as a deviation from the mean of the distribution, then divide each county deviation by the standard deviation of the distribution. Some of the Z-scores will be negative in sign because some of the scores will be smaller than the mean. These standardized values reflect a distribution with a mean of zero and a standard deviation of one. The Z-score for infant mortality for a county in a health service area thus becomes:

$$Z_{county/HSA} = X_{county/HSA\ infant\ mortality} - \langle X \rangle_{av\ infant\ mortality} / S_{infant\ mortality}$$

$$Z_{county/HSA} = (10.220 - 26.540)/20.360$$

$$Z_{county/USA} = -.802$$

This process is continued in each county of the health service area for as many mortality rates as one wishes to include in the health status index. At this point, the health planner can weight the mortality rates equally or weight the individual mortality rates in terms of the judged importance as derived weights, using known standards. The sets of weighted or unweighted standard scores obtained by this method are then summed in the Z-score additive model as follows:

$$D_j = \sum_{i=1}^{K}$$

where: D_j = the sum of all weighted or unweighted standard scores for each disease for that county (j), giving a health status index value for that county (j)

Z_{ij} = the weighted or unweighted standard score for each disease (i) for that county or health service area (j)

K = the number of diseases used in determining the health status index

The results obtained from this model are expressed as Z-scores. The final results are shown in Table 7-13[17] and Figure 7-3.

Table 7-13 General Index of Black Health Status as Determined by an Unweighted Z-Score Additive Model Ranked by Service Area, 1972

	Rank Order	Service Area	Index Value	
	1	6	1.683	Low Health Status
	2	7	1.047	
	3	2	1.044	
	4	4	.832	
	5	8	.572	
Above State Index	6	17	.331	
	7	22	.328	
	8	9	.303	
	9	5	.285	
	10	3	.239	
	11	1	.228	
	12	21	.197	
	13	15	.103	
	14	16	.058	
STATE INDEX			.000	
	15	11	−.041	
	16	12	−.052	
	17	13	−.094	
Below State Index	18	19	−.220	
	19	20	−.282	
	20	23	−.314	
	21	10	−.396	High Health Status
	22	14	−.565	
	23	18	−.979	

Note: Index value is a standardized Z-score computed for each service area.
Source: Nonwhite Disease Patterns—Black Health Status in Georgia, Health Services Research and Statistics Section, Division of Physical Health, Georgia Department of Human Resources, Atlanta, Georgia, February 1975, p. 20.

Figure 7-3 General Index of Black Health Status as Determined by a Nonweighted Z-Score Additive Model

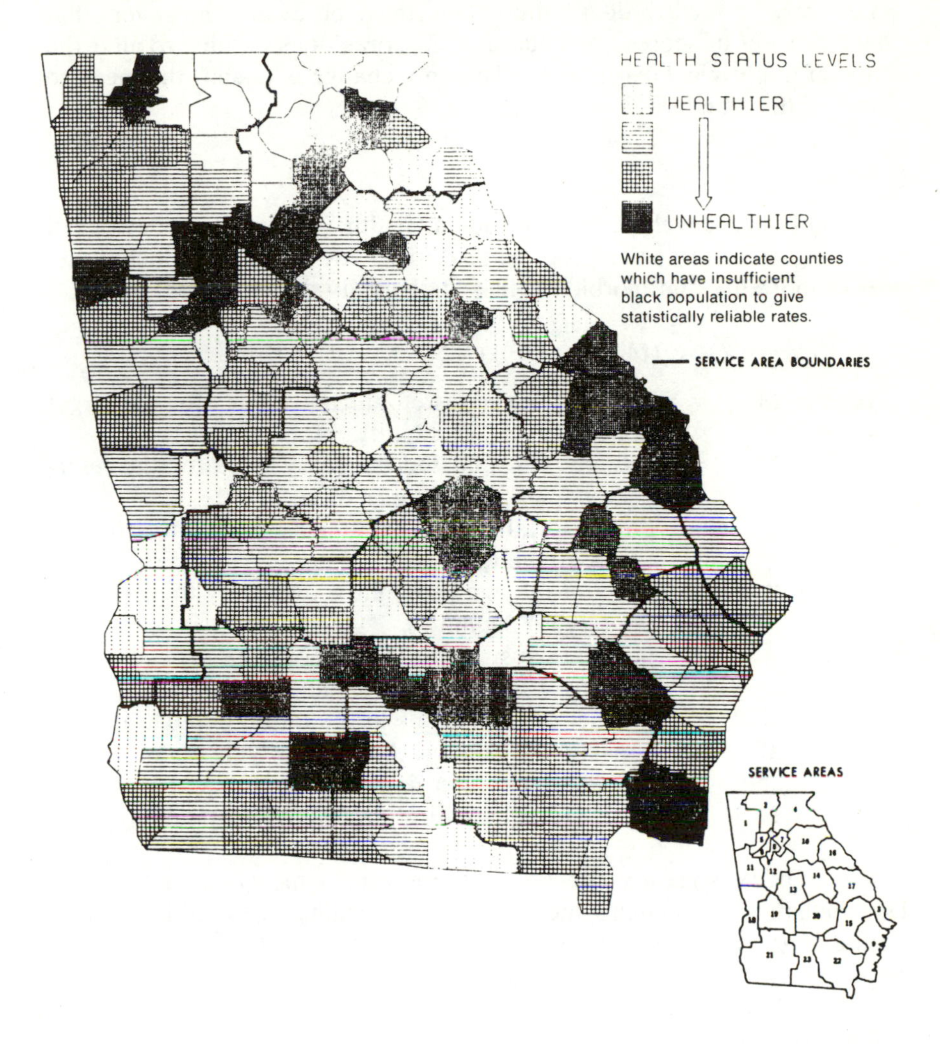

Source: Nonwhite Disease Patterns—Black Health Status in Georgia, Health Services Research and Statistics Section, Division of Physical Health, Georgia Department of Human Resources, Atlanta, Georgia, February 1975, p. 18.

The model is relatively simple and easily applied. It is meaningful in the interpretation and comparison of geographic areas concerning disease, manpower, or facility distribution. One must be aware, however, that changing a set of scores to standard or Z-scores does nothing to alter the shape of the original distribution. The only change is to shift the mean to zero and the standard deviation to one.

Q Index

The Q Index, developed by the Indian Health Service,[18] has been used by management to decide program priorities. The index combines measures of mortality and morbidity. It is statistically defined as follows:

$$Q = [(Mi/Ma)\ (DP)] + (274\ A + 91.3\ B)/N$$

Where:

Mi	=	age- and sex-adjusted mortality rates for the target population (HSA, county, etc.).
Ma	=	age and sex adjusted mortality rates for the reference population (state, nation).
D	=	crude mortality rate (per 100,000 population) for the target population.
P	=	years of life lost using life expectancy to age 65 for the target population.
A	=	hospital days for the target population.
B	=	outpatient visits for the target population.
N	=	number of individuals in the target population
274 and 91.3	=	constants to convert A and B to years per 100,000 population; i.e., three outpatient visits are equated in time to one hospital day.

The Q index is greatly affected by the mortality measures of D and P. Donabedian has shown that the rankings of mortality by D and P are quite similar to the ranking of mortality in the Q index.[19] Thus, the dominant measurement in the Q index is mortality, with the exhibited activity having little influence on the rankings.

Because of these problems, and because HSAs often have difficulty in obtaining data on hospital days and outpatient visits, it is recommended that an alternative form of the Q index be used:

$$Q = (Mi/Ma)\ (DP)$$

One could apply this formula using only age- and sex-adjusted mortality rates for the HSA and the state and using the crude mortality rate plus years of life lost.

When Q is computed by either method for each of the several diseases, the rank order of the most important diseases may be determined. One should be constantly reminded that final program priorities must weigh political and community attitudes. (The G index,[20] although not discussed here, is based on the same rationale as the Q index.)

Life Expectancy and Weighted Life Expectancy

Variation in life expectancy is a result of variation in the relative impact of disease and death. Thus, variation in life expectancy may be used as a measure to demonstrate variation in health status[21] (see Figure 7-4).

Life-expectancy data also may be used as a dependent variable in a regression model to analyze the determinants of health status or to identify areas of need for programs such as urban or rural health initiatives.

A weighted life expectancy is demonstrated in Table 7-14. This is based on a prorated age-specific disability value which may be determined from survey findings. For this reason, it may be difficult for an HSA to apply this index in local-area analysis. The major advantage of a weight value for life expectancy is that it can represent either individuals or populations.

Regression Analysis

Disease variables and their respective values may be subjected to a multiple regression analysis. The purpose of this approach is to determine the interrelationship of the diseases as a measure of the existing health status. In this process, the regression coefficients are used as weights and applied to the Z-score value of all diseases for each of the areas under consideration. The method provides a weighted score for each area:

$$H_j = W_1Z_{1j} + W_2Z_{2j} + \ldots\ldots + W_iZ_{ij}$$

where: H_j = weighted score measuring the relative health status of area j.

W_1 = the regression coefficient or b value used as a weight for the first mortality rate in the equation.

Z_{1j} = the mortality rate for the first disease (1) for the county or HSA (j).

j = notation for a real unit (county, HSA).

W_2Z_{2j} = the weight and mortality rate for the second disease (2) in the county or HSA (j).

The result is a ranked priority score which attempts to evaluate objectively the health status of an area in terms of selected, weighted disease

Figure 7-4 Life Expectancy at Birth, 1970

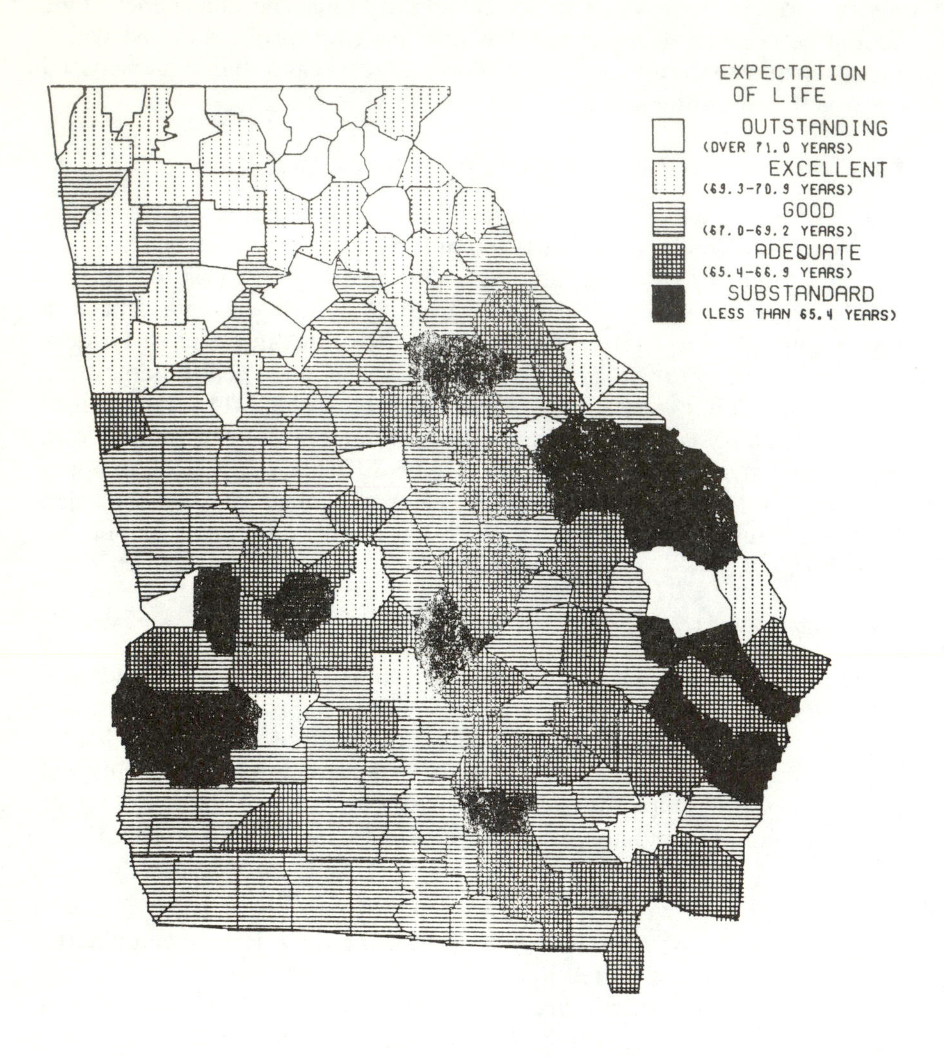

Source: Life Expectancy: Current Trends and Potential Gains, Health Services Research and Statistics Section, Division of Physical Health, Georgia Department of Human Resources, Atlanta, Georgia, January 1976, p. 7.

Table 7-14 Weighted Life Expectancy Table

Ages	Hypothetical Average Value of Life	Weighted Life-Years
0– 4	0.91	3.64
5–14	0.94	9.40
15–24	0.93	9.30
25–44	0.90	18.00
45–64	0.88	17.60
65–74	0.85	8.50
75+	0.80	. . .
		66.44

Note: The total of 66.44 weighted life-years represents the value of life expectancy for an individual with a 75-year life expectancy at birth. It is equivalent to saying that the value of 74 years of life with the average amount of infirmity and disability is roughly equal to 66.44 years of a fully healthy life. Similarly, a life expectancy of, say, 24 years under these circumstances would be equal to (.91 × 4) + (.94 × 10) + (.93 × 10), or 22.34 years of healthy life. This type of weighted life expectancy is based on current experience. That is, life and disability tables are created from the current death and disability rates in given age ranges.

Source: R. L. Berg, "Weighted Life Expectancy as a Health Status Index." Reproduced with permission from *Health Services Research,* Vol. 11, No. 4, p. 335. Copyright 1976 by the Hospital and Educational Trust, 840 N. Lake Shore Drive, Chicago, Illinois 60611.

categories. For example, each of the variables listed in Table 7-15 was subjected to a multiple regression technique to derive appropriate weightings. Life expectancy at birth was used as the dependent variable because it is an accepted indicator of health status. The five independent variables, classified as morbidity/mortality indicators and median household buying power, proved to be significantly related to the dependent variable. To arrive at a weighted measure, the morbidity/mortality measures were transformed into standardized Z-scores, multiplied by their respective weights, and summed. The values were rank-ordered from 1 to 159 (the number of Georgia counties). Thus, for each county, the following morbidity/mortality measure was developed:

$$W_1Z_{1j} + W_2Z_{2j} + W_3Z_{3j} + W_4Z_{4j} + W_5Z_{5j} + W_6Z_{6j}$$

where: W_1 = regression weight for mortality rate (1).
Z_{1j} = standardized Z-score for mortality rate (1), county (j).

Table 7-15 Health-Status Indicators Used in Developing Priority Ranking for a Health-Status Index

Health Index	Independent Variables	Health Status Indicators
MORBIDITY/ MORTALITY	Z_1	Infant mortality, 1970–74
	Z_2	Age-adjusted death rates from motor vehicle accidents, 1970–74
	Z_3	Age-adjusted death rates from acute myocardial infarction, 1970–74
	Z_4	Live birth rates, 1975
	Z_5	Immature birth rates, 1970–74
	Z_6	Median household buying power, 1974

Source: C. M. Plunkett and G. E. A. Dever, Division of Physical Health, Georgia Department of Human Resources, Health Services Research and Statistics, Atlanta, Georgia. Adapted from "Rural Health Initiative," 1977, p. 3.

As an example of the approach used, each county's ranking for morbidity/mortality was derived as follows:

$$[-.2931\ (.726)] + [-.1682\ (-.168)] + [-.1790\ (1.97)]$$
$$+ [-.1788\ (.868)] + [-.2633\ (-.021)] + [.2138\ (-.767)]$$
$$= -.2128 + .0283 \quad -.1915 \quad -.1522 + .0055 \quad -.1640$$
$$= -.6897 \text{ (ranks 27th among 159 counties)}$$

The priority groups one through five were derived by dividing the county ranks into five approximately equal groups of 32 each (31 in group five). Group one represented counties with the highest priorities.

The priority scores represent a quantitative input into the decision-making process for the need and location of primary health care centers. In conjunction with other more subjective criteria, they can provide priorities related to health status.

Factor Analysis

Factor analysis is a statistical technique used to deduce relationships among diseases in such a way that highly interrelated diseases are combined to form a new factor.[22,23] The basic purposes of factor analysis are:

1. to delineate a distinct cluster of interrelated health status data,

2. to group interdependent disease variables into descriptive health status categories, and
3. to provide weightings by dividing health status characteristics into independent sources of variations so that each factor becomes a method for applying weights to the original values of each variable.

The result is a composite index for each observation (health service area, county) on each of the factors.

To map the pattern of variations uncovered by factor analysis, the weights provided by the factor-score coefficient matrix are multiplied by the Z-scores of the original values on each variable. This yields a weighted score for each observation. The model is as follows:

$$H_j = W_1 Z_{1j} + W_2 Z_{2j} + \dots + W_i Z_{ij}$$

where: H_j = the magnitude of the health status indicator in county j for the factor in question.
W_1 = the factor score coefficient (weight) for the first disease (1) of the factor in question.
Z_{1j} = the standard score for the first disease (1) in county j.

The computation of an index using factor analysis is a rather complicated task. However, statistical computer packages employing standard software simplify the actual calculations.[24] Critical aspects of this approach are in satisfying the assumptions of the statistical test and in understanding the significance of the results. Examples of the index's output are demonstrated in Table 7-16 and Figure 7-5.

Mortality Index

In 1951, Yerushalmy introduced the mortality index (MI) as an alternative to techniques which can be unduly influenced by composition and which summarize absolute rather than relative differences in specific rates.[25] For a comparison of schedules of age-specific rates, Yerushalmy proposed a simple unweighted average of ratios which assigns equal weight to the ratio at each year of life and which summarizes the relative difference in weights (Table 7-17).

The MI can be expressed by the formula:

$$MI = \sum \left[n_i (c_i / c_{si}) \right] / \sum n_i$$

where: n_i = the number of years in the ith age interval.
$c_i c_{si}$ = the ratio of specific rates.

Table 7-16 Composite Index of Black Health Status as Determined by Factor Analysis, Factor 2, Ranked by Service Area, 1972

	Rank Order	Service Area	Index Value	
	1	2	2.034	Low
	2	9	.639	Health
Above	3	15	.477	Status
State	4	8	.355	↓
Index	5	17	.272	
	6	21	.265	
	7	7	.182	
	8	22	.098	
STATE INDEX			.000	
	9	13	−.011	
	10	4	−.012	
	11	3	−.015	
	12	6	−.021	
	13	1	−.088	
	14	19	−.115	
	15	12	−.185	
	16	18	−.228	
	17	5	−.239	
Below	18	16	−.254	
State	19	10	−.259	
Index	20	11	−.260	
	21	14	−.284	High
	22	20	−.295	Health
	23	23	−.323	Status

Source: Nonwhite Disease Patterns—Black Health Status in Georgia, Health Services Research and Statistics Section, Division of Physical Health, Georgia Department of Human Resources, Atlanta, Georgia, February 1975, p. 55.

Figure 7-5 Black Health Status in Georgia as Determined by Factor Analysis, Factor 2

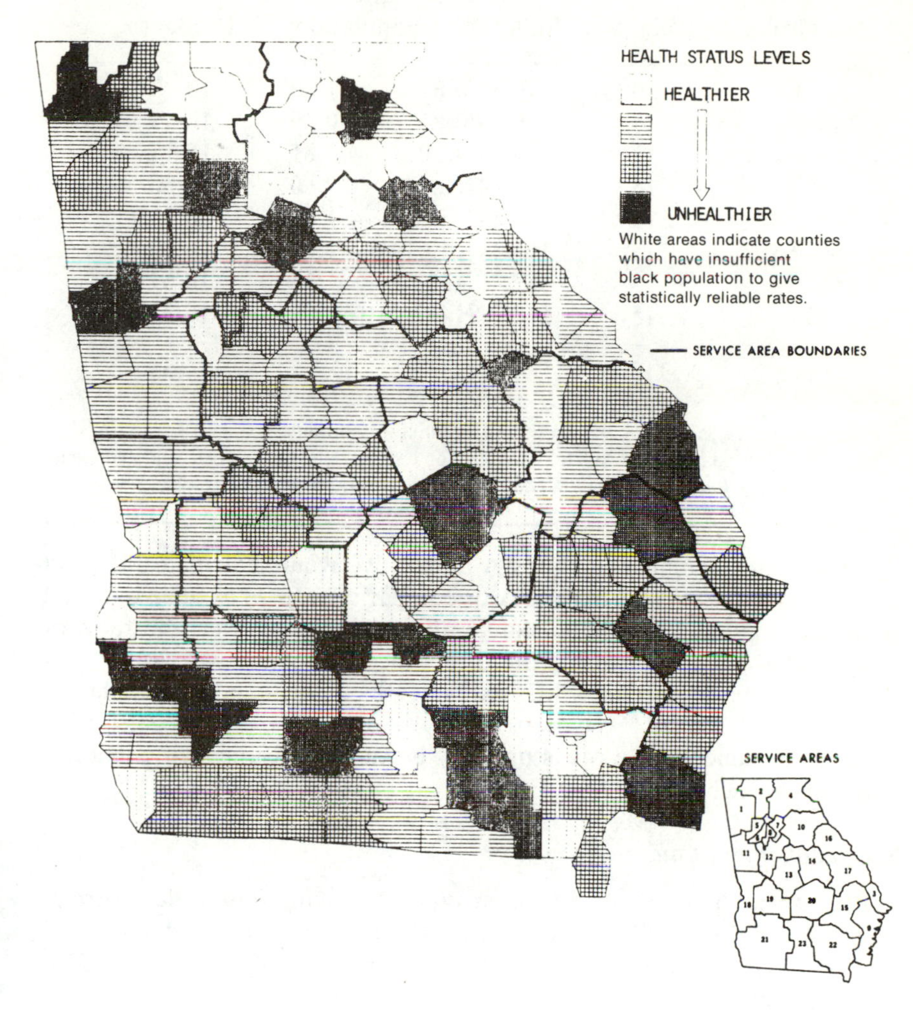

Source: Nonwhite Disease Patterns—Black Health Status in Georgia, Health Services Research and Statistics Section, Division of Physical Health, Georgia Department of Human Resources, Atlanta, Georgia, February 1975, p. 54.

Table 7-17 A Mortality Index Using an Unweighted Average of Ratios

Age Group	Weights	Specific Ratios Male/Total Population		Product
< 10	10	0.81/0.81	= 1.00	10.00
10–24	15	0.59/0.85	= 0.69	10.35
25–34	15	4.54/4.50	= 1.01	15.15
35–44	15	14.81/16.48	= 0.90	13.50
45–54	15	47.11/43.32	= 1.09	16.35
55–64	15	161.11/149.19	= 1.08	16.20
65–74	15	482.49/434.48	= 1.11	16.65
75+	15	1548.37/1417.44	= 1.09	16.35
Sum	115			114.55

Note: MI = 114.55/115 = 0.99: no sex differential in mortality.
Source: J. Yerushalmy, "A Mortality Index for Use in Place of the Age-Adjusted Death Rate," *American Journal of Public Health* 41 (Aug. 1951), pp. 901–908.

If we want to compare Groups A and B, we would calculate MI_A and MI_B and take the ratio as our index of comparison. If we used an external standard population, it would not be difficult to show that the ratio of age-adjusted death rates using the direct method for the two groups has the same form as the ratio of MIs using deaths in the standard population as weights.

Full acceptance of the MI is unlikely because it assumes an equal importance to each year of life.

Socioeconomic Status Index

This index can be applied to mortality rates using rank-order correlation.[26] From the 1980 U.S. Census, data are available on median education, median income, and occupation for each geographical unit. In 1970, these variables were operationally defined as follows:

1. Median education: years of school completed by males and females, 25 years old and over, in 1970.
2. Median income: the median income of families and unrelated individuals in 1970.
3. Occupation: the ratio of employed professional, technical, and kindred workers, managers, and administrators to the total work force in 1970.

Data on education, income, and occupation may be mathematically combined to determine the socioeconomic status index for each geographical unit. The method used to obtain the index score follows the approach used by Nagi and Stockwell[27] and Donabedian et al.[28]

Since education, income, and occupation have different ranges, it is necessary to standardize the three variables (or any others selected) so that all scores are treated with equal weight. If the scores are not standardized, income would carry more weight than education and occupation because it is measured in thousands. In contrast, occupation is measured as a percentage and education in a range of scores from 0 to 16+ school years. Scores may be standardized by the following formula:

$$\text{Standardized score} = (M_v - L_v)/(H_v - L_v) \times 100$$

where: M_v = the individual county score for median education, median income, or occupation.
L_v = the lowest score for the variable being standardized.
H_v = the highest score for the variable being standardized.

An example of standardized scores of three variables for a selected county in Georgia is presented in Table 7-18.The three standardized scores are added together and divided by three to obtain the combined score for a socioeconomic status index for the county. Thus:

$$S_c = (E + I + O)/3$$

where: S_c = socioeconomic status index
E = standardized score for education
I = standardized score for income
O = standardized score for occupation

Therefore, from Table 7-18, the combined score for the socioeconomic status index is:

$$(35.42 + 21.70 + 25.83)/3.00 = 27.65$$

This method may be followed for all county units, with 100 the maximum score and 0 the minimum score.

Rank-Order Correlation Analysis

Spearman's rank-order correlation can be used to test the hypothesis that as the socioeconomic status index of the counties increases, mortality

Table 7-18 Standardizing Scores for a Selected County, Georgia

Variables	Median Scores (M_v)	Highest Scores (H_v)	Lowest Scores (L_v)
Education	9.5 years	12.6 years	7.8 years
Income	$5,284	$12,137	$3,384
Occupation	15.24	34.75	8.45

Variables	Calculations	Standardized Scores
Education (E) =	$\frac{9.5 - 7.8}{12.6 - 7.8} \times 100$	= 35.42
Income (I) =	$\frac{\$ 5,284 - \$3,384}{\$12,137 - \$3,384} \times 100$	= 21.70
Occupation (O) =	$\frac{15.24 - 8.45}{34.74 - 8.45} \times 100$	= 25.82

Source: Socioeconomic Analysis of the Disease Patterns of the 70s, Division of Physical Health, Georgia Department of Human Resources, Health Services Research and Statistics, Atlanta, Georgia, August 1977, pp. 3–4.

rates for those counties also increase, that is, they show a direct corresponding relationship with socioeconomic status.

Spearman's rank-order correlation focuses on the differences (D_i) between paired rankings of two variables (X_i and Y_i). Thus, the equation $D_i = X_i - Y_i$ measures the extent to which the paired rankings of mortality rates and socioeconomic statuses depart from a perfect direct or inverse correlation.

The formula for determining Spearman's rank-order correlation is:

$$r_s = 1 - 6\sum D_i^2/n(n^2 - 1)$$

where: r_s = the r values of Spearman's rank-order correlation
$\sum$ = the sum of

D_i^2 = the difference between the socioeconomic status rankings (X_i) and the mortality rate rankings (Y_i) for the counties, squared. D_i is squared because some of the differences will be negative.

n = the number of observations or counties.

Using Spearman's rank-order correlations, a perfect direct relationship between a mortality rate and socioeconomic status will yield an r_s value of +1, while a perfect inverse relationship will yield an r_s value of −1. The procedure for testing r_s for significance depends on the sample size. The statistic $Z = r_s \sqrt{n-1}$ is computed and compared with appropriate values of the standard normal distribution.

Socioeconomic scores may have to be normalized by transforming the scores to the log 10 to ensure that all scores fall under a normal curve. This computation permits the data falling on the extreme ends of the distribution to be collapsed into a more normal curve. The score results may be divided into five socioeconomic groups (Figure 7-6).

Figure 7-6 Breakdown of Socioeconomic Groups

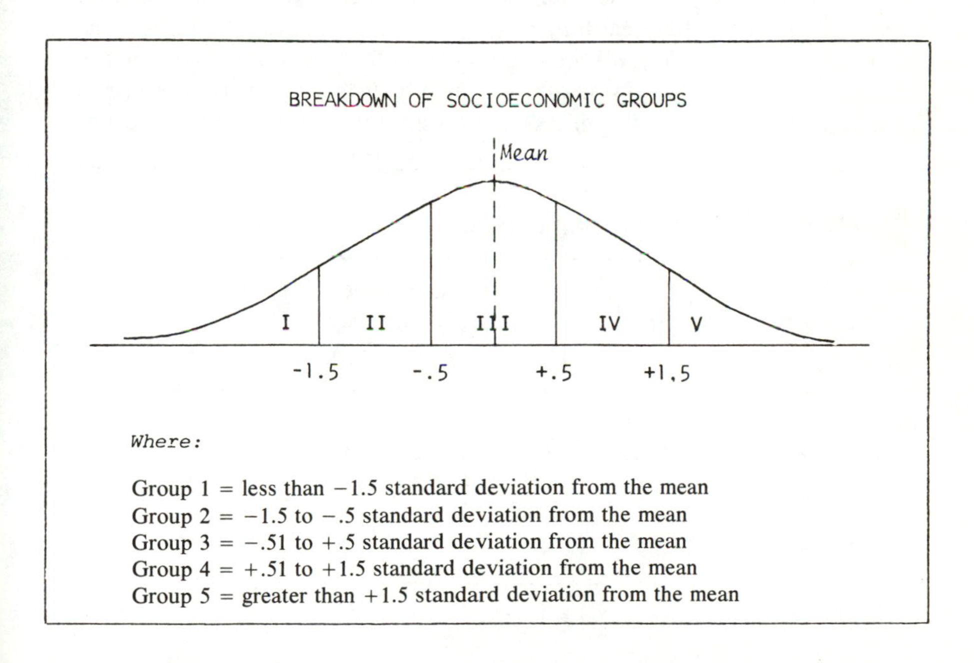

Source: Health Services Research and Statistics, *Socioecomomic Analysis of the Disease Patterns of the '70s,* Series 2, Vol. 4 (Aug. 1977), p. 51.

Table 7-19 characterizes each socioeconomic group in terms of education, income, and occupation. For example, Group 3 has 9.4 median school years completed, a median income of $6,395, and 15.7 percent of its occupations classified as professional.

Table 7-20 indicates that not all of the 11 mortality variables correlated directly with socioeconomic status when analyzed by Spearman's rank-order correlation coefficient. Of the 11 mortality categories, 9 correlated at the .05 level of significance or better. Two of the nine significant mortality variables were direct correlations, as hypothesized: ischemic heart disease and cancer of the trachea, bronchus, and lung. The two causes of mortality showing no significant relationship to socioeconomic status using Spearman's rank-order correlation coefficient were acute myocardial infarction (except for occupation) and other forms of heart disease.

Figure 7-7 shows the results for motor vehicle accidents. Interestingly, a low socioeconomic index is related to this mortality rate for motor vehicle accidents.

Overview

This section has presented ten health-status indexes: (1) the wellness appraisal index, (2) the health hazard appraisal index, (3) standard scores (Z-score additive model), (4) the Q index, (5) life expectancy and weighted life expectancy, (6) regression analysis, (7) factor analysis, (8) the mortality index, (9) the socioeconomic status index, and (10) rank-order correla-

Table 7-19 Socioeconomic Status Index Levels by Variables

Variable	Mean	Socioeconomic Groups				
		1	2	3	4	5
Median Education	9.5	7.9	8.5	9.4	10.3	11.9
Median Income	$6,526	$3,766	$4,038	$6,395	$8,089	$10,035
Occupation (Professional)	15.7	11.4	13.0	15.7	18.9	25.6
SES Score	32.7	14.8	21.1	31.7	45.3	70.1

Source: Socioeconomic Analysis of the Disease Patterns of the '70s, Health Services Research and Statistics, Division of Physical Health, Georgia Department of Human Resources, Atlanta, Georgia, August 1977, p. 9.

Table 7-20 Spearman's Rank-Order Correlation Coefficients of Mean Mortality Rates, Combined Socioeconomic Index, Median Education, Median Income, and Occupation, Georgia, 1969–1972

Mortality Categories	Combined Socioeconomic Status		Median Education		Median Income		Occupation	
	"r" Value	Significance	"r" Value	Significance	"r" Value	Significance	"r" Value	Significance
Total Mortality	−.6203	.001	−.5001	.001	−.7233	.001	−.2561	.001
Other Accidents	−.3630	.001	−.3271	.001	−.4515	.001	−.1590	.05
Motor Vehicle Accidents	−.3250	.001	−.3542	.001	−.2936	.001	−.2326	.01
Infant Mortality	−.2762	.001	−.1772	.05	−.3357	.001	−.1611	.05
Ischemic Heart Disease	.2116	.01	.2424	.01	.1376	NS	.1866	.05
Influenza and Pneumonia	−.1885	.05	−.1917	.05	−.2193	.01	−.0498	NS
Cancer of the Trachea, Bronchus, and Lung	.1812	.05	.1657	.05	.0936	NS	.2189	.01
Cerebrovascular Disease	−.1754	.05	−.1116	NS	−.2472	.01	−.0400	NS
Homicide	−.1581	.05	−.0961	NS	−.2350	.01	−.0292	NS
Acute Myocardial Infarction	−.1461	NS	−.1000	NS	−.1482	NS	−.1615	.05
Other Forms of Heart Disease	.0186	NS	.0066	NS	−.0070	NS	.0457	NS

NS = Not significant.

Source: Socioeconomic Analysis of the Disease Patterns of the 70s, Health Services Research and Statistics, Division of Physical Health, Georgia Department of Human Resources, Atlanta, Georgia, August 1977, p. 10 (slightly modified).

tion analysis. The health planner should be encouraged to use these indexes—some very simple, others very complex—together with the population-based approach to planning to promote sensible planning and index application.

The holistic and wellness approach to health-status analysis will guide a health agency to a conceptual framework and a clearer understanding of what should be included in an index. The basic difficulty in measuring health status stems from the fact that sensitive data have been lacking, not because the methodology by which data are applied is lacking.

Figure 7-7 Mean Death Rate by Socioeconomic Status Group for Motor Vehicle Accidents

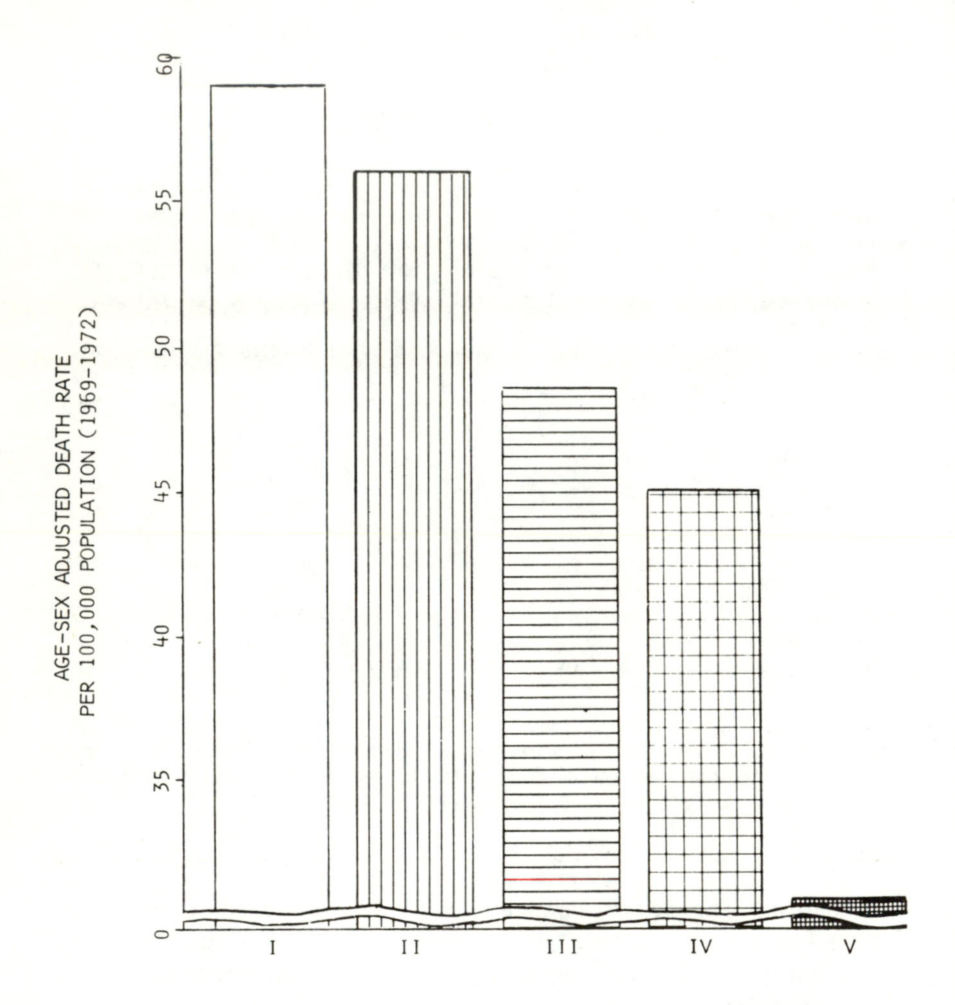

Source: Socioeconomic Analysis of the Disease Patterns of the '70s, Health Services Research and Statistics, Division of Physical Health, Georgia Department of Human Resources, Atlanta, Georgia, August 1977, p. 24.

SUMMARY

Community health-status assessment is of utmost importance and of tremendous value to those who make program decisions. Health-status indicators and indexes are thus crucial to the development and evaluation of health plans. Health planners should determine goals and objectives as a basis for developing indicators and indexes. Data needs and the criteria for selecting a health status indicator or index will suggest the future needs as well as present requirements. The development and application of health-status indicators and indexes can be either a simple or sophisticated process. Whatever the reason for selecting the indicator or index—for monitoring, evaluating, planning, community diagnosis, or any other reason—the approach should be that which is most aligned with the health planner's personal and potential skills. Clearly, the health planner will not be able to apply the indicator or index directly in all cases. The planner is encouraged, however, to use the ideas presented above and, where warranted, to develop them further.

NOTES

1. G. E. Alan Dever, *Considerations in the Measurement of Health Status,* HEW Contract #HRA 232-78-0109 (Houston, Texas: Region VI Center for Urban Research, June 1978), p. 46.
2. Bureau of Health Planning and Resource Development, *Guidelines Concerning the Development of Health Systems Plans and Annual Implementation Plans,* U.S. DHEW (Dec. 23, 1976), p. 22.
3. Ibid., p. 26.
4. U.S. DHEW, "The Conditions of Health and Health Care: Context for Goals and Standards," in *Baselines for Setting Goals and Standards,* HRA 77-640 (January 1977), pp. 47–51.
5. H. L. Blum, *Planning for Health—Development and Application of Social Change Theory* (New York: Human Sciences Press, 1974), p. 622.
6. Ibid., pp. 223–224.
7. National Center for Health Statistics, Clearinghouse on Health Indexes, *Correlated Annotations, Oct. 1973–Dec. 1974,* DHEW Pub. No. (HRA) 76-1225, 1976. NCHS volumes are extremely helpful to anyone involved in the issues of health status measurement. At present, this publication is free, p. 45.
8. J. E. Miller, "Guidelines for Selecting a Health Status Index: Suggested Criteria," in *Health Status Indexes,* R. L. Berg, ed. (Chicago: Hospital Research and Educational Trust, 1972), pp. 243–244.
9. For an excellent discussion on the different levels of measurement, see S. Siegel, *Nonparametric Statistics for the Behavioral Sciences* (New York: McGraw-Hill, 1956), pp. 21–34.
10. Georgia Dept. of Human Resources, Div. of Physical Health, Health Services Research and Statistics, *Infant Health Status, a Quality of Life Analysis,* series 2, vol. 2 (January 1976), p. 37.

11. G. E. A. Dever and M. R. Lavoie, "Data Base—Identification of Needs" in *A Companion to the Life Sciences,* Stacey B. Day, ed. (New York: Van Nostrand Reinhold Co., 1979), pp. 16–19. See also G. B. Hill and J. M. Romeder, "Health Statistics in Canada" (paper presented at the Society for Epidemiological Research, Toronto, Ontario, June 18, 1976), p. 11.
12. D. M. Smith, *The Geography of Social Well-Being in the U.S.: An Introduction to Territorial Social Indicators* (New York: McGraw-Hill, 1973), 144 pp.; K. C. Land and S. Spilerman, *Social Indicators Models* (New York: Russell Sage Foundation, 1975), 411 pp.; Environmental Protection Agency, *The Quality of Life Concept—A Potential New Tool for Decision Makers,* Office of Research and Monitoring, Environmental Studies Division (March 1973), 300 pp.
13. J. C. Kleinman, "Mortality," in *Statistical Notes for Health Planners,* no. 3, National Center for Health Statistics (NCHS) (Feb. 1977), p. 16, and Kleinman, "Infant Mortality," in *Statistical Notes for Health Planners,* no. 2, NCHS (July 1976), p. 14.
14. U.S. DHEW, *A Data Acquisition and Analysis Handbook for Health Planners,* Health Planning Information series no. 4, vol. 1 (Oct. 1976), pp. 142–143; and D. O. Rutstan et al., "Measuring the Quality of Medical Care," *New England Journal of Medicine* 229, no. 11 (March 14, 1974): 603–610.
15. J. W. Travis, M.D., *Wellness Workbook for Health Professionals* (Wellness Resource Center, 42 Miller Ave., Mill Valley, CA), 1977, p. 49.
16. Fulton County Health Department, *Risk Analysis Detection and Reduction (RADAR),* acknowledgments are made to St. Louis and Lake County Health Departments, Minnesota; *Miami Herald,* Feb. 27, 1977; American Heart Association; and "Operation Life Style, Life Style Profile," *Georgia's New Health Outlook* (April 1977), p. 4.
17. Georgia Dept. of Human Resources, Div. of Physical Health, HSRS, *Nonwhite Disease Patterns—Black Health Status in Georgia,* series 2, vol. 1 (February 1975), pp. 18, 20; and Dever et al., *Cripplers and Killers—A Profile of Georgia* (1974), pp. 65–72.
18. J. E. Miller, "An Indicator to Aid Management in Assessing Program Priorities," *Public Health Reports* 85, no. 8 (April 1970): 725–731.
19. Avedis Donabedian, *Aspects of Medical Care Administration: Specifying Requirements for Health Care* (Cambridge, Mass.: Harvard Univ. Press, 1973), p. 649.
20. M. K. Chen, "The G Index for Program Priority," in *Health Status Indexes,* R. L. Berg, ed. (Chicago: Hospital Research and Educational Trust, 1973), pp. 28–39.
21. Georgia Dept. of Human Resources, Div. of Physical Health, HSRS, *Life Expectancy, Current Trends and Potential Gains,* series 2, vol. 3 (January 1976), p. 7; and R. L. Berg, "Weighted Life Expectancy as a Health Status Index," *Health Services Research* (Summer 1975), pp. 153–156.
22. Georgia Dept. of Human Resources, *Disease Patterns,* p. 99.
23. W. L. Hightower, "Development of an Index of Health Utilizing Factor Analysis," *Medical Care* 16, no. 3 (March 1978): 245–255.
24. The most common statistical package is SPSS (Statistical Package for the Social Sciences); BMD (Biomedical) is also usually available. An excellent example of the application of factor analysis to derive an index is in J. C. Maloney, *Social Vulnerability in Indianapolis* (Community Services Council of Metropolitan Indianapolis, Ind., July 1973), p. 53.
25. J. Yerushalmy, "A Mortality Index for Use in Place of the Age-Adjusted Death Rate," *American Journal of Public Health* 41 (August 1951): 901–908. Also, some of the material presented in this section is modified from Course No. 401 of the Applied Statistical Training Institute, Washington, D.C.
26. Georgia Dept. of Human Resources, Div. of Physical Health, Health Services Research and Statistics, *Socioeconomic Analysis of the Disease Patterns of the '70s,* series 2, vol. 4 (August 1977), p. 51.

27. M. H. Nagi and E. G. Stockwell, "Socioeconomic Differences in Mortality by Cause of Death," *Health Services Reports* 88, no. 5 (May 1973): 449–450.
28. Avedis Donabedian et al., "Infant Mortality and Socioeconomic Status in a Metropolitan Community," *Public Health Reports* 80, no. 12 (December 1965): 1083–1094.

Chapter 8

Health Resource Analysis

Recognizing the importance of an expanded concept of epidemiology to include holism and wellness in determining community health status, we must also realize that, at present and also in the future, health must be lived and can only in small part be delivered. It becomes clear, therefore, that the various aspects of the health care delivery system must be analyzed in accordance with the epidemiological model for health planning and analysis.

Federal legislation has mandated the analysis of the health care delivery system in six areas: accessibility, availability, acceptability, quality assurance, cost containment, and continuity. At present, the federal government has placed the most emphasis on cost containment, that is, reduced or controlled hospital costs and physician fees. Within the framework of the federal mandates, the health care delivery system must be examined, with specific emphasis on patient-origin studies and on accessibility, resource analysis, location, and allocation analyses. These areas impose recurring requirements on health systems agencies (HSAs), state health planning and development agencies (SHPDAs), hospitals, and public health departments. Techniques used in each of the six areas will, when applied, facilitate plan development and lead to efficiency in service delivery.

DEFINING PROBLEM AREAS

Various techniques can be applied to the following specific operational problems involving resources, patient-origin, location, allocation, and accessibility:[1]

1. *Defining planning subregions*. What are the appropriate geographic units for developing a community health profile, for analyzing sub-

regional variations in health status and system performance, and for identifying other important characteristics such as demography and social indicators?

2. *Creating new regional capability.* This issue has gained importance in relation to burn-treatment centers, neonatal intensive care units, CAT (computer axial tomography) scanners, radiation therapy units, renal dialysis units, and other expensive services. The questions of best location (accessibility to population) and desired capacity (utilization levels) and the possibility of coordination between HSA and state are relevant here.
3. *Reorganizing services.* Reorganizing services, one of the goals of the federal planning legislation, poses complex questions regarding location and districting, particularly in the emergency medical service area. There planners have been concerned with determining which hospital should provide what level of services for what geographic areas, with assessing the problem of triage of emergency patients involving assignment to the most appropriate treatment site, and with minimizing distance in order to increase ambulance-response time in emergencies.
4. *Reducing duplication of services.* The problem of redundancy has been experienced most acutely in inpatient hospital services, particularly obstetric care because of the declining birth rate and the emphasis on reducing neonatal mortality. Planners have attempted to incorporate considerations of travel time, utilization levels, and consumer preference into decisions to keep facilities in service.
5. *Meeting increasing demands.* Projecting future demands for a health service is a recurring problem in community health planning. When the service has a seemingly unbounded growth potential, as in renal dialysis, the problem is particularly difficult. Facility location and allocation are dependent on forecasts of demand and severity of condition by subregion, as well as on travel time and network considerations.
6. *Reviewing certificate-of-need requests.* The agency decision in this case is a reaction to a proposal rather than a planning initiative. Often, the planning agency will be faced with provider-generated proof, possibly contradicting agency forecasts, of the "community need" for service initiation or expansion. The agency must be prepared to examine the assumption behind the provider's analysis, especially as it relates to demand considerations, subarea analysis, service area definitions, or market-penetration expectations.
7. *Adjudicating competing proposals for the same service or service area.* This is a special project review problem that occurs when a

service need has been previously established and the planner must decide, among other things, which of the two or more proposed locations or services is preferable.

Each of these decision problems requires study, focusing on the definitions of accessibility, facility location and allocation, and delineation of service areas and utilizing patient-origin analysis. Planning for community health care delivery specifically requires the delineation of service areas to reflect either the market penetration of the health service or the consumer's preference for the facility.

DETERMINATION OF HEALTH SERVICE AREAS

The establishment of health service areas is important in determining the market share of patients for hospitals. In many cases, a hospital's market base is necessary to justify its needs in terms of beds, radiation therapy units, CAT scanners, or other special services. The hospital must show from its population base or utilization rate that it has sufficient usage to justify the new service. On the other hand, the health planning agency must determine service areas to meet its planning needs and to justify its decisions to support or reject hospital applications for new services. For these reasons, the health planner must recognize the potentials and limitations of the various methods for determining service areas. Among these methods are the following:

Consumer Surveys

Direct Method

In this method,[2] a consumer is asked, via questionnaire or interview to specify where the health care is obtained. In this type of survey, the health planner should consider the following:

1. Knowledge of survey design, sampling, and sampling errors is required.
2. The method is expensive.
3. Results can indicate potential needs and demands.
4. The method is very similar to the health interview survey.
5. A telephone survey may accomplish similar results.
6. This method's results are similar to those from relevance or commitment indexes.

Indirect Method

The following points should be noted with regard to this method.[3]

1. Hospital patient records can be reviewed to obtain patient-origin information.
2. Specific services (that is, discharge diagnoses) may be used with this method.
3. Specific knowledge of record sampling, time frames, and seasonal variations (adjustments), is required.
4. The method is relatively inexpensive, compared to the direct method.
5. Results reflect demand (morbidity and mortality).
6. Results yield fairly accurate locations.
7. Difficulties may arise when relating patient-origin data with social, economic, and demographic data.
8. For urban areas (Standard Metropolitan Statistical Areas), either census tracts, planning districts, or five-digit zip codes can be used.
9. For rural areas (where census data are available), the county or, in some instances, the enumeration district can be the geographic unit.

The use of the indirect method for analyzing patient-origin data, using five-digit zip codes, is illustrated in a study of 23 acute care, short-term hospitals in the Baltimore, Maryland, area.[4] The service areas were established by distributing the admissions across hospitals in direct proportion to the population of the zip code area. The demographic characteristics of each portion of a postal zone were assumed to be identical with those of the entire zone and were weighted according to the proportion of the zone's admissions to a given hospital's total admissions. For example, if 40 percent of the admissions generated in zip code area 31303 were admissions to Johns Hopkins Hospital, 40 percent of the zip code area's population ($50,000 \times .40 = 20,000$) would be allotted to the Johns Hopkins Hospital market service area. Likewise, if 20 percent of all the admissions to Johns Hopkins Hospital were from zip code area 31303, 20 percent of the characteristics of the hospital's market service area would be derived from the characteristics of zip code area 31303. This would be continued until all zip code areas were allocated. Mutually exclusive market service areas could be determined by assigning each zip code zone to the hospital receiving the highest percentage of its residents as patients. This method can be very useful for determining population-based planning results. It should be noted that the service area is not important in a geographic sense, but only in a population sense. A hospital using this method of apportionment and following stated, related assumptions can determine the total population which it serves and, in accordance with federal guidelines in Section 1501 of P.L. 93-641, can apply population-based standards.

Provider Surveys

In using a provider survey,[5] the following aspects should be considered:

1. The provider is asked to define the service area by listing the communities from which the patients originate.
2. The survey may be administered to the population of providers rather than to a sample of consumers.
3. The provider must estimate the percentage of patient visits coming from the communities listed on a questionnaire.
4. The list of communities should, according to federal guidelines, represent all incorporated places within a specified time distance (30 minutes). Other requirements may also apply.
5. Total patient visits would be recorded.
6. Such a survey involves primarily a rural state approach and would be most difficult to accomplish in an urban area.
7. The following calculations are possible: (1) the number of patient visits each community makes to each provider; (2) the number of patient visits each community makes, with each community having one or more providers; (3) the utilization rates for each community; and (4) overlapping service areas.
8. Complete enumeration is essential. For example, if only one rural provider fails to participate, inaccurate utilization rates will result.
9. Utilization rates can be calculated on the basis of the population of the community and the patient visits from that community.

Determination of Mental Health Catchment Areas

In mental health terminology, "catchment" area rather than "service" area is used to define market penetration. To determine catchment areas, the following assumptions apply:

1. Adoption of a community standard population ranging from 75,000 to 200,000.
2. Easy access to all facilities in the catchment area.
3. Omission of political boundaries.
4. Uniform distribution of mental health problems among all population groups in the catchment area.

5. Application of the catchment area concept can vary. For example, Illinois bases its catchment area on the distance from the mental health hospital, Pennsylvania adheres strictly to county boundaries, while Arizona bases its catchment area on geographic area and distance from the mental health center.

The following considerations relate to the determination of mental health catchment areas:

1. Because census data are based on political boundaries, boundaries of a population-based catchment area are difficult to determine.
2. Population shifts require boundary adjustments.
3. The problem of area definition in sparsely or densely populated places must be solved.

Birth and Death Record Analysis

When using birth and death records for service area determination, the following points should be considered:[6]

1. Information on birth and death certificates indicates place of residence, place of occurrence of the event, and hospital of occurrence, if applicable.
2. Such information identifies movement of patients to hospitals.
3. Service areas may be determined from birth and death records.
4. Birth records provide a most reliable means of justifying obstetrical services.
5. Birth records also provide crude estimates of demographic characteristics of the population (mothers).
6. Although they can provide estimates of patient movement, death certificates are obviously less reliable in providing a complete picture for service area analysis.
7. Information from birth and death records may have to be combined with a survey.
8. Given time constraints, birth and death record analysis may be the most appropriate method for the first year of the program.

Hierarchical Structuring (Population Threshold)

This method is based on population levels. The following aspects should be noted:

1. The minimum population required for providing categorical services to effectively support a specific resource must be determined.

2. The method provides services which are delivered within a hierarchical structure.
3. Primary, secondary, and tertiary services require a minimum population before they can be supplied.
4. An important variable is the minimum or the maximum distance people are willing to travel for the service.

Combining population and distance with administrative characteristics results in a functional/spatial organization of health services.[7] Examples include the functional/spatial organization of health care in the U.S.S.R. (Figure 8-1), in Sweden (Figure 8-2), and in England and Wales (Figure 8-3).[8] A domestic application for Rhode Island is shown in Table 8-1.[9] In addition, Table 8-2 provides a guide demonstrating the population base necessary to provide health services of various types.[10]

Figure 8-1 Spatial/Functional Organization of Health Care in the U.S.S.R.

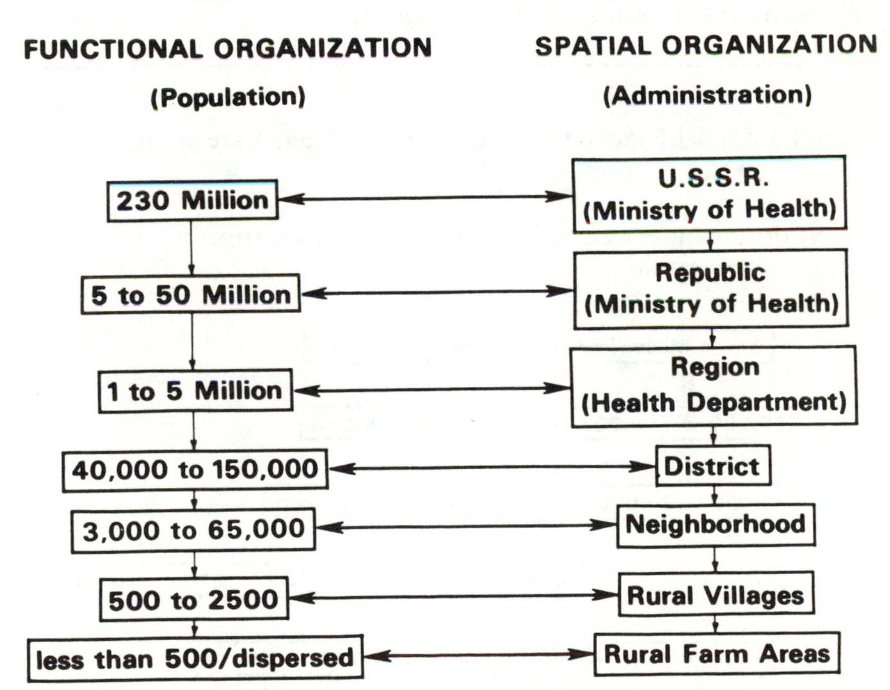

Source: G. W. Shannon and G. E. Alan Dever, *Health Care Delivery—Spatial Perspectives* (New York: McGraw-Hill Book Co., 1974), p. 15.

Figure 8-2 Spatial/Functional Organization of Health Care in Sweden

FUNCTIONAL ORGANIZATION (Population) **SPATIAL ORGANIZATION**

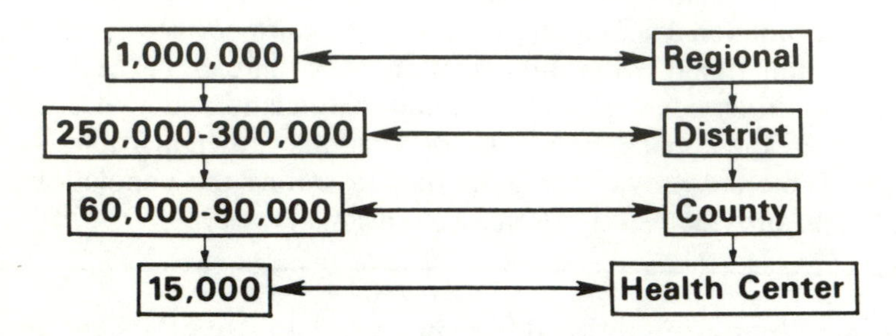

Source: G. W. Shannon and G. E. Alan Dever, *Health Care Delivery—Spatial Perspectives* (New York: McGraw-Hill Book Co., 1974), p. 20.

Figure 8-3 Spatial/Functional Organization of Health Care in England and Wales

FUNCTIONAL ORGANIZATION (Population) **SPATIAL ORGANIZATION**

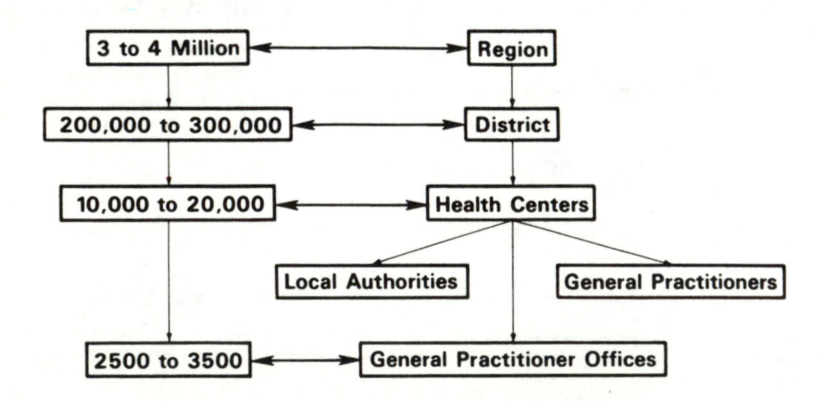

Source: G. W. Shannon and G. E. Alan Dever, *Health Care Delivery—Spatial Perspectives* (New York: McGraw-Hill Book Co., 1974), p. 20.

Table 8-1 Criteria for Delineating Health Service Planning Subarea Boundaries

1. A set of health service planning subareas (HSPSs) includes primary, secondary, and tertiary areas.
2. Primary HSPSs should have a minimum population of 30,000. Secondary HSPSs should have a minimum population of 100,000. Tertiary HSP areas should have a minimum population of greater than 1,000,000. Exceptions may be made in cases where a geographical (e.g., mountains, poor roads, water) or an economic barrier exists or where extreme isolation pertains.
3. HSPSs should conform to a hierarchical distribution in space, i.e., primary HSPSs should be nested within secondary HSPSs, which in turn should be nested within tertiary HSP areas.
4. At any one level (i.e., primary, secondary, or tertiary) HSPSs should be mutually exclusive. Mutually exclusive HSPSs should cover the whole population of the state.
5. Service area boundaries should be contiguous with (i.e., they should not violate) city or town boundaries and with human service district boundaries. Regional or area planning groups or advisory councils should also be reflected in HSPS designation.
6. HSPSs should reflect to some extent current utilization patterns as well as existing roads, transportation systems, and geographical barriers.

Source: Rhode Island Dept. of Health, "Proposed Health Services Planning Subareas for Rhode Island," Health Planning and Resources Development, Tech. Report No. 7, March 1977, p. 30.

Hierarchical structuring has the following advantages: It requires minimum data (population, sometimes distance); it is easily understood; it involves a minimum of analysis; and it establishes service areas based on what should be rather than what exists. Its disadvantages include the fact that utilization patterns (that is, behavioral considerations) are ignored and that no attempt is made to deal with accessibility (travel time and distance).

Poland-Lembcke method

This method[11] has been widely used. The following issues are pertinent:

1. Patient-origin data are required.

Table 8-2 Survey of Minimum Population Bases for Tertiary Health Services

Service(s)	Population Base	Source of Suggested Population Base
Swedish Regional Hospital	1,000,000	Arthur Engel, *Perspectives in Health Planning* (London: The Athlone Press, 1968), pp. 75–76. Services provided include plastic surgery, thoracic surgery, and neurosurgery.
Level III (High Risk) Perinatal Center	670,000–1,000,000	Committee on Perinatal Health, *Toward Improving the Outcome of Pregnancy: Recommendations for the Regional Development of Maternal and Perinatal Health Services* (White Plains, N.Y.: The National Foundation—March of Dimes, 1976) p. 1. The population base is derived from the recommended regional number of births (8,000–12,000) and an assumption of a birth rate of 11.9 births per 1,000 population (the 1975 birth rate in Rhode Island). New Jersey and Wisconsin have adopted the midpoint (10,000 births) of the Committee's range as a standard.
Comprehensive Hemophilia Care Center	6,000,000	World Federation of Hemophilia standard quoted in: Petit and Klein, *Hemophilia, Hemophiliacs, and the Health Care Delivery System* (National Heart and Lung Institute, 1975) p. 51.
	2,000,000	Health Plan Development Services, New Jersey Department of Health, *Proposed Standards and General Criteria for the Planning and Certificate of Need for Regional Hemophilia Care Centers,* 1976, p. 8.
Renal Transplant Center	1,500,000	Division of Health Policy and Planning, State of Wisconsin, *Planning Standards for End Stage Renal Disease Kidney Transplantation and Dialysis* (Madison, Wisconsin, 1976) p. 3.
	750,000	DHEW minimum cited in: Michigan Department of Public Health, *Minimal*

Table 8-2 continued

Service(s)	Population Base	Source of Suggested Population Base
		Criteria and Guidelines for Kidney Transplantation Services (Lansing, Michigan, March, 1972) p. 17.
	2,000,000	Roger Platt, "Planning for Dialysis and Transplantation Facilities, *Medical Care* (May–June, 1973) p. 209.
	2,000,000	Kidney Advisory Committee, "Optimal Criteria for End-Stage Renal Disease Care," *Journal of the American Medical Association* 226 (October 1, 1973) p. 47.
End-Stage Renal Disease Network	3,500,000	Social Security Administration, Department of Health, Education and Welfare, "End-stage Renal Disease Conditions for Coverage," *Federal Register,* Volume 40 (July 1, 1975), Washington, D.C., p. 27786. The proposed ESRD network would include at least two transplant centers to allow for patient choice and sufficient peer review.
Burn Center	4,500,000	Division of Health Policy and Planning, State of Wisconsin, *Planning Standards for Burn Centers* (Madison, Wisconsin, 1975) p. 3.
CAT Scanning	465,000	Health Planning and Resources Development, Rhode Island Department of Health, *The Acquisition and Use of Computer Assisted Tomography in Rhode Island* (January, 1976) p. 14. Prepared for RIDH by Health Planning Council, Inc., this report proposes there to be an initial need for two CAT scanning units in Rhode Island.

Source: "Proposed Health Planning Subareas for Rhode Island," Rhode Island Department of Health, Health Planning and Resources Development, Technical Report Number 7, March 1977, pp. 45–46.

2. Postal addresses are allocated to geographic units (townships or minor civil divisions) to match rural census data.
3. Determinations are made manually in rural areas.
4. Metropolitan areas may use ADMATCH or UNIMATCH in association with DIME (see the Chapter on Computer Graphics).

From the patient-origin study, data on admissions to each geographic unit are used to calculate the percentage of admissions to each hospital. The following possibilities may result:

1. If 50 percent or more of the admissions from one geographic unit are to one hospital, the geographic unit is in the service area.
2. If less than 50 percent of the admissions are not to one hospital, the geographic unit is not in the service area.
3. If several hospitals draw large proportions from the geographic unit but none gets 50 percent or more, the service area line passes through the geographic area.
4. No admissions are from the geographic unit.

Given these possibilities, the following rules for setting boundaries apply:

1. There must be one continuous service area boundary line which cannot cross another line.
2. The geographic unit in which the hospital is located is, with rare exceptions, assigned to the hospital.
3. Drawing service area lines through the geographic unit is a matter of judgment. If a population center exists in a township, the line should be drawn through the center to indicate it is not clearly in the hospital's service area.

Relevance and Commitment Indexes

By far the most popular, relevance and commitment indexes are probably the easiest to apply because they are based on patient-origin data, they reflect behavioral and distance components, and they are based on the premise of a gravity model (to be illustrated in a subsequent method).

Relevance and commitment indexes have also been labeled resident dependency (RD), provider dependency (PD), or market penetration (MP).

The following steps are required to create relevance and commitment indexes:

1. Formulate a matrix of admissions to each hospital by geographic unit, as in Table 8-3.
2. Compute relevance index (RI):

$$RI = \frac{\text{Tract A}^{\text{Adm}}}{\text{Total Tract Adm.}}$$

$$RI = \frac{\text{Admissions from Tract A to Hospital 3}}{\text{Total Admissions to All Hospitals from Tract A}}$$

$$RI = \frac{TA^{A}}{TA} = \frac{30}{100} = .30 \times 100 = 30\%$$

The relevance Index for Tract A to Hospital 3 is 30 percent, representing the percentage of total admissions from Tract A which go to the study hospital (Hospital 3). The complete set of RIs show the tendency of each tract to use the study hospitals.

3. Compute the commitment index (CI):

$$CI = \frac{\text{Tract A}^{\text{Adm}}}{\text{Total Hospital}^{\text{Adm}}}$$

$$CI = \frac{\text{Admissions from Tract A to Hospital 3}}{\text{Total Hospital Admissions from All Tracts}}$$

$$CI = \frac{TA^{\text{Adm}}}{\text{Total Hosp.}^{\text{Adm}}} = \frac{30}{70} = .43 \times 100 = 43\%$$

Commitment Index for Hospital 3 to Tract A is 43 percent, representing the percentage of total hospital admissions (Hospital 3) from Tract A.

4. Identify tracts by various levels of relevance to identify service areas (Figure 8-4).
5. The service area population for the study hospital can be determined by multiplying the population of each tract by the RI for that tract. For example:

Tract population	= 20,000
RI	= 30%
Service area population for Hospital 3	= 20,000 × .30 = 6,000 people

Table 8-3 Matrix of Admissions to Hospitals

Tract \ Hospital	1	2	3	4	5	6	Total per Tract
A	10	20	30	10	20	10	100
B			10				
C			10				
D			0				
E			20				
Total per Hospital			70				Total Admissions

Source: Modified from P. Reeves, Applied Statistic Training Institute, Executive Series IV, Myrtle Beach, South Carolina, December 1978, p. 16.

SERVICE AREA DELINEATION

The Three-Tiered System

An approach used in Ontario, Canada, uses patient-origin information and the concept of hierarchical structuring or, as it is called in Ontario, the three-tiered system.[12] Relevance and commitment indexes are calculated, and these in turn are related to the community, district, and regional centers. Service areas for each hospital center are then delineated on the basis of this three-tiered system. Thus, while a community center is surrounded only by a community service, the regional center is surrounded by all three areas. The three tiers are defined as follows:

1. Community centers, usually containing hospitals with less than 100 beds, handle maternity cases, less complicated medical cases, and surgical cases of a relatively minor nature.
2. District centers, generally containing hospitals with 100 to 500 beds can render more complicated care because of their more specialized staff and facilities. These centers supply their own needs on the community level and also accept some referral cases from nearby community hospitals.

Figure 8-4 Hospital Service Area, Clinton Regional, by Patient Origin and Time/Distance Accessibility

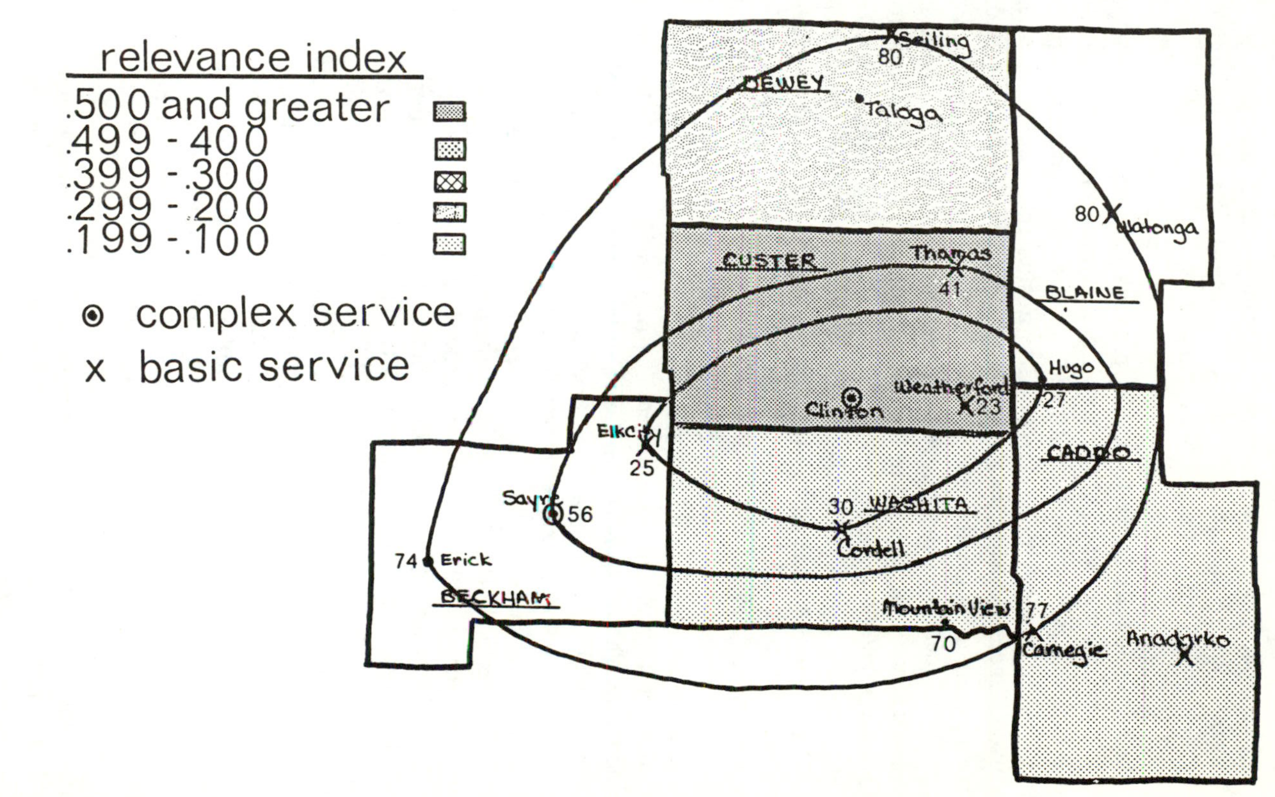

Source: Facilities and Service Task Force Report, Oklahoma Health Systems Agency, April 1979, p. 11.

3. Regional centers are usually university teaching centers. Hospitals in these centers are equipped and staffed to provide very specialized treatment, such as heart surgery, brain surgery, and cancer clinic work and are thereby able to accept cases referred from both community and district hospital centers.

The admission-discharge forms for patients discharged from hospitals are of primary importance in the above delineation. From information on these forms, it is possible to learn the origin and destination of patients being moved, the present referral pattern, and the volume of patients involved. Each township area (that is, the municipal township and the urban communities located within each) is considered individually. Population is allocated on three levels to the hospital centers serving each township area, in proportion to the actual patterns of use; the total township area population is assigned to each of the three levels.

The Ontario experience indicates that, in general, 80 percent of the total active-treatment needs can be provided on the community level, with the remaining 20 percent divided equally between the district and regional levels. The normal planning standard of five beds per 1,000 population designated for active-treatment care (excluding active psychiatric cases) is therefore divided into a community component of four beds per 1,000 and district and regional components of one-half bed per 1,000 for each component. The overall standard of five beds is based on 1,550 days of care per 1,000, and on an assumed occupancy rate of 85 percent. If the population of any area utilizes hospital facilities at a rate higher than this, the demand for beds will be greater than the number indicated as necessary when normal planning standards are used.

Tables 8-4, 8-5, and 8-6 show the delineation of hospital service areas in three sample township areas. In each table, the hospital centers to which township area cases go are listed at left. The number of township residents separated from each center are listed in the first column as a percentage of total township separations. Adjacent columns show, in parentheses, the unadjusted percentages and, without parentheses, the percentages related to the regional, district, and community levels of care. In each instance, the percentage not accounted for on one level is transferred to the next, since regional centers are able to provide care on the district and community levels as well as the regional, and district centers can provide care on both community and district levels. For example, in Township Area 1, Regional Center A provides district as well as regional care, while District Center B provides community as well as district care. Table 8-7 presents the extent of service areas, population service, and beds needed in Regional Center A.

Table 8-4 Delineation of Hospital Service Areas, Township Area 1, Population 15,000

Hospital Centre		% of Total Twp. Separations	Regional Level %	District Level %	Community Level %
Regional	Centre A	12.0	(10.0) 100	(2.0) 20	
District	Centre B	12.8		(8.0) 80	(4.8) 6
Community	Centre C	24.8			(24.8) 31
Community	Centre D	50.4			(50.4) 63
Township Total		100.0	(10.0) 100	(10.0) 100	(80.0) 100

Source: Modified from a letter from Dr. Frank Houser, District Health Officer, Georgia Department of Human Resources, Dalton, Georgia, 1978.

Table 8-5 Delineation of Hospital Service Areas, Township Area 2, Population 20,000

Hospital Centre		% of Total Twp. Separations	Regional Level %	District Level %	Community Level %
Regional	Centre A	10.0	(10.0) 100		
District	Centre B	26.0		(10.0) 100	(16.0) 20
Community	Centre C	33.6			(33.6) 42
Community	Centre D	30.4			(30.4) 38
Township Total		100.0	(10.0) 100	(10.0) 100	(80.0) 100

Source: Modified from a letter from Dr. Frank Houser, District Health Officer, Georgia Department of Human Resources, Dalton, Georgia, 1978.

Because it has been found that more care is required by those in the older age categories, modifications are made in the active standards to take into account the age structure of the population of the specific hospital service area under consideration. Thus, the five beds per 1,000 have been subdivided, based on experience in the province as a whole, to show the number of beds per 1,000 population which are required for each age group. Bed standards per 1,000 population increase as the general age level of the population increases (for ages 0–14, 2.6 beds per 1,000 population; for ages 65 and over, 14.7 beds per 1,000 population). These "age refined" standards are then applied to the particular age composition of the service area under study. In an area where the population is relatively

Table 8-6 Delineation of Hospital Service Areas, Township Area 3, Population 25,000

Hospital Centre		% of Total Twp. Separations	Regional Level %		District Level %		Community Level %	
Regional	Centre A	30.5	(5.0)	50	(25.5)	31	(22.4)	28
Regional	Centre E	5.0	(5.0)	50				
District	Centre B	54.9			(54.9)	69	(48.0)	60
Community	Centre C	6.4					(6.4)	8
Community	Centre D	3.2					(3.2)	4
Township Total		100.0	(10.0)	100	(80.4)	100	(80.0)	100

Source: Modified from a letter from Dr. Frank Houser, District Health Officer, Georgia Department of Human Resources, Dalton, Georgia, 1978.

Table 8-7 Extent of Service Areas, Population Served, and Beds Needed in Regional Centre A

Township Area	%	Regional Population	%	District Population	%	Community Population
I	100	15,000	20	3,000	—	—
II	100	20,000	—	—	—	—
III	50	12,500	31	7,750	28	7,000
Total Population		47,500		10,750		7,000
Active Standard		0.5/1000		0.5/1000		4.0/1000
Active Bed Needs		23.75		5.38		28.00

Total active need, excluding psychiatric—57.13 beds.

Source: Modified from a letter from Dr. Frank Houser, District Health Officer, Georgia Department of Human Resources, Dalton, Georgia, 1978.

much older than the provincial average, more beds are required when needs are weighted to age; where the population is younger, fewer beds are needed.

The flexibility of this system must be emphasized. Since service areas are delineated according to actual use, they may vary with changing conditions. The opening of a new hospital, the addition of a new wing, an expansion to provide a greater range of services—all may contribute to produce a shift in service areas. For example, allowance is made for hospital centers situated at provincial boundary points to take into account the needs of out-of-province residents who regularly use hospital facilities in Ontario. If Ontario residents indicate that they prefer to go to hospitals located outside the province, the population of the local hospital service area is reduced.

Flexibility is important in another way as well. If a district center provides more than the usual district level services, allowance is made for this through the allocation of some regional level beds to the district center, in proportion to actual patterns of use.

The Nearest Neighbor (Proximal) System

This is probably the simplest way to define a service area.[13] It is based simply on the nearest place that has the medical service being analyzed. In this system, area boundaries do not reflect patient behavior in seeking health care. The geographic unit utilized will be dependent on population density: A high-density population will use a small unit; a low-density population will use a larger unit, probably a county. With this method, distances to all surrounding places are calculated, and the area is assigned to the nearest place having the service. Other measures which may be computed are the average and the maximum distances between people and the service if data are available for small geographic units (townships, enumeration districts). A computation of this sort would include these steps:

1. Calculate the distance from the center of each area to its nearest service.
2. Multiply by the area's population.
3. Sum the result for each area unit in the service area.
4. Divide the total by the total population of the service area.

If only those communities having a particular health care resource are known, proximal areas may be determined graphically, using either of two procedures:

Procedure 1. Construct perpendicular bisectors between two adjacent points having the resource and assign the region to the closest point. The result is a series of "theisson polygons" (see Figure 8-5).

Procedure 2. Use cartesian *(X, Y)* coordinates and calculate the distance from consumers to various resource centers. Assign consumers to their closest resource center. The population is assigned in proportion to area served (usually determined by grid squares or planimeters).

Figure 8-5 Graphic Delineation of Service Areas

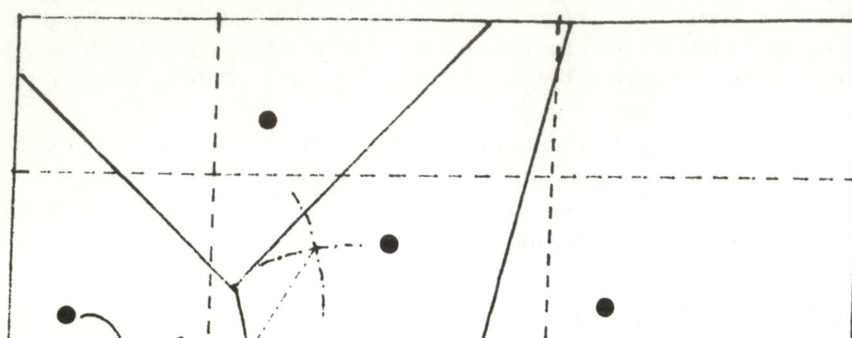

Source: Meneley et al., *Methodologies for Delimiting Health Service Areas,* Iowa City, Iowa, Health Services Research Center, University of Iowa, January 1977, p. 3.

Gravity Models

The primary use of gravity models[14] to determine service areas has been in rural areas; there has been only limited application to urban areas. The major hypothesis of the gravity model is that the interaction between two places is directly proportional to the mass of the two places and inversely proportional to the distance between the two places. Thus:

$$I_{ij} = P_i \, P_j / D_{ij}^{b}$$

where:
- I_{ij} = the interaction between two places (i and j)
- P_i = mass of city i
- P_j = mass of city j
- D_{ij} = distance between two places (i and j)
- b = empirically estimated exponent

With basic modifications, the gravity or interaction model may be changed to:

$$P_{ij} = (A_j^{s}/D_{ij}^{b}) / \sum_{j=1}^{m} A_i^{s}/D_{ij}^{b}$$

where: P_{ij} = the probability that a person in the ith area will use services in the jth place (this is equivalent to the proportion of people in the ith area who will be in the service of the jth place).

i = 1, 2, ... n (areas for which demographic data exist: enumeration districts, townships, counties).

j = 1, 2, ... m (area where health services exist, or hospitals, beds, occupancy rates, or some other attraction force).

A_j = attraction of health resources at the jth place.

D_{ij} = distance from the ith to the jth place.

b = function of distance for utility of place.

s = the rate of increase in attraction of place j with an increase in health resources.

The above equation is used to compute expected probabilities of the use of a given center by each geographic unit in the local area. The size and shape of the service area depends on three factors: (1) the health resources (quantity) at the center and at other competing centers around the tributary area, (2) the attraction influence of additional health resources, and (3) the effect of distance as a deterrent factor.

Patient-Origin Studies

Many of the methods used to delineate hospital service areas are based on patient-origin studies. The following describes some of the advantages and disadvantages of such studies.

1. *Advantages*

   a. The patient-origin study is a reasonable way to gather data about the existing medical market.
   b. Data can be used to make location and allocation decisions (informally using maps and charts and estimating the most logical locations and patterns).
   c. Indexes derived from patient-origin studies can be incorporated into formal decisions (rules).
   d. Data can be used as input to more sophisticated problems of location or allocation.
   e. Areas based on actual flow of medical trade will be identified; that is, the association between location of supply of medical services and the demand for them.

f. Ratios of resource to population will reflect more accurately the existence of shortages or surpluses since they will be based on actual demand for services by the population at risk.
g. Given sufficient data resources, areas can be developed for different types of diagnostic categories (service specific).
h. Planning of facilities can be based on known characteristics of the population being served.
i. A rationale can be developed for determining an adequate mix of services needed in an area, based on patient commuting behavior patterns.

2. *Disadvantages*
   a. Patient-origin studies are not equally useful for all kinds of health services or communities.
   b. In general, tertiary and specialized types of care (not geographically constrained as with primary care) lend themselves to this approach.
   c. Data for dense inner cities are less meaningful than data for communities of "average" population density.
   d. The approach is not suitable for providers who serve populations not geographically contained (HMO members).
   e. Distortion in demand for services may appear because of the absence of resources in a particular area, causing the need to go elsewhere.
   f. Social, psychological, and economic dimensions of seeking health care may divert demand out of local area.
   g. Selected population groups (nonusers of services) may be omitted from data used to determine areas.
   h. The necessary data resources depicting community patterns may be more difficult to obtain on a uniform basis.
   i. Other data resources, for example, sociodemographic characteristics, may not be available in desired geographic units.
   j. Problems may occur because of lack of congruence with other planning areas based solely on geopolitical boundaries.

No single method, of course, can be applied perfectly to all hospital service areas. The planner must make an informed choice and clarify for decisionmakers assumptions about each method. Within this context, the mechanics of a patient-origin study are quite important. A good patient-origin study includes several steps and should involve several members of a team. Also, patient-origin data must be updated as shifts occur in the population and as people change their patterns of seeking care. Physicians' affiliations and locations will also contribute to changing patterns.

Steps to Complete a Patient-Origin Study

Selection of the Data Elements of Interest. The geographic identifiers used to describe patient residence must be delineated at an early stage. Frequently used geocodes include county, zip, municipality, and census tract. It is often desirable to collect multiple geocoded data at different levels of aggregation or, if one wants cross-checks on the geocoding, at the same level of aggregation. The patient-origin study is often used to collect other related information, such as patient's age and sex, length of inpatient stay, and mode of payment. These additional elements should be defined and justified early in the study.

Selection of the Mode of Capturing Data. Preferably, data should be captured in "real time" from all providers in the area. In inpatient studies, data questionnaires should be completed upon discharge for all inpatients discharged during the sample period. Similarly, in the case of ambulatory services, data questionnaires should be completed upon discharge for all outpatients and emergency patients treated during the sample period.

Determination of Sampling Method and Sample Size. The most statistically valid method of patient sampling is with the simple random sample. Other commonly used sampling methods are cluster and systematic sampling. The differing effects of these sampling techniques, that is, how they affect the reliability of the results, should be considered before the survey starts. Equally important is the question of sample size, which determines the probable error range in the resulting data. It may be desirable to consult a statistical expert on these issues so that data gathered during the patient-origin study will be as statistically valid as possible, given cost and other constraints.

Design of Data Questionnaires. Data questionnaires should be designed to make them easy to complete and to manipulate in the data processing task that follows. If the data are to be tabulated manually, keypunched, and then processed through automated means, the requirements for the data questionnaire design will be quite different from those needed if the data are to be read on optical scanning equipment.

Design of Administrative Procedures for Management of the Survey Process. It is important to have well-defined procedures for securing and managing the flow of data from the completion of the survey form through the data processing stage, particularly in a project collecting data on a large scale. Potential problems in data collection and processing should be defined at an early stage, refined through discussion with others who have conducted similar surveys, and further refined in the study pretest. Written procedures are necessary, not only to assure the efficient flow of survey forms during the study, but also to assure that the data collection forms are completed in a consistent manner and that questions arising during the data collection process are answered in a consistent manner.

Securing Provider Cooperation and Orienting Participants. Providers must be informed at an early stage about the survey to be conducted. Provider cooperation must be secured to assure complete survey coverage. The active participation of the local hospital council in survey design and study development can also facilitate this task. Once their cooperation has been secured, the providers should be fully oriented as to the nature of the study to be conducted, their role in data collection, and their individual and cooperative benefits from the study. The latter is particularly important in patient-origin studies conducted by planning agencies. The providers must realize the study is being conducted not only to aid the regional planners but also to help the providers reach a better understanding of their relationships to their particular communities and to each other (thus facilitating their individual market analyses).

Pretest Data Collection Method. Even with careful presurvey planning, it is imperative that the data collection scheme be pretested with a limited number of providers. This will confirm the feasibility of the method as designed and act as an aid in identifying weaknesses in the surveying instruments and accompanying administrative procedures. The results of the pretest should be used to redesign survey instruments and alter administrative procedures to increase the probability of a successful survey.

Processing and Storing of Information. The scale of the study and the type of processing system employed will dictate the requirements for processing and storage. If automated data processing is used, computer programs should be written before the survey begins. Arrangements for keypunching or optical scanning must also be made at an early point. Data processing procedures and contracts should be completed at the time data are ready to be keypunched or scanned; the processing should not be delayed by inadequate preparation. The mode of storage—whether on hard copy, punched cards, optical scan forms, or magnetic tape—should also be defined prior to the receipt of completed data forms.

Design and Generation of Output Reports. At the time that the data elements are identified, the basic output reports desired from the study should begin to take shape. If fundamental output needs are described at an early point, the computer programming necessary in an automated data processing system for the production of output reports can be completed before data capture. The computer programs can then be pretested, revised, and readied for report production when the data processing is complete. Information from at least the basic descriptive output reports should be made available for use by providers and planners as soon as possible.[15]

Summary

The patient-origin study is a useful tool to gather data about patient-to-provider flow patterns, thus helping the health planner to conceptualize the health care delivery system for a geographic area. The study can also be used to gather data tangential to the basic purpose of the patient-origin study, thus providing a cost-effective way to generate data valuable for other health planning or research purposes.

ACCESSIBILITY ANALYSIS

Standards and Guidelines

Increased accessibility to health services is a major consideration for most health advocates. Public Law 93-641 suggests guidelines and standards in planning for health services which may be adjusted in terms of accessibility. The standards are both mandatory and discretionary. Discretionary adjustments, in turn, may be generic or standard-specific. The major generic adjustment which can be made in applying national standards (but only if relevant situations cannot be avoided through standard-specific or mandatory adjustments) would result in the denial of access by area residents to necessary health services. Generic adjustments may also significantly increase costs of care for a substantial number of patients in the area and deny care to persons with special needs stemming from moral and ethical values. Such adjustments must be supported by detailed analysis and justification.

Many variables can justify standard-specific adjustments: time and distance to service (accessibility), seasonal changes in use of service, high-risk areas, geographic remoteness (accessibility), and age of the population (see Table 8-8). Standard-specific adjustments must be based on analysis. The level of analysis will depend upon the adjustment proposed. At the very least, however, the agency must: (1) determine the data required for analysis, (2) retrieve such data, (3) analyze and interpret the data, and (4) produce a justifiable base of the results. As indicated by the federal guidelines, it is apparent that, on the one hand, accessibility is a very important factor in the determination of an adequate number of

Table 8-8 Standard-Specific Adjustments

Category	Standard	Basis for Adjustments	Criterion, If Any
General hospital beds	4 beds/1000 population	Age	Persons over 65 constitute more than 12% of population
		Seasonal population fluctuations	"Large" seasonal variations
		Rural areas	"Reasonable" access time
		Urban areas	Variations within an SMSA
		Referral hospitals	Beds utilized by referral patients residing outside area
	80% occupancy	Seasonal population fluctuations	"Large" seasonal variations
		Rural areas	"Normal fluctuations" in admissions
Obstetrical services	Regional planning	None	None
	1500 births per year in level II and level III units	Varying range of service	None
		Moral and ethical preference	None
	75% occupancy in units with greater than 1500 births/year	None	None
Neonatal units	Regional planning	None	None
	4 beds/1000 live births	High rate of high risk pregnancy	None
	15 beds/level II or III units	Travel time	None
Pediatric services	20 beds/unit in urbanized area	Travel time	More than 30 minutes for 10% or more of the population
	Occupancy rates by unit size	None	None
Open heart surgery	200 procedures per year in adult units	None	None
	100 procedures	None	None

Table 8-8 continued

Category	Standard	Basis for Adjustments	Criterion, If Any
	per year in pediatric units		
	Minimum operating levels prior to opening new units	None	None
Cardiac catheter-ization	300 procedures per year in adult units	None	None
	150 procedures per year in pediatric units	None	None
	No new units in facilities not performing open heart surgery	None	None
	No new adult units unless existing units have 500 procedures per year	None	None
Radiation therapy	300 cases per year in an area with 150,000 population	Geographic remoteness	None
	No new units unless existing units performing 6000 treatments per year	Geographic remoteness	None
CT Scanners	2500 medically-necessary procedures per year operating goal	Multi-scanner installations	Average of 2500 scans/machine
		Clinical trials	None
		Specialized applications	Seriously sick or pediatric patients
	No new scanners unless existing scanners are operating at 2500 per year levels	Same as above	Same as above

Source: Application of the *National Guidelines for Health Planning* and *Application and Adjustment Procedures Manual,* Midwest Center for Health Planning, September 1978, p. 4.

facilities, but that, on the other hand, attempts must also be made to contain health care costs. The methodology presented here can aid health planners in dealing with the factors of accessibility, availability, and cost of the health care system.

Because accessibility is one of the major factors in health care, it makes sense to analyze the relationship between time and distance to the service, the type of facility and service, and the population served. The primary goals are to minimize the travel time or distance to the health service and to maximize the proportion of the population to be served by the facility. During project review, health planners are faced with the basic question, Is there a need for a new facility or service, such as radiation therapy units, CAT scanners, or obstetrical service?

In a completely interactive system, accessibility analysis is critical to the analysis of bed needs. The analysis outlined below can show that a new service or facility may not be required because travel time and distance are not changed and the population to be served is not increased. The results have cost implications; the advantages of developing a new service or facility do not change either accessibility or availability. In this case, by rejecting the new proposal, costs are kept under control.

Steps in Accessibility Analysis[16]

First, a base map of the area to be analyzed must be digitized. Digitizing is done for every link in the transportation network, that is, distance is determined between each population center and is weighted according to the type of road. For example, a major four-lane highway is assumed to have a value of one, with 55 miles equaling one hour of travel time. Another possible approach is to use the Department of Transportation's time zones which are generated from a small sampling of the distance links traveled to determine the approximate travel time. From the sample, all distances are assigned time values. The correlation between the two methods is so high that either will give quite accurate results. The result is a time/distance matrix which can be used to calculate average accessibility to the service.

Second, population data are required for every town or city that is coded or given a time/distance value. Towns of less than 2,500 population are assigned to a central point in the county.

Third, the facility data must be assigned to one of the many towns in the network. Thus, if 26 CAT scanners are needed, they would be assigned to their respective 26 locations. In this step, urban areas should be analyzed separately from the state analysis.

Fourth, because of the potential for travel by individuals outside the state for service, buffer zones outside or surrounding the state or area being analyzed must be determined, based on the above three steps.

Finally, an algorithm is used to calculate the shortest distance from each town (or node) to the town (or node) that has the service being analyzed. These distance values may be summed for the entire county. The result is a value representing average accessibility in the county to the service being analyzed. The procedure can be done for each census tract or other geographic unit where population data are available.

Graphing Analytical Output

The output from the above analysis (Figures 8-6 and 8-7) shows in graphic and tabular form the following: (1) average accessibility, by county, to each service or trade area defined by accessibility limits (which can be specified by the user); (2) unserved nodes (that is, those towns beyond the specified maximum distance); (3) node assignment and distance (for example, Node 1, population 2,134, is assigned to Node 173, population 37,331, which is the nearest node in terms of time/distance); (4) spatial arrangement of each node to the closest service center (allowing one to define trade areas for the service being analyzed); (5) cumulative proportions reflecting the proportion of population being served with each increment of time/distance to the service for the first, second, third, and fourth nearest locations. (See Figures 8-8 and 8-9.)

These results may be updated using new population estimates, and the process may be repeated when an agency is asked to review an application for a new service at a new location. For instance, a new map or graph can give the project review officer information showing that the requested service increase does nothing to increase accessibility positively or to serve a greater proportion of the population. If these two objectives have not been attained, the new service location would increase medical care costs without improving accessibility or availability. Thus, the trade-off between a new facility or service on the one hand and accessibility and availability on the other can be made quite clear.

Trade-Off Analysis

Eaton and others suggest that in a trade-off analysis of a set of objectives one can describe how much of one objective must be sacrificed to achieve given values of other objectives.[17] Such an analysis produces trade-off curves that can be very helpful to a project review office. The trade-off curve is a statement of the change in the rate at which one

Figure 8-6 Accessibility to Oklahoma Hospitals Providing CAT Scanner Services

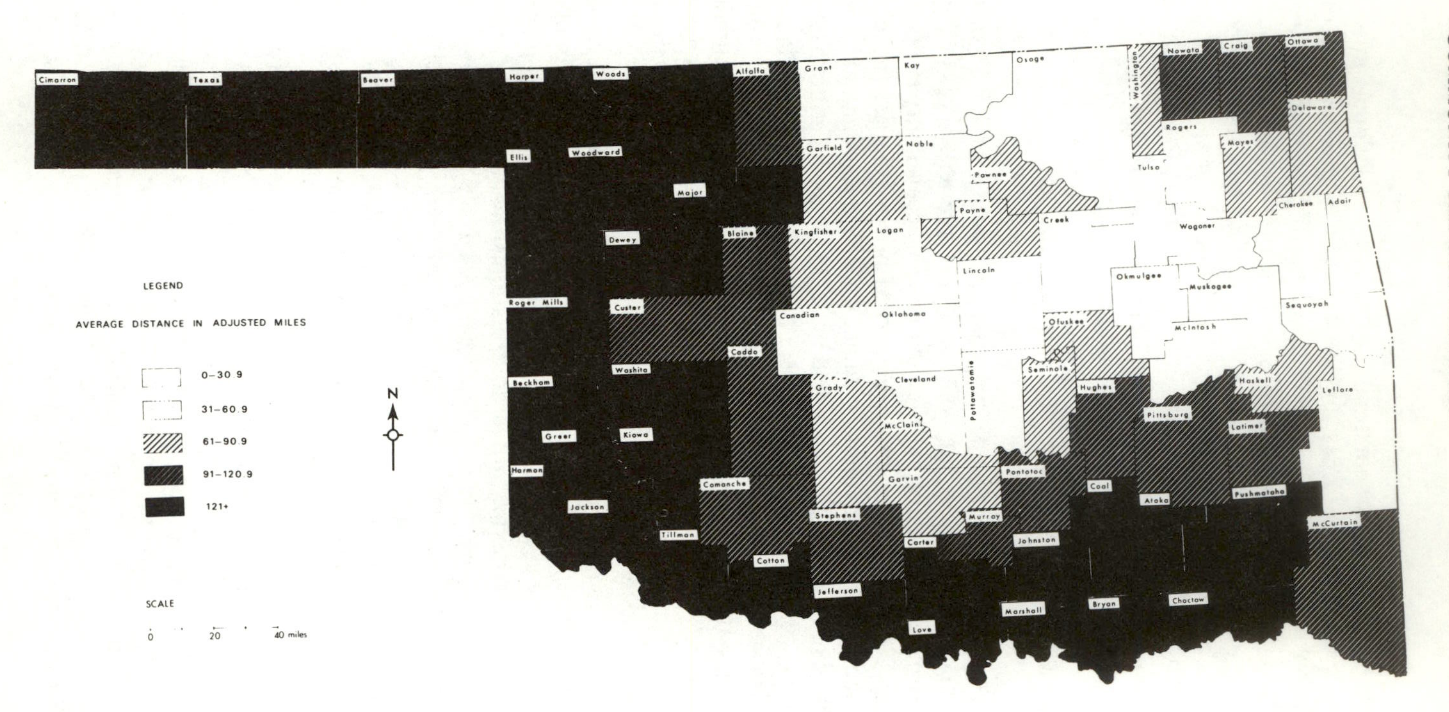

Source: Oklahoma Health Systems Agency, Health Services Analysis, Inc., Atlanta, Georgia, Health Services Research Center, Iowa, 1978.

Figure 8-7 Accessibility to Oklahoma Hospitals Providing Radiation Therapy

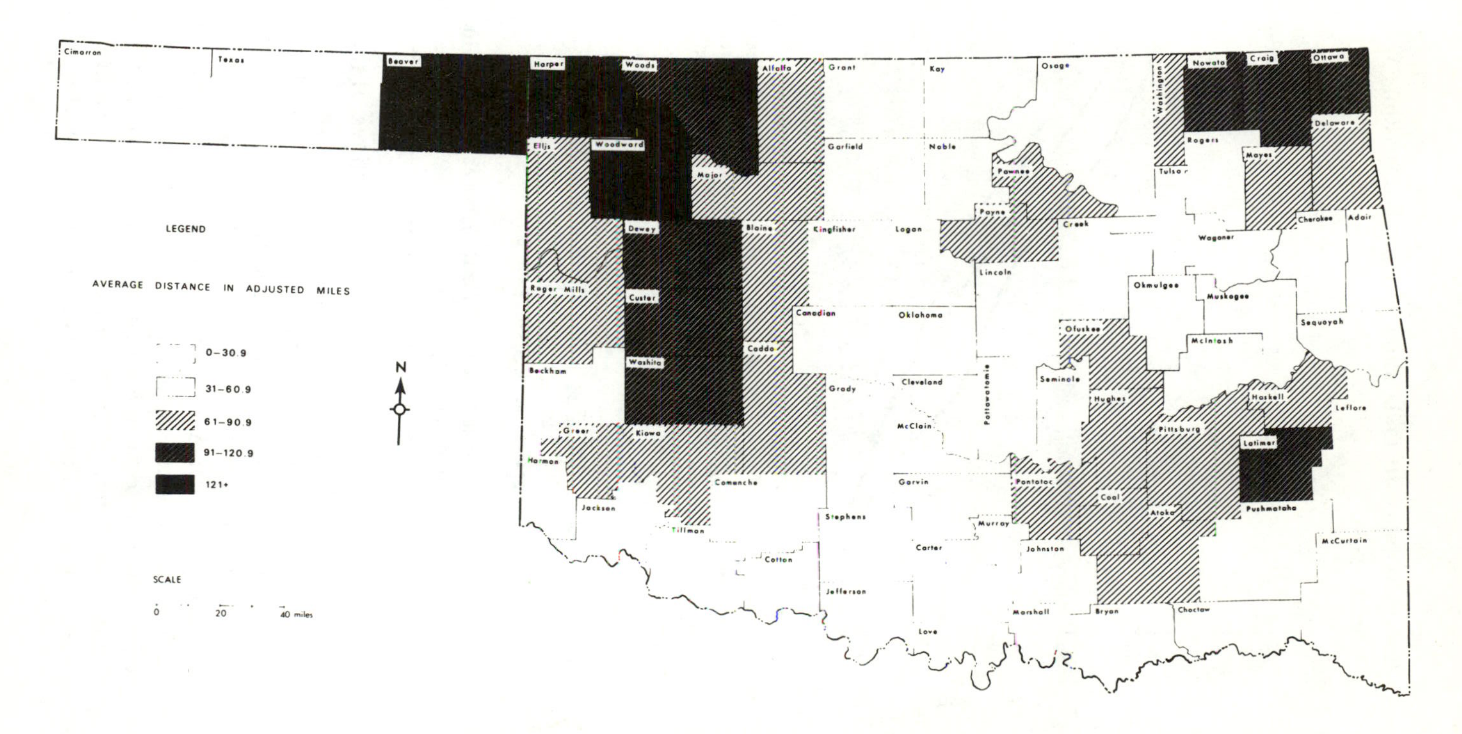

Source: Oklahoma Health Systems Agency, Health Services Analysis, Inc., Atlanta, Georgia, Health Services Research Center, Iowa, 1978.

Figure 8-8 Accessibility to Oklahoma Hospitals Providing CT Scanner Services

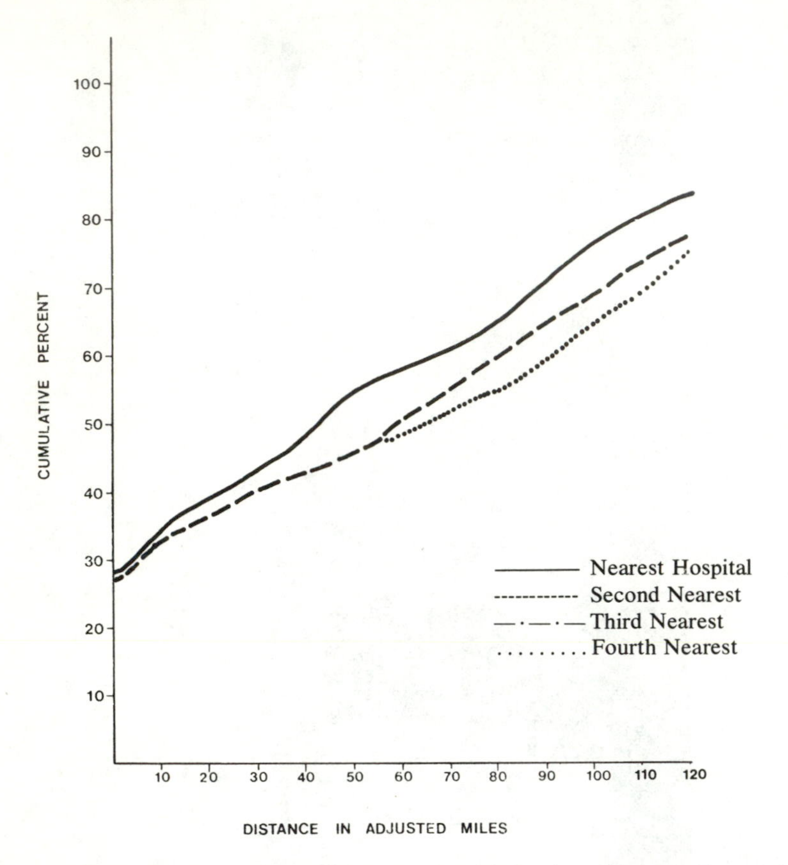

Source: Oklahoma Health Systems Agency, Health Services Analysis, Inc., Atlanta, Georgia, Health Services Research Center, Iowa, 1978.

objective is improved at the expense of other objectives. If there are two objectives, the trade-off function appears as a curve. In Figure 8-10, the trade-off is between accessibility (time/distance) and availability (number of facilities). Accessibility may be defined as the proportion of the population served within a time/distance constraint (the graph gives a value of two hours, that is, S = 2). Availability may be defined as the maximum number of facilities/services needed to achieve the access. For instance, one objective might be to have enough facilities to provide 90 percent of the population access within 120 minutes. From the curve in Figure 8-10, it can be seen that 12 facilities can cover 100 percent of the population in

Figure 8-9 Accessibility to Oklahoma Hospitals Providing Radiation Therapy

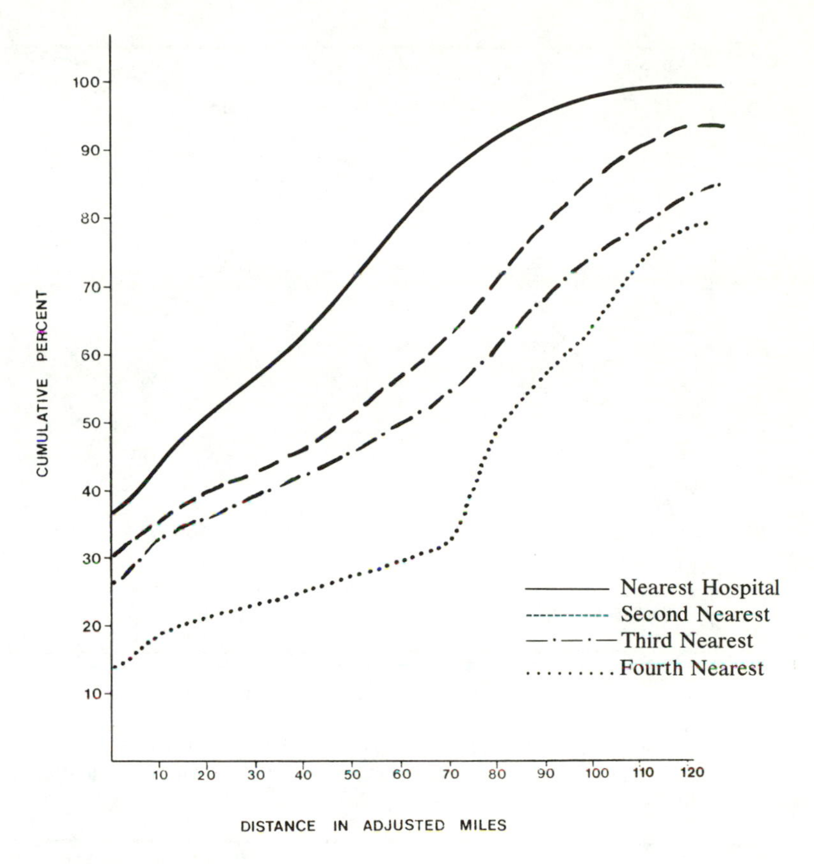

Source: Oklahoma Health Systems Agency, Health Services Analysis, Inc., Atlanta, Georgia, Health Services Research Center, Iowa, 1978.

120 minutes, while one facility can serve only about 30 percent of the population. Thus, a trade-off occurs between accessibility and availability.

The trade-off curve shows that point A is not feasible and that point B is inferior to some other point on the curve, such as C. Consequently, only points on the curve represent plausible policy alternatives. The curve makes explicit the implication of any course and, therefore, can help one to arrive at a decision. For instance, by adding one facility to the existing two facilities, accessibility increases from 46 to 57 percent or 11 percent. The first increases in population covered are less costly than later in-

Figure 8-10 A Trade-Off Curve Between Accessibility and Number of Facilities

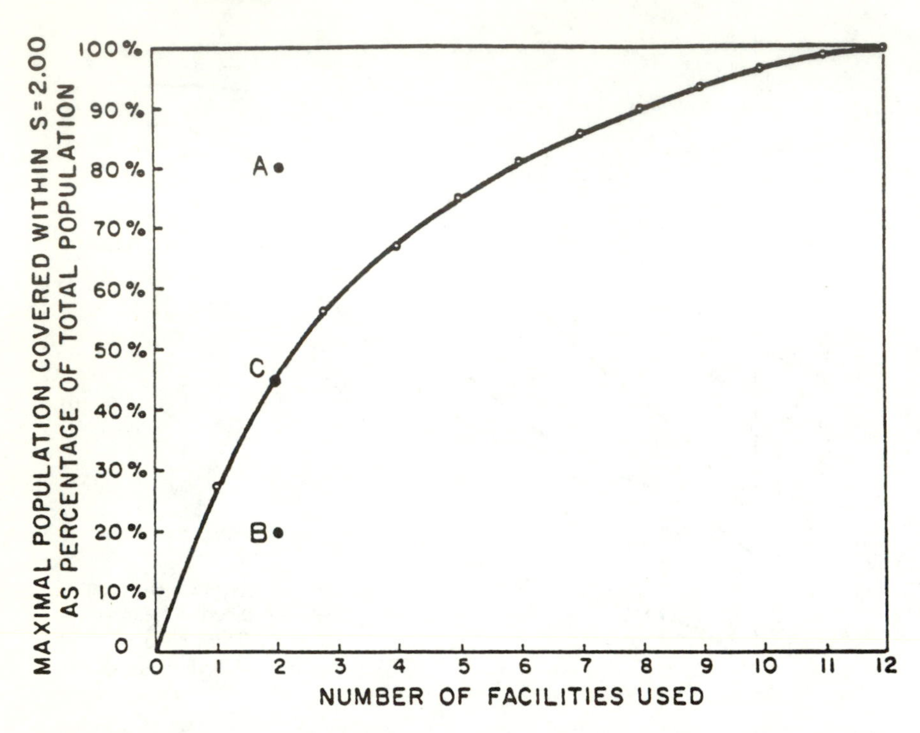

Source: D. Eaton, R. Church, and C. Revelle, "Location Analysis: A New Tool for Health Planners," Agency for International Development (A.I.D.), Washington, D.C. (mimeo), No. 53, May 1977, p. 5.

creases, that is, an increase from 11 to 12 facilities increases the gain only 2 percent (98 percent to 100 percent). The planner and policy analyst thus can gain insight about the cost-effectiveness of establishing a new facility or service.

Figure 8-8 (accessibility to CAT scanners) represents 10 facilities with CAT scanners. From the figure we can determine that 10 facilities within 120 minutes travel time serve about 80 percent of the population. A new location for a CAT scanner would increase the number of facilities to 11. If the accessibility were reanalyzed with the additional CAT scanner, we would be able to determine what percentage changes would occur in the population served and the time/distance to the service. Several runs of the analysis at various locations could aid in determining what locations would have the most cost benefits to the population.

Rushton et al. have produced a series of trade-off curves showing the effect of adding new centers for primary medical care (Figure 8-11).[18] The results suggest that after 20 minutes travel time, the options for centers range from 64 to 101 sites. Over 90 percent of the population is served by each service plan; after this point the increase is minimal (the curves flatten out). Clearly, to satisfy the two objectives, it would be best to choose the 64 sites to control the rising health care costs.

Although only the rudiments of trade-off analysis are presented here, the methodology can become quite complex so as to include alternative plans, sites, facilities, and services based on patient behavior, health resource index (required if a new service can only be located where services presently exist), and an accessibility index. The interplay of these factors results in compromise plans by trading off the accessibility index with the resource index. The results of the accessibility analysis and the trade-off function analysis may determine reasonable standard-specific adjustments based on accessibility, efficiency, and level of care.

HOSPITAL PLANNING

Demand-Based Planning

The prediction of future bed needs is based on current levels and trends in service utilization. The disaggregation of data can be very detailed but still not increase the precision of the estimate. Factors such as age, sex, and type of service may have to be separated out for a more specific analysis. An illustration of the use of demand-based methodology is given by McClure:

> As a simple example, suppose a community of 50,000 population currently uses 1400 patient days per 1000 population. Current "demand" is then (50,000 persons × 1400 days per 1000 persons) or 70,000 patient days. Now further suppose that the population is growing 1% per year and the use rate is increasing 0.2% per year (these are approximately national average growth rates). In five years, the population will increase 5% and the utilization rate by 1%. Then future demand in five years can be projected as (50,000 × 105%) × (1400 days per 1000 persons × 101%) or 74,235 patient days. If we apply an average occupancy factor, utilization can be converted to bed needs. Suppose current occupancy is 75%, and it is desired to increase

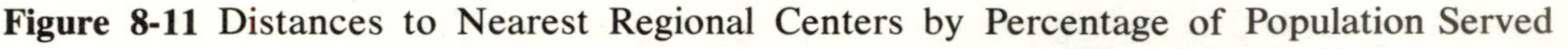

Figure 8-11 Distances to Nearest Regional Centers by Percentage of Population Served

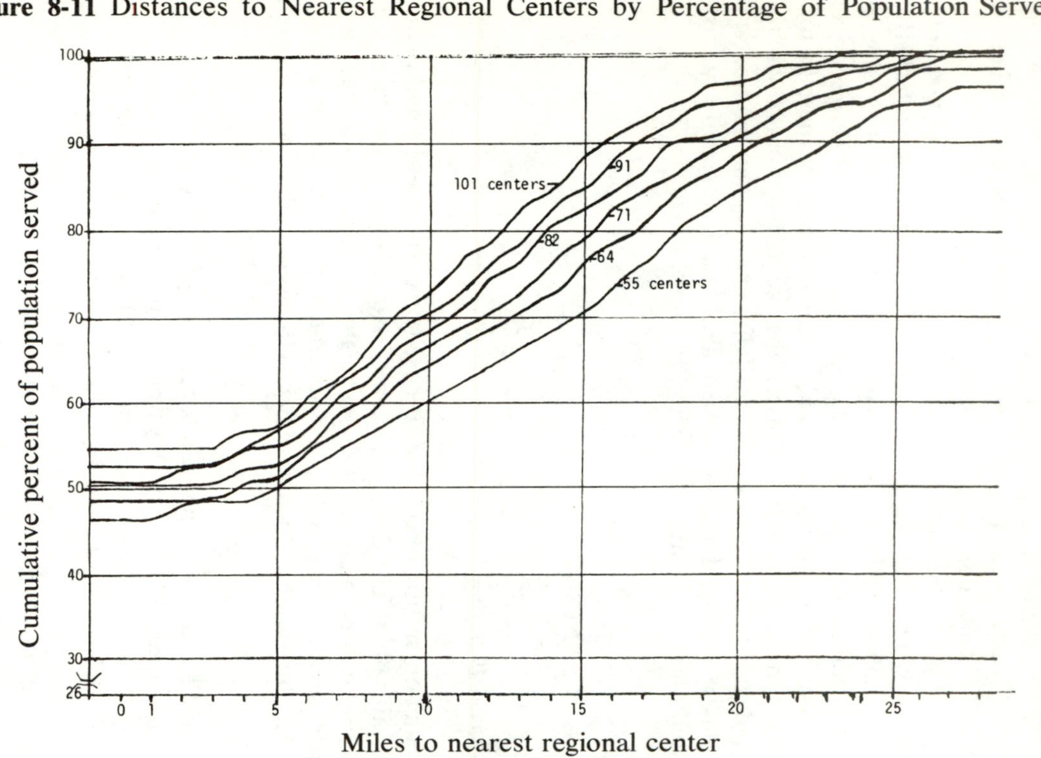

Source: G. Rushton et al., *A Statewide Plan for Regional Primary Medical and Dental Care Centers in Iowa*. Institute for Urban and Regional Research and Health Services Research Center, University of Iowa, Iowa City, Iowa, August 1976, p. 53.

> occupancy to 77% in five years. The current bed supply is given by (70,000 patient days ÷ by 365 days per year ÷ 75% occupancy) or 256 beds. This is a bed rate of (256 ÷ 50,000 persons) or 5.1 beds per 1000 persons. Similarly, the future bed need is (74,235 patient days ÷ 365 days per year ÷ 77% occupancy) or 264 beds. This would be a bed rate of (264 beds ÷ 52,500 persons) or 5.03 beds per 1000 persons. According to this simple demand-based method then, this community with a current bed rate of 5.1 beds per 1000 persons would need eight new beds in five years.[19]

McClure also notes that a review of the literature on demand-based planning reflects four approaches or models: formula models, regression models, stochastic approaches, and simulation. His position is that demand-based planning is self-fulfilling and inflationary and that planning should shift toward a population-based approach, requiring population-based data systems as well as training and improved methods for planners.

Population-Based Planning

Population-based planning is a major tenet of PL 93-641. Basically, one sets objectives or goals reflecting a population-based rate, that is, the rate is expressed using a population figure as the denominator. Population-based planning proceeds on the assumption that need is determined by health status and demography and that these population characteristics may be translated into general standards for utilization and capacity rates (that is, four beds per 1,000 population).[20] The purpose is to determine the best allocation of services (utilization and capacity) to population groups so that maximum equity and efficiency in availability, accessibility, and cost can be achieved. McClure illustrates this approach using the same information as in the demand-based model. Assume:

> . . . a typical community of 50,000 persons with a utilization rate of 1400 patient days, and a bed rate of 5.1 beds per 1000 population. (For simplicity, we assume this community has typical age, sex, and other risk characteristics, so that such adjustments can be ignored for the moment.) The research evidence shows that for such a typical population, the range of acceptable medical practice varies from an uncertain minimum of 600–800 patient days to an uncertain maximum 1600–1800 patient days per 1000 population. Since the research evidence shows that comparable

> health levels are achieved anywhere within this range, then from a health standpoint the policymaker may arbitrarily choose any utilization rate standard within this range as the planning target for the community. If he is interested only in patient and provider convenience, he might choose a higher rate, say 1500 patient days per 1000 persons. But if he is interested in cost containment, he will choose a lower rate, say 1300 patient days per 1000 persons or less. (He could equally well choose 1200 or 1000 days or less; all are equally safe from a health standpoint. He can choose arbitrarily on the basis of whatever is politically and pragmatically feasible to obtain.) At the specified occupancy of 77%, a goal of 1300 patient days translates to 4.6 beds per 1000 persons. Thus, this population-based assumption would produce a reduction in existing capacity down to 241 beds or less. This is in contrast to the increase to 264 beds projected by the demand-based assumptions. . . .[21]

McClure makes it quite clear that the population-based planning approach should set overall use and capacity rates and then monitor these variables to see that goals are achieved.

> We know, for example, that hospital use rates exceeding 600–800 patient days per 1000 population are more than sufficient to produce the optimum health levels achievable by well organized medical care. But as we work down to specific services there are fewer rigorous studies to guide us, and planning judgments become more subjective. For example, we are less certain how many of these hospital days should be intensive care unit days. The important finding that different types of beds are substitutable for each other . . . protects us from reasonable errors in planning judgment and also obviates the need for community health planning at too detailed a level. *Except for extremely high cost services, such detailed planning is better left to individual hospitals*. . . .[22]

This allows the planner to analyze the problem in terms of the total number of beds, not the various types of beds. Many times the health planner stalls the analysis or does an incomplete analysis because data by bed type are not available. Or, worse, hospital administrators and physicians criticize the methodology because bed types were not accounted for. On this point, McClure is correct in stating that the determination of overall bed needs should be based on population-based planning, letting the hospital administration determine bed mix, except of course in the case of very high cost services.

The results of population-based planning by health planners are poor but improving. Data systems at the local level are ineffective and inadequate to provide knowledge about utilization, capacity, and expenditures. With publication of federal guidelines, standards, and reasons for adjustment to the standards, however, the health planner can proceed rapidly with population-based planning.

Demand/Population-Based Planning

Obviously, data constraints preclude the development of a true population-based planning model. For this reason, it is necessary to combine the demand-based model with the population-based approach. For example, occupancy rates (percentages) and average length of stay per 1,000 population may be used in a demand-based model. Other criteria might be patient days and beds per 1,000 population. McClure illustrates this approach with the following example:

> . . . . Suppose a state averages 1300 patient days and 4.75 beds per 1000 persons, based on 160 admissions per 1000 persons, 8.1 days length of stay, and 75% occupancy. Suppose the five-year demand-based projection states utilization will rise to 1360 days due to a rise in admissions to 170 offset by a slight fall in length of stay to 8.0 days. At 75% occupancy, this would require an increase in the bed rate to 4.97 beds per 1,000 persons. But suppose the state now makes the easily understood, simple argument that 75% occupancy represents costly, excess underutilized capacity and proposes an occupancy goal of 85%. At the projected use rate of 1360 patient days, only 4.4 beds per 1000 persons will be required. Another simple argument, with lots of research to support it, is that length-of-stay is excessive and could be lowered from 8.0 to 7.8 days (the national average). Then the five-year demand-based projection would be modified to 1325 patient days, which at 85% occupancy would require only 4.25 beds per 1000 persons. Thus, with two simple, defensible arguments—efficient occupancy and length-of-stay standards—the state could justify a reduction in its demand-based projected bed rate from 4.75 to 4.25 beds per 1000 persons, a decline of 10%. The reduction in current bed rate will produce about a 4% decline in use. Then, over five years, this reduction in capacity, if achieved, should in fact produce a fall in patient

> days from 1300 to 1250 days per 1000 persons—considerably less than original modified demand projection of 1325 days. At this use and bed rate, occupancy would rise to only 80%. Since 85% remains the occupancy target, 1250 patient days will require only 4.0 beds per 1000 population, permitting a further reduction in projected bed needs.[23]

The purpose of this approach is to aid communities in determining where reduction in capacity should be given high priority. In Oklahoma, the reduction of hospital capacity is based on both accessibility analysis and the above type of analysis, particularly, in the latter case, on the demand/population-based planning approach. The Oklahoma program is quite unique, with a tremendous potential for driving down, or at least controlling, the cost of hospital care.

Hospital Planning—The Oklahoma Example[24]

Hospital planning in Oklahoma is based on a four-part analysis. The analysis produces (1) utilization estimates, (2) estimates of hospital performance and bed needs, (3) an identification of hospital location based on accessibility criteria, and (4) estimates of the effects of reallocation of capacity and beds due to possible closure of a hospital. The results are relevance indexes based on demand estimates and population-based estimates, such as beds per 1,000 population and patient-origin data.

Utilization Estimates

In the Oklahoma program, two primary objectives were specified, each focusing on the determination of utilization rates. The first projected the number of discharges by county, service area, and state for 1977 and 1985, utilizing patient-origin data from 1976. The second projected the number of patient days by county, service area, and state for 1977 and 1985, utilizing the above discharge estimates and different estimates of average length of stay (ALOS). The following data were required for this process:

1. Patient-origin data for 1976
2. County populations for 1976, 1977, and 1985
3. Service area boundaries and nodes (towns) within the service areas
4. Current ALOS
5. An estimated ALOS for 1985

Once this part of the model is operational, the health planner can vary the ALOS. That is, if from current literature an appropriate standard can be gleaned, the agency can use that standard as a targeted objective such as ALOS per 1,000 population. Of course, if data are available on different discharge diagnoses, they can also be used.

Utilizing patient-origin data and population estimates, the health planner aggregates total discharges by county service area and state and divides by 1976 population to produce 1976 discharge rates by county, service area, and state. Thus:

1. 1976 County Discharge Rate = Total County Discharges from All Hospitals/1976 County Population × 1,000
2. 1976 Service Area Discharge Rates = Total Service Area Discharges from All Hospitals/1976 Service Area Population × 1,000
3. 1976 State Discharge Rate = All Discharges/1976 State Population × 1,000

The resulting discharge rates (1976) are applied to the 1977 and the 1985 population projections to estimate new discharges. These discharges are multiplied by current ALOS to provide patient days for 1977 by county, service area, and state. In addition, two estimates of patient days for 1985 are calculated, using two estimates of ALOS multiplied by the estimated number of discharges. The products from this step in the analysis, formatted as a table, would be generated three times: once for 1977, using current ALOS, and twice for 1985, using two estimates of ALOS. The results from this step serve as input to the next part of the four-part methodology.

Hospital Performance and Bed Need Estimates

Whereas the focus in the first part of the methodology was on the geographic unit (county, service area, and state), the focus in this part is on the institution (hospital). The primary objective here is to estimate present and future bed needs for the state. There are several subobjectives in this phase of the methodology:

The first subobjective is to estimate discharges by hospital for 1977 and 1985. To accomplish this subobjective, the patient-origin data are used to establish a relevance index matrix which provides relevance indexes for each hospital in 1976. Hospital relevance indexes from 1976 applied to estimated county discharges in 1977 will furnish estimated discharges by hospital for 1977. Similarly, 1985 hospital relevance indexes are applied to northeast service area hospitals and 1976 hospital relevance indexes to the remaining hospitals to estimate hospital discharges in 1985. This step is done three times, in order to account for the impact on the surrounding hospitals of a new hospital, City of Faith, that Oral Roberts in Tulsa, Oklahoma, will be building. Three cases are identified. In Case A, Oklahoma residents represent 10 percent of City of Faith discharges, in Case B they represent 30 percent, and in Case C they represent 70 percent. The results of the analysis of Cases A, B, and C are shown in four tables developed for 1977 and 1985.

The second subobjective is to estimate hospital performance, that is, expected occupancy rates, given projected utilization and total number of beds for 1977. The utilization estimates from the first part of the methodology by county, service area, and state will now be used. In addition, hospital utilization rates (patient days) will be calculated by multiplying the projected number of hospital discharges (Subobjective 1) by the three estimates of ALOS. Based on this information, expected occupancy rates by hospital can be calculated. The "givens" are the number of beds and projected number of patients for all hospitals, service areas, and the state. Obviously, occupancy rates on a county level are meaningless in this situation, given the methodology for determining county patient days. To obtain the expected occupancy rates, the projected patient days must be divided by 365, resulting in an average daily census (ADC). The ADC is divided by the number of beds, giving the expected occupancy rate by hospital. To get expected occupancy rates by service area and state, the individual hospitals are aggregated. The results will be portrayed seven times: once for 1977 and six times for 1985 (three estimates of City of Faith Hospital times two ALOS).

The third subobjective is to calculate the number of beds needed and the number of beds underutilized, by hospital service area, county, and state. The occupancy rate used will be the standard of 80 percent plus median occupancy rates, by size of hospital and service area. To calculate the number of beds needed, the projected patient days are divided by 365 to give an ADC. Then the ADC is divided by the standard occupancy rate. The result is the number of beds needed. By comparing this value to the number of beds currently available, overutilization or underutilization will be shown. By varying the occupancy rates and the projected patient days (based on ADCs), the methodology becomes interactive. Specifically, if a hospital provides a value reflecting a certain ALOS and occupancy rate, the number of beds to add or delete can be determined.

The fourth subobjective is to estimate bed/population ratios after excess beds are subtracted. Bed/population ratios are calculated by hospital, county, service area, and state. It is possible that the first reduction in beds is too large (that is, more beds have been subtracted than is necessary), and the bed/population ratio will be well below the federal guidelines of 4.0 per 1,000 population. At this point, successive runs can be made utilizing different bed/population ratios in association with various standard occupancy rates. This provides maximum flexibility for the project review officer to determine new beds or services for the hospital. The results of this analysis are critical to development of the third part of the methodology.

Identification of Hospital Locations Based on Accessibility Criteria

The major objective in this part of the analysis is to determine the best location for cutting the number of underutilized beds. Some constraints, however, must be considered before beds are eliminated. A major constraint is that beds (or hospitals) cannot be cut if accessibility to the hospital meets the criteria specified in the accessibility analysis. Also preference will be given to locations with higher levels of service and performance based on relevance indexes and occupancy rates. Thus, if a hospital or bed were dropped, it would not change the accessibility criteria, and the relevance index and occupancy rates would be low. Here, a decision rule must be established, for example, 30 minutes travel time, a relevance index of .25, and an occupancy rate of .45. Any hospital or hospital beds meeting these criteria could potentially be deleted. The results of this analysis will provide values or locations and potentials to reduce the number of beds.

Effects of Bed Closure and Reallocation

The basic objective in the final part of the analysis is to estimate the effects of bed or hospital closure and of the subsequent reallocation of utilization to their remaining locations. This analysis may be approached in two ways. The first method uses information regarding underutilized beds and the results of an accessibility analysis (see the previous section). The procedure is as follows:

1. Add together all underutilized beds which are not exempted due to accessibility criteria by service area and subtract them from the total number of available beds in that service area.
2. Recalculate a projected service area occupancy rate for the remaining beds, utilizing total patient days for the service area as estimated previously for the years specified.
3. Compare this total occupancy rate with the standard rate applied in part two of the methodology. Then compare the resulting total beds per population ratio with federal guidelines to assess compliance.

The second method is essentially the same as the first except that it is more detailed and institution-specific. The procedure is as follows:

1. Subtract excess beds by node and institution based upon specified criteria.
2. Develop revised relevance matrices, utilizing institutions which remain following the cut in Step One. Reallocate total discharges by county over the remaining hospitals and calculate new relevance indexes.
3. Reestimate the total number of patient days per hospital, utilizing the new estimates of hospital discharges calculated in Step Two and multiplied by the specified ALOS. Next, recalculate projected hospital performance utilizing the new bed complement and new utilization estimates to produce projected occupancy rates by institution. At this point, compare the resulting occupancy rates with the standard imposed in part two to see if the elimination of underutilized beds has brought the state into compliance with the federal guidelines criteria. If expected occupancy rates are not in compliance with the standard imposed in part two, the process can be repeated until occupancy rates and bed/population ratios satisfy these guidelines.

Hospital Planning under Rural Conditions

The national guidelines' standards provide for adjustment of occupancy and bed supply targets under rural conditions.[25] Criteria for adjustment are "rural areas where a majority of the residents would be more than 30 minutes travel time from a hospital" and "rural areas with a number of small (fewer than 4,000 admissions per year) hospitals." Both provisions imply an adjustment of occupancy (and thus the bed supply) targets.

By ensuring "accessibility," an area's utilization is distributed over several small facilities rather than concentrated in one single large facility. If a single large hospital can operate more efficiently than several small ones, the expected occupancy of one large facility will be greater than the aggregated occupancy of several small facilities. For example, if one were to apply the Poisson statistical estimate (at the 99 percent confidence level) to an area with an ADC of 100, the beds needed in one single facility would be $100 + 2.33\sqrt{100} = 124$ beds. If the ADC were equally distributed in four institutions, the beds needed would be $4(25 + 2.33\sqrt{25}) = 4 \times 37 = 148$ beds. The expected occupancies would be 80.0 percent and 67.5 percent, respectively.

Acceptance of occupancy targets due to the size of the facilities is shown in the allowance of a lower occupancy for a large number of hospitals with less than 4,000 admissions per year. The Poisson statistical estimate at the 99 percent confidence level (an assurance that the ADC will not exceed the beds available 99 out of 100 days) does not permit an 80 percent occupancy level until the ADC is 88. An average daily census of less than 88 would mean a lower occupancy target using the Poisson statistical estimate (at the 99 percent confidence level). An ADC of more than 88 would permit an occupancy of more than 80 percent.

Thus, an adjustment for rural conditions is, first, an adjustment to the occupancy target and, second, an adjustment to the bed-supply target. The methodology outlined below uses the Poisson statistical estimate for determining an optimal occupancy in an area.

Step One

Project the ADC for institutions or service areas using whatever methodology is employed by the state C/N standards to forecast bed need.

Admissions/1,000 population × ALOS = patient days/1,000 population

Patient days/1,000 population × population (thousands) = patient days

Patient days ÷ by 365 = ADC

Note: It is assumed that all states use a form of Hill-Burton to project ADC. This form takes current use for a current population and forecasts future use depending upon increases or decreases in the population. Some states also make assumptions about changes in the use rate regardless of population changes, but this does not really affect the basic concept.

Step Two

Apply the Poisson statistical estimate to the ADC to determine the number of beds needed.

$$\text{ADC} + Z\sqrt{\text{ADC}} = \text{beds needed}$$

Z refers to a confidence level (or interval) that statistically estimates, on the basis of the Poisson distribution, the number of days that the ADC will not exceed the beds needed. Health planning agencies have some flexibility in setting this figure.

Z	Confidence Level	# Times ADC ≤ Beds Needed
1.65	95%	95 out of 100
2.33	99%	99 out of 100

Step Three

Determine individual hospital or service area occupancy targets.

ADC/beds needed = Occupancy

Step Four

Determine HSA occupancy target by aggregating individual hospital or service area ADCs and the number of beds needed.

HSA ADC/HSA beds needed = HSA occupancy

Barring other discretionary adjustments, this becomes the national-guideline, ''adjusted'' occupancy target.

Step Five

Adjust the bed supply target (4.0 beds/1,000 population) to reflect the adjusted occupancy target.

Bed supply target × Occupancy target/Adjusted occupancy target = Adjusted bed supply target

Barring further discretionary adjustments, the adjusted bed supply target will be the target used to compare with number of beds needed. For example, there are six hospitals in HSA 1, one in each of the six planning subareas. All of them are considered to be needed to ensure reasonable accessibility. The bed need forecasting methodology is as follows:

Current pt. days/Current population × Projected population/365 = Projected ADC

The area population is expected to increase 10 percent, from 75,000 to 82,500 in five years. The analysis and target adjustment would appear as shown on the chart on the next page.

The beds needed per 1,000 population in the following example are not equal to the adjusted bed supply target (4.25) because the anticipated use rate of the population is 1,332 days of care per 1,000 persons. Adjustment to the occupancy and/or bed supply target for other conditions (for exam-

	Step 1				Step 2	Step 3
Hospital	1977 ADC	1977 Pop. (000s)	1982 Pop. (000s)	1982 ADC	1982 Beds Needed	1982 Occ.
A	20.7	10	11	23	35	66%
B	42.3	10	11	47	63	75%
C	91.8	20	22	102	126	81%
D	50.4	15	16.5	56	74	76%
E	31.5	10	11	35	49	71%
F	34.2	10	11	38	53	72%
Total	290.9	75	82.5	301	400	Step 4

Step 4. 301/400 = 75.3% = Adjusted Occupancy Target

Step 5. 4.0 beds/1,000 pop. × .80/.753 = 4.25 beds/1,000 pop. = adjusted bed supply target.

ple, age, seasonal population fluctuations) might be possible and would bring the bed supply target closer to the beds-needed figure.

The Poisson statistical estimate is an adjustment for size, a condition implied by the "rural," standard-specific conditions. It may only be used where state C/N bed-need methodologies include it as part of the formula for determining bed need or where a bed-need projection formula does not exist. Formulas for projecting bed need which include or state an occupancy target directly would apparently not allow the use of the Poisson statistical estimate or any other adjustment for rural conditions unless specifically provided for in the formula.[26]

METHODS FOR DETERMINING RESOURCE REQUIREMENTS

Below are four methods (provided by the Region IV HPDC) for determining health resource requirements.[27] The four methods, which do not exhaust the list of available approaches, are summarized in Table 8-9 in terms of data requirements and general applicability to the resource standards of the initial national guidelines. Appendix 8A presents additional methods for determining resources for several of the standards noted in the national guidelines.

Table 8-9 Data Requirements of the Four Basic Methods and Applications

Method	Basic Data Requirements: Current Population	Projected Population	Resource Ratios	Standard of Service Use by Time	Production Capacity	Health Status Indices	Disease Counts	Volume of Treatment	Duration of Aggregate Services	Annual Service Production Capacity	Annual Use Rates	To Initial National Specific Standard	Applications Guidelines	Resources Concerns General
1. Resource/ Population Ratio Method	X	X	X									• Acute care pediatric hospital beds	1. General hospital beds 2. Neonatal intensive/ intermediate care 3. Pediatric beds	
2. Service Target Method	X	(X)		X	X							• CT scanner equipment	1. Radiation therapy units 2. Renal dialysis units 3. CT scanner units 4. Cardiac catheterization/ open heart surgery	

3. Health Needs Approach						X	X	X	X	X		• Radiation therapy equipment	1. Radiation therapy units 2. Renal dialysis units 3. CT scanner units 4. Cardiac catheterization/ open heart surgery
4. Effective Demand Approach	X	X									X	• General hospital bed capacity and occupancy rates	1. General hospital bed capacity 2. Neonatal intensive/ intermediate care 3. Pediatric beds

Source: William E. DeBardlaben, "Basic Methods for Determining Community Resource Requirements," *Methodological Approaches to Address the National Guidelines for Health Planning in Local and State Health Plan Development, A Workbook for Planners,* Health Planning/Development Center, Inc., Atlanta, January 1979, p. 62.

Resource/Population Ratio Method

The resource/population ratio method determines resource requirements by multiplying population by a selected ratio:

Resource requirement = Population × Selected ratio

Current requirements are calculated by multiplying present population by the selected ratio; future requirements, by multiplying projected population by the same selected ratio. For this calculation, the planner would need the following:

1. Current population in pediatric age group (<15)	227,063
2. Projected 1983 pediatric age population	233,100
3. Current selected ratio of beds/population	1.3/1,000
4. Desired selected ratio of beds/population	1.0/1,000

With the above data set, the computation is:

Current status = 1.3/1,000 × 227,063 = 295
Present requirements = 1.0/1,000 × 227,063 = 227
Future requirements = 1.0/1,000 × 233,100 = 233

Thus, based on the desired selected ratio of 1.0 beds per 1,000 population, the HSA in 1983 would require 233 acute care, pediatric hospital beds. The following comment on this method is noted:

> The simplicity of the method is its greatest advantage. Relative to other methods, data requirements are minimal, and the statistics are easily obtained; the estimates can be prepared in short order at low cost; the methodology requires only modest staff expertise. It is useful as a descriptive device, as an input to more sophisticated methodologies, as a validation of estimates derived by other means, and as an initial datum to be used in producing more thoughtful judgments within the community.
>
> The weaknesses of the method are serious and may be overriding. Inevitable changes in the future involving socioeconomic conditions, technological and biomedical advances in health care and the configuration of the delivery system are ignored, although they affect the amount of services the population demands and the amount of services health personnel will provide. To ignore these changes and focus on population growth may be feasible in the very short run, but is perilous for long-term projections.[28]

Service-Target Method

The service-target method focuses on the service produced and the volume of the resources as the central determinant of resource requirements. Occasionally referred to as the "normative approach," this method has as key parameters the norms or standards of the services required by the community and of the services produced by health resources. Thus, the methodology quantifies the public's health demands and the health care system's resource outputs:[29]

Resource requirement = Population × Services per person/
Resource productivity (average output per unit of time)

In a mathematical format, the formula is:

$$R_t = \frac{V \times P}{q \times a} \quad \text{or} \quad \frac{N}{q \times a}$$

where: R_t = resource requirement for year t
V = standard or norm for quantity of service required per year, per person
P = population, current or projected
N = $V \times P$ = total number of services per year for a given population
a = optimal standards of resource performance or production capacity
q = maximum production capacity of a specific resource

A typical problem facing an HSA might be the determination of projected requirements for CAT scanners for a health service area by 1983. By obtaining the following inputs, the planner can apply the model to estimate the number of CAT scanners needed:

1. Projected area population in 1983 (total) = 888,000
2. Service target = .03116 scans per person per year
3. An assumed optimal scanner utilization rate of 85 percent (with allowance for down-time, institutional peculiarities, and so forth)
4. An assumed maximum theoretical capacity per scanner of 4,000 procedures per year, 16 procedures per day, and 250 days per year.

Given the above information, the planner applies the formula as follows:

$$R_t = \frac{V \times P}{q \times a}$$

where: V = .03116 scans per person per year (based on national estimates of 6.7 million scans per year)
P = 888,000 projected population, 1983
a = 85% optimal utilization (task force consensus)
q = 4,000 production capacity (theoretical)

then: R_t = .03116 × 888,000/4,000 × .85 = 8.1 scanners
R = 8 scanners by 1983 (assuming optimal utilization of existing capacity)

The results suggest that eight scanners will be sufficient by 1983. It should be noted that the method has nothing to do with the location of the scanners based on availability standards (see the section on accessibility analysis which demonstrates the process of planning facilities in optimum locations).

The service-target method has been described in the following terms:

> The strength of the service target approach to estimating requirements is its focus on the central issue of providing services and, therefore, on the importance of the efficient and effective functional organization of the delivery of care, not spatial. Attention is directed to utilization and its impact on productivity. The implications of work flow and referral patterns can be studied, allowing the planner to theoretically test the effect of alternative mixes on resource requirements.
>
> The search for understanding of the underlying factors and relationships that are required in the service target approach is one of its greatest strengths. The planner is faced with the Achilles' heel of this method when he attempts to quantify the variables dealing with service targets and productivity. He will almost certainly find important data gaps. Should he decide to collect primary data, he must be prepared for a long-term effort, considerable expense, and the need for expert technical assistance. The planner should be wary of the temptation to elaborate the study to such an extent that the detailed findings are only of academic interest and of no practical value in the light of his community's actual policy options.
>
> By far the greatest danger of this method is the use of improper criteria for setting the service standards, in terms of the demand for services and the productivity of the resource. If the standards

used are not valid, the estimates may be grossly unrealistic. (Eight scanners would not reflect the present emphasis on cost containment) . . .[30]

Health-Needs Method

A more sophisticated approach to resource requirements employs the biologic needs of the community as the fundamental determinant of resource requirements. The starting point is to identify and quantify the community's health care needs, using normative judgment of what constitutes good health care. Reflecting its basic orientation, the health-needs approach has been labeled the "biologic care" and "professional standards" method. Thus,

> [w]hen asked, "how much and what types of health resources do you need to provide optimal care for your community," the planner turns to the health needs approach. His concern is with what "ought to be" and what "might be," not with "what is" or "what is likely to be." As a planner, he is thinking in terms of the ultimate goal and highest target of health care planning to assure that level of preventive, diagnostic, or therapeutic care which will obtain the optimal health status for the community. . . .
>
> The health needs approach may be viewed as a particular application of the service target method, in which the standard for consumer demand for services is set by professional judgment of the care needed. These standards can be set at any level: optimal, minimal, or acceptable care somewhere in between. . . .[31]

The health-needs method is based on the following formula:

$$\text{Resource requirements} = R_t = P \times C \times V \times D/W$$

The computations are as follows:

R_t = resource requirements in year t
P = population that needs a given type of care for a specific health problem in year t
C = the average number of specific conditions per year per person
V = the average number of a given kind of service per person/per condition/per year, based on need
D = average time duration required per unit of service
W = average annual operating time of a given resource

A problem the agency may be required to solve is, What are the required resources projected for radiation therapy for a health service area by 1983? Utilizing the above formula,

where: P = 1,332 cancer patients in need of treatment (obtained by assuming a total projected population base is 888,000 for 1983, a crude annual average incidence rate of .003 cases per person, and a 50% rate of new cases needing radiation therapy)

C = one condition

V = 30 treatments for each new case per year

D = 11 minutes per treatment

W = 115,200 minutes per year (based on 8 hours per day, 5 days per week, 48 weeks per year)

then:

$$R_t = P \times C \times V \times D/W$$
$$= 1{,}332 \times 1 \times 30 \times 11/115{,}200$$
$$= 3.8$$

Thus: R = 4 radiation therapy units in 1983.

The following further comment on this method is noted:

> The logical coherences of the health needs approach—that needs are determined by health care required—are very satisfying for health resources planners. One can easily conceptualize the analytical framework: types of health conditions, such as acute, chronic, preventive; required types of care, such as ambulatory, hospital based, long term; and health professionals providing the care, such as physicians, nurses, therapists. When the community's needs are the proper criteria, and data on health status and appropriate treatment are obtainable, this approach is excellent.
>
> The planner should be aware that the technical difficulties in defining and quantifying health needs, "acceptable" modes of care, and resource output are formidable but not insurmountable. Professionals do not agree; the health status of a population changes over time; medical practices advance; and last, but not least, published statistics are out of date, inapplicable, or incomplete.
>
> Most serious of all, criticism is directed at the method's failure to take into account the patients' willingness to seek care in the first place and the community's ability to pay for health services.

The assumption is that there are no financial, psychological, or social constraints to seeking care. The concept of "demand as need" has the inherent danger of overestimating requirements.[32]

Effective-Demand Method (Population-Based)

This dynamic approach assumes that the composition as well as the size of the population are major determinants of the types and quantity of services used. In turn, it is the population's demand for particular services that creates resource requirements.[33] The effective demand method is expressed in the following formula:

$$R_t = \sum R_{tp} = \sum V_{tp} \times N_{tp}$$

where: R_t = resource quantity needed in target year t

$\sum_{p=1}^{n}$ = sum over the n population cohorts (≤15, 15–44, 45–64, ≥65)

R_{tp} = resource quantity needed in target year by the pth cohort

V_{tp} = utilization rate of the service in the target year by the pth cohort

N_{tp} = number of individuals (1,000s) in the target year in the pth cohort

Since we assume that utilization rates, by cohort, remain constant over time:

$$V_{tp} = V_{bp} = R_{bp}/N_{bp}$$

where: V_{bp} = utilization rate of the service in the base year by the pth cohort

R_{bp} = resource quantity utilized in base year by the pth cohort

N_{bp} = number of individuals (1,000s) in the base year by the pth cohort

Substituting this in the first formula:

$$R_t = \sum_{j=1}^{n} [(R_{bp}/N_{bp}) \times N_{tp}]$$

The determination of projected requirements for hospital beds by age and sex for the health service area by 1983 is a major problem for a health agency. The above formula, applied in the following manner, can provide an estimate of bed needs in 1983 (Table 8-10).

$$R_t = R_{bp}/N_{bp} \times N_{tp}$$

$$= 40{,}787 + 105{,}632 + 124{,}971 + \ldots + 193{,}435 = 1{,}013{,}545$$

Hospital beds = 1,013,545 (patient days)/365 (days) × .80 (optimal occupancy) = 3,471 beds

Thus, 3.5 beds per 1,000 population will be required by 1983.

These comments on the effective-demand method are relevant:

> The strong suit of this method is its reliance on measures of effective demand—the utilization rate—and its detailed study of the behavior of groups of people seeking health care. The degree of disaggregation inherent in this method permits the planner to base resource estimates on the health care demands of each

Table 8-10 Population and Patient Days for the Health Service Area, 1977 and 1983

Age-Sex Cohorts	Base-Year Population (1977) (N_{bp})	Base-Year (1977) Demand (R_{bp})	Average Annual Utilization Rate (V_{bp}) ($V_{bp}=R_{bp}-N_{bp}$)	Projected Year (1983) Population (N_{tp})	Project Year (1983) Demand ($V_{bp}XN_{tp}$) (Total Days)
MALES					
<15	115,564	39,731	343.8	118,637	40,787
15–44	180,266	102,896	570.8	185,059	105,632
45–64	81,570	121,735	1,492.4	83,738	124,971
65>	36,676	149,455	4,075.0	37,651	153,428
FEMALES					
<15	111,499	30,439	273.0	114,463	31,248
15–44	195,836	213,109	1,088.2	201,043	218,775
45–64	91,430	141,506	1,547.7	93,861	145,269
65>	52,159	188,424	3,612.5	53,546	193,435
TOTAL	865,000	987,295	1,141.38	888,000	1,013,545

Source: William E. DeBardlaben, "Basic Methods for Determining Community Resource Requirements," *Methodological Approaches To Address The National Guidelines for Health Planning in Local and State Health Plan Development, A Workbook for Planners,* Health Planning/Development Center, Inc., Atlanta, January 1979, p. 58.

segment of the population, reflecting the cultural and physical characteristics of each group of people. This estimate represents the change likely to occur as a result of one important factor, namely, the change in population over time.

However, the assumption that other important economic factors, such as income, price, and third-party financing, remain unchanged is very limiting and unlikely to represent reality. The assumption that population and the demand for services are so related that a change in population brings a proportionate response in the demand for services is very restrictive and needs to be validated. Furthermore, the assumption that present utilization patterns are the proper standard for the future is questionable, since we realize that there are many unmet health needs in our country as well as inappropriate uses of limited health resources.[34]

Summary

Clearly, the selection of a method to determine resource needs should be approached cautiously. There is no standard method, but there are standard guidelines. Thus, the assumptions underlying the methods should be critically examined and thoroughly explained to the individuals who make the decisions. None of the four methods approaches the problem of optimum utilization through optimum geographical distribution of services. For this reason, the methods require one further step, illustrated in the question, If the need is for eight CAT scanners, where should they be located? The accessibility analysis and the hospital performance analysis reviewed earlier are needed to complete this final step.

LOCATION AND ALLOCATION ISSUES IN HEALTH PLANNING

Location and allocation issues may be subdivided into four problem categories: (1) locational problems, (2) allocation problems, (3) location-then-allocation problems, and (4) allocation-then-location problems.[35] The main concern in locational problems is to locate one or more health services or facilities in the most desirable place. This procedure can involve running or relocating a facility in the existing system. The major concern in allocational problems (relatively rare in health planning) is to have boundary lines which tie consumers to specific service sites or providers. In this case, the federal guidelines concerning obstetrics and neonatal services suggest that regionalization of the services must be considered. Location-then-allocation problems are concerned with which sites are selected and with the way consumers or the population are "districted" for the new sites. This type of planning has been prevalent in school districting. The concern in allocation-then-location problems, the reverse of the location-then-allocation problem, is to first draw the districts and then to define the best location for the services or providers within the district.

The first requirement is a set of points, consumers or population, distributed in a geographic area. A weighted value may be attached to each point that would make the location more or less desirable. A set of facilities without predetermined locations must then be located within the geographic area. The major objective in this process is to find locations for the central facilities and to allocate each of the points (consumers or population) to one of the facilities. The destination points may represent counties, communities, census tracts, or neighborhoods. The weights used may be estimates of demand, for example, the population may be used as the demand value. The central facilities would be either hospitals, primary care centers, emergency facilities, obstetrical services, or neonatal services.

Location/allocation problems are solved by optimization or heuristic techniques. If the issues represent an optimization problem, optimization techniques can solve the problem. The major purpose of this approach is to identify an objective function which will be maximized or minimized. If heuristic techniques are applied to an optimization problem, the results will be suboptimal. Optimization techniques include linear programming, integer programming, and the tree-searching method (branch and bound). Each method will produce the best solution based on the stated objective function and constraints. Solving by optimization techniques, however, is not always feasible. There are three reasons for this: First, many problems cannot be expressed as a series of linear equations because of too many complex relationships among the variables. Second, the techniques may require too much data or inaccessible data. Third, some optimization problems are so complex that excessive and expensive computer time is needed to determine an optimal solution.

Heuristic methods provide potential alternatives to optimization methods. The solution of optimization problems heuristically requires a set of decision rules (algorithms) to find good solutions; optimality is not guaranteed. The practical side of this approach is that it reflects more of "real world" constraints. The results from heuristic methods are quite satisfactory and hold the greatest promise for health planners.

Many issues complicate location, allocation, and accessibility problems. First, primary, secondary, and tertiary service areas must be determined for hierarchical services. Second, multiple services with different travel distance requirements can be obtained from the same facility. Third, different distance and travel measures may be used, for example, straight-line, actual, time, cost, and subjective. Fourth, location and allocation problems may be formulated as static problems (these assume that location/allocation assignments can be implemented immediately) or as dynamic problems (these provide for phasing in the implementation). Finally, in both static and dynamic models, there is a conflict between short-run and long-run solutions. A brief listing of significant contributions to the solution of location and allocation problems is provided in Appendix 8B.

SUMMARY

Health care resources analysis involves methods for determining appropriate service areas and trade-off functions, for doing accessibility and location/allocation analysis, and for hospital planning (demand-based, population-based, and a combination of the two). By applying these resource analytical methods to problems facing our country, the health planner can be greatly rewarded. The need to reduce health care costs and to find more equitable and efficient solutions poses a continuous challenge to health care planners.

APPENDIX 8A*
DETERMINATION OF RESOURCE NEEDS BY VARIOUS METHODS

Details of eight methods to determine health resource needs are presented below.[36]

Table 8A-1 Calculations for Short-Stay Hospital Bed Requirements for 1983, Resident Population

A) *Indigenous Urban Population*

P = 829,056

PD = 829,056 × 1,141.38/1,000 = 946,268

W = 1 percent of patient days

Q = .80

$$N = \frac{D - W}{365 \times Q} = \frac{946{,}268 - 9{,}463}{365 \times .80} = 3208$$

B) *Indigenous Rural Population*

P = 55,944

PD = 55,944 × 1,141.38/1,000 = 63,853 patient days

W = 1 percent of patient days

Q = .70

$$N = \frac{D - W}{365 \times Q} = \frac{63{,}853 - 639}{365 \times .70} = 247 \text{ beds}$$

Source: This entire appendix is from William E. DeBardlaben, *Methodological Approaches to Address the National Guidelines for Health Planning in Local and State Health Plan Development, A Workbook for Planners,* Health Planning/Development Center, Inc., Atlanta, January 1979.

Table 8A-1 continued

C) *HMO Population*

P = 3000

PD = 3000 × 856.0

W = 0

Q = .80

$$N = \frac{D - W}{365 \times Q} = \frac{2{,}568 - 0}{365 \times .80} = 9 \text{ beds}$$

D) *Referral Population*

D = 30,000 patient days

W = 0%

Q = 80%

$$N = \frac{D - W}{365 \times Q} = \frac{30{,}000 - 0}{365 \times .80} = 103 \text{ beds}$$

E) *Transient Population*

P = 25,000 annual average visitors

D = 25,000 × 570.69/1,000 = 14,267

W = 0

Q = .80

$$N = \frac{D - W}{365 \times Q} = \frac{14{,}267 - 0}{365 \times .80} = 49 \text{ beds}$$

F) *Total Beds Needed* = 3,208 + 247 + 9 + 103 + 49 = 3,616

P = Population
PD = Patient Days
W = Wellness Factor
Q = Occupancy Standard
N = Number of Beds

Figure 8A-1 Short-Stay Hospital Bed Requirements for 1983

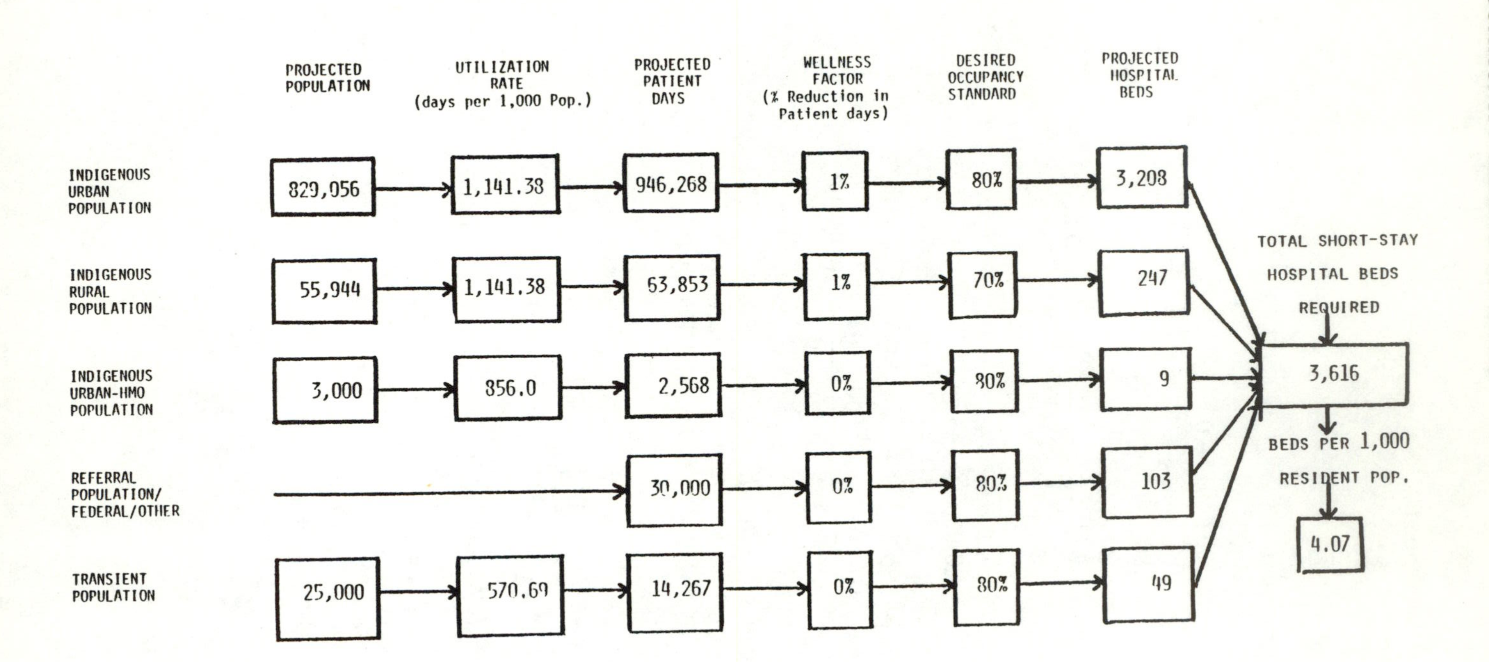

Table 8A-2 Calculations for Obstetrical Resource Requirements, 1983

RESIDENT POPULATION

A) *Indigenous Urban Population*

Projected Child-bearing Population = 186,970

Projected Birth Rate = 66.0 per 1,000 pop.

$$\text{Projected Births} = \frac{186{,}970 \times 66.0}{1{,}000} = 12{,}340$$

$$\text{Projected Admissions} = 12{,}340 + (.02 \times 12{,}340) = 12{,}587$$

$$\text{Projected Beds} = \frac{4 \times 12{,}587}{365 \times .75} = 184$$

B) *Indigenous Rural Population*

Projected Child-bearing Population = 14,073

Projected Birth Rate = 60.0 per 1,000 pop.

$$\text{Projected Births} = \frac{14{,}073 \times 60.0}{1{,}000} = 844$$

Projected Admissions = 844

$$\text{Projected Beds} = \frac{4 \times 844}{365 \times .60} = 15$$

NON-RESIDENT POPULATION

Projected Births = 1200

$$\text{Projected Admission} = 1200 + (.02 \times 1200) = 1224$$

$$\text{Projected Beds} = \frac{4 \times 1224}{365 \times .75} = 18$$

Total Projected Beds = 217

Figure 8A-2 Obstetrical Resource Requirements for 1983, Health Service Area 1

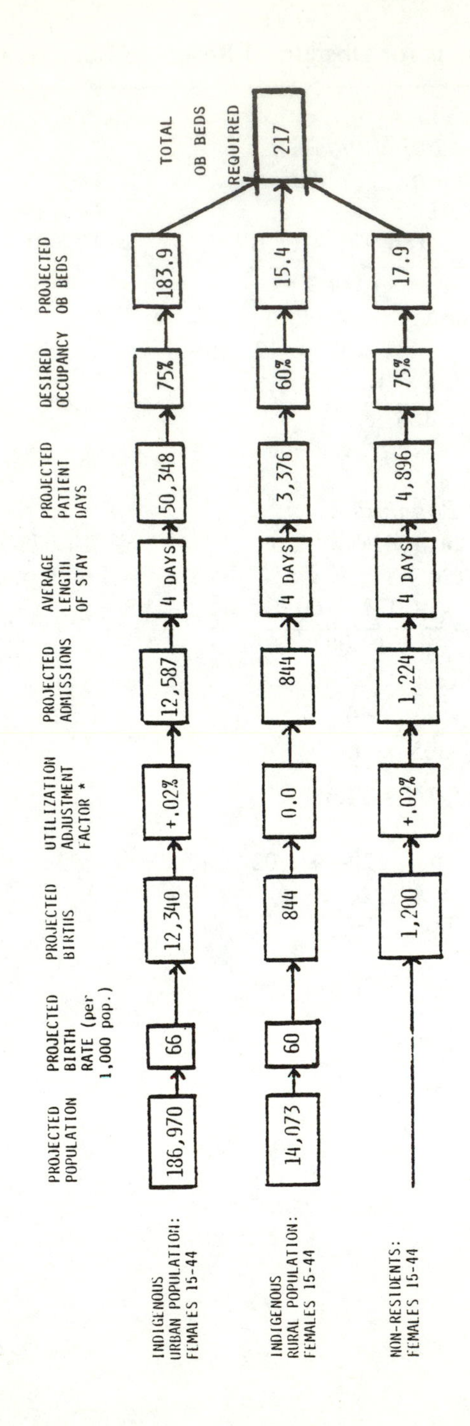

* Adjustment for Alternate Delivery Modes, False Pregnancies, Observation of High Risk Patients, etc.

Table 8A-3 Calculations for Neonatal Special Care Resource Requirements, 1983

RESIDENT POPULATION

Projected Births = 12,340
Low Weight Birth Rate (per 100 live births) = 7.5

$$\text{Projected Admissions} = \frac{7.5 \times 12{,}340}{100} = 926$$

$$\text{Projected Neonatal Beds} = \frac{12 \times 926}{365 \times .75} = 41$$

NON-RESIDENT POPULATION

Projected Births = 844
Low Weight Birth Rate (per 100 live births) = 7.5

$$\text{Projected Admissions} = \frac{7.5 \times 844}{100} = 63$$

$$\text{Projected Neonatal Beds} = \frac{12 \times 63}{365 \times .75} = 3$$

HIGH RISK NEONATES

Projected Admissions = 85

$$\text{Projected Neonatal Beds} = \frac{30 \times 85}{365 \times .90} = 8$$

Total Neonatal Beds = 51

Figure 8A-3 Neonatal Special Care Resource Requirements for 1983

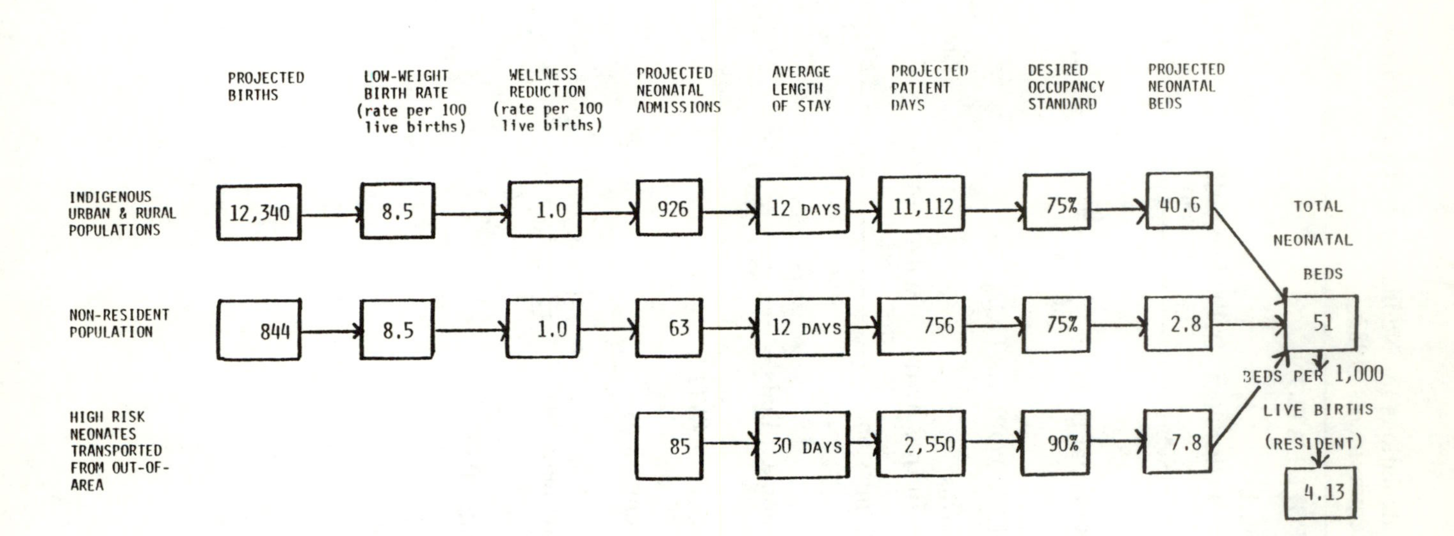

Table 8A-4 Calculations for Pediatric Bed Requirements, 1983

A. INDIGENOUS URBAN AND RURAL (EXCLUSIVE OF HMO ENROLLEES)

Population = 232,311

Patient Days = $\frac{309.03 \times 232{,}311}{1{,}000}$ = 71,791

Wellness Factor = .01 × 71,791 = 718

Occupancy Factor = 70%

Beds = $\frac{71{,}791 - 718}{365 \times .70}$ = 278.17

B. HMO POPULATION

Population = (26.3%) × 3,000 = 789

Patient Days = $\frac{789 \times 309.03}{1{,}000}$ = 244

Wellness Factor = .25 × 244 = 183

Occupancy Factor = 70%

Beds = $\frac{244 - 61}{365 \times .70}$ = .71

C. REFERRAL POPULATION

Patient Days = 10,450

Occupancy Factor = 100%

Beds = $\frac{10{,}450}{365 \times 1}$ = 28.63

D. TOTAL BEDS

278.17 + .71 + 28.63 = 307

Figure 8A-4 Pediatric Bed Requirements for 1983, Health Service Area

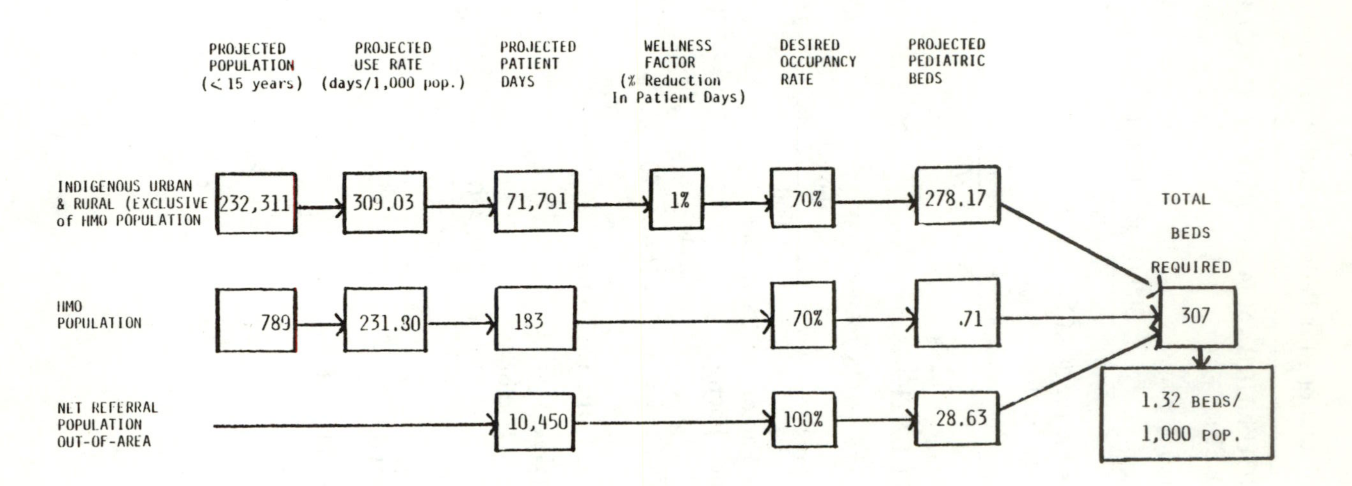

Table 8A-5 Calculations for Cardiac Catheterization Requirements, 1983

A. RESIDENT POPULATION (≥15 years)

Population 15 years and older	=	654,900
Resource Level	=	1.25 Labs/300,000 pop.

$$\text{Resource Requirements} = \frac{1.25 \times 654{,}900}{300{,}000} = 2.73 \text{ units}$$

B. RESIDENT POPULATION (≤15 years)

Population under 15 years	=	233,100
Resource Level	=	1 Lab/300,000 pop.

$$\text{Resource Requirements} = \frac{1 \times 233{,}100}{300{,}000} = .78 \text{ units}$$

C. REFERRAL POPULATION (out of area, all ages)

Population (from studies)	=	800
Resource Level	=	1 Lab/600 patient studies

$$\text{Resource Requirements} = \frac{1 \times 800}{600} = 1.33$$

D. TOTAL RESOURCE REQUIREMENTS

$2.73 \times .78 + 1.33 = 4.84$ units

Figure 8A-5 Cardiac Catheterization Requirements for 1983, Health Service Area 1

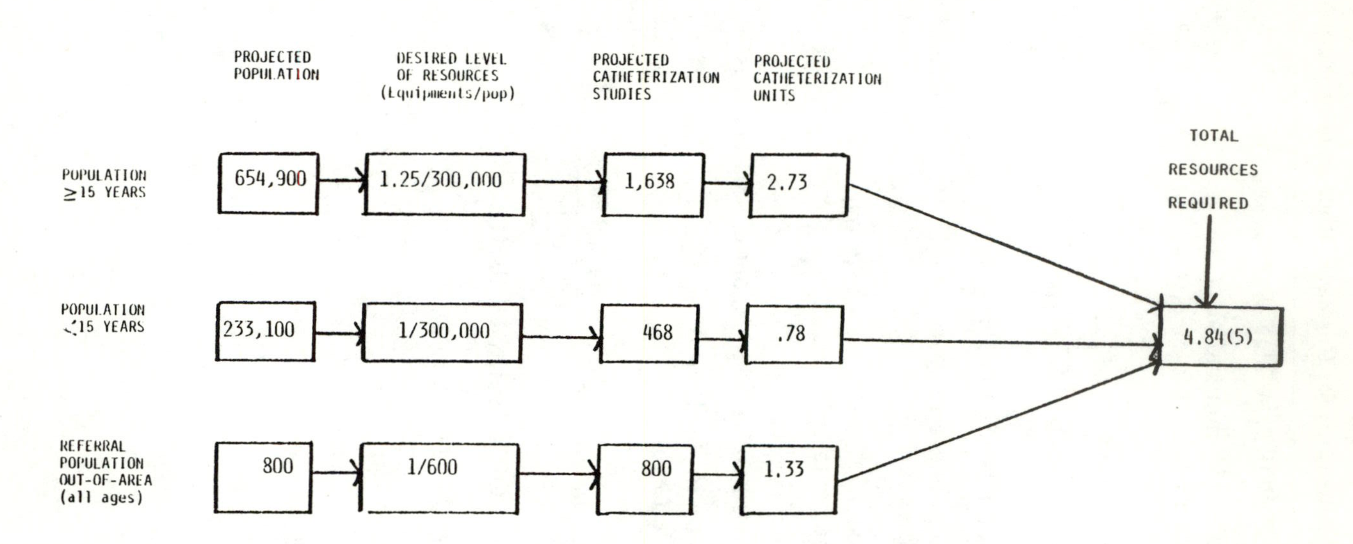

Table 8A-6 Calculations for Open Heart Surgery Requirements, 1983

A. RESIDENT POPULATION (≥15 years)		
Projected Cath Procedures		= 1,638
Open Heart Procedures Generated per Cath Study		= 1 per 4
Number of Open Heart Procedures generated	= .25 × 1,638	= 410
Maximum Number of Open Heart Units	$= \frac{410}{350}$	= 1.17
B. RESIDENT POPULATION (<15 years)		
Projected Cath Procedures		= 468
Open Heart Procedures Generated per Cath Study		= 1 per 4
Number of Open Heart Procedures Generated	= .25 × 468	= 117
Maximum Number of Open Heart Units	$= \frac{117}{130}$	= .90
C. REFERRAL POPULATION		
Projected Cath Procedures		= 800
Open Heart Procedures Generated per Cath Study		= 1 per 4
Number of Open Heart Procedures Generated	= .25 × 800	= 200
Maximum Number of Open Heart Units	$= \frac{200}{350}$	=.57
D. TOTAL OPEN HEART UNITS		
1.17 + .90 + .57 = 3 units		

Figure 8A-6 Open Heart Surgery Resources Requirements for 1983, Health Service Area 1

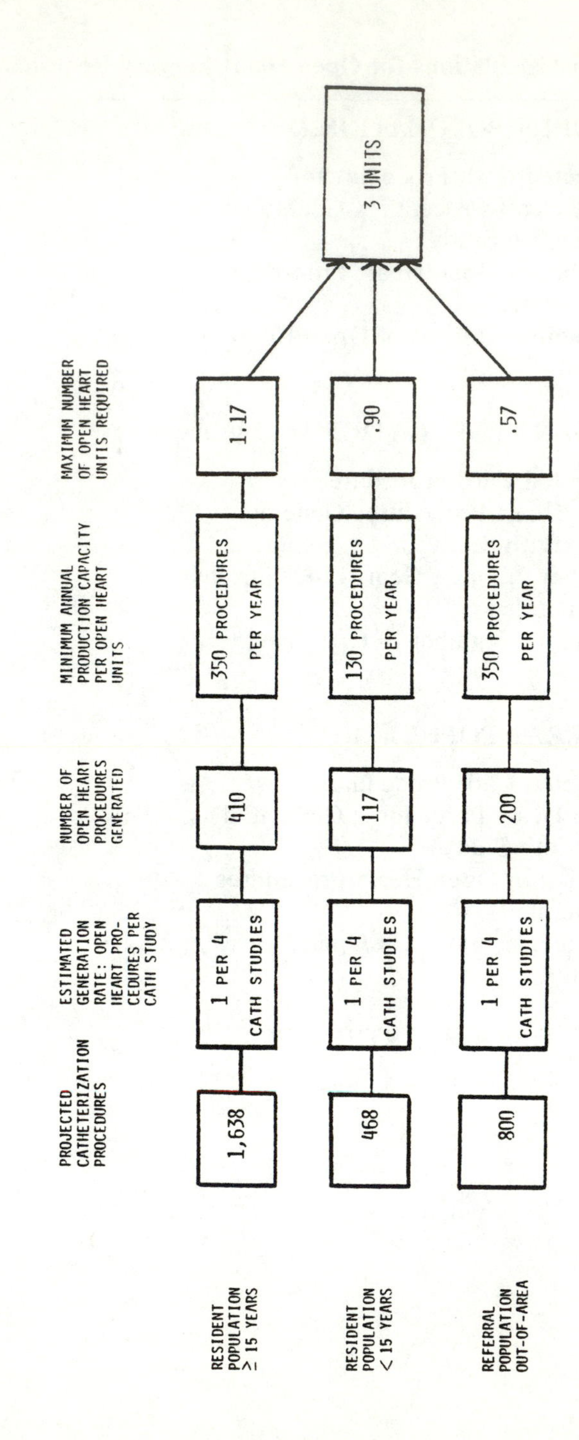

Table 8A-7 Calculations for Radiation Therapy Requirements, 1983

A. RESIDENT POPULATION

Population		= 888,000
New Cancer Patients	$= \frac{3 \times 888,000}{1,000}$	= 2,664
Patients Requiring Treatment	$= .50 \times 2,664$	= 1,332
Projected Number of Treatments	$= 30 \times 1,332$	= 39,960
Maximum Number of Megavoltage Units	$= \frac{39,960}{10,000}$	= 3.99 or 4

B. REFERRAL POPULATION

Patients Requiring Treatment		= 333
Projected Number of Treatments	$= 30 \times 333$	= 9,990
Maximum Number of Megavoltage Units	$= \frac{9,990}{10,000}$	= .99 or 1

C. TOTAL UNITS REQUIRED

$4 + 1 = 5$ units

Figure 8A-7 Radiation Therapy Requirements for 1983, Health Service Area 1

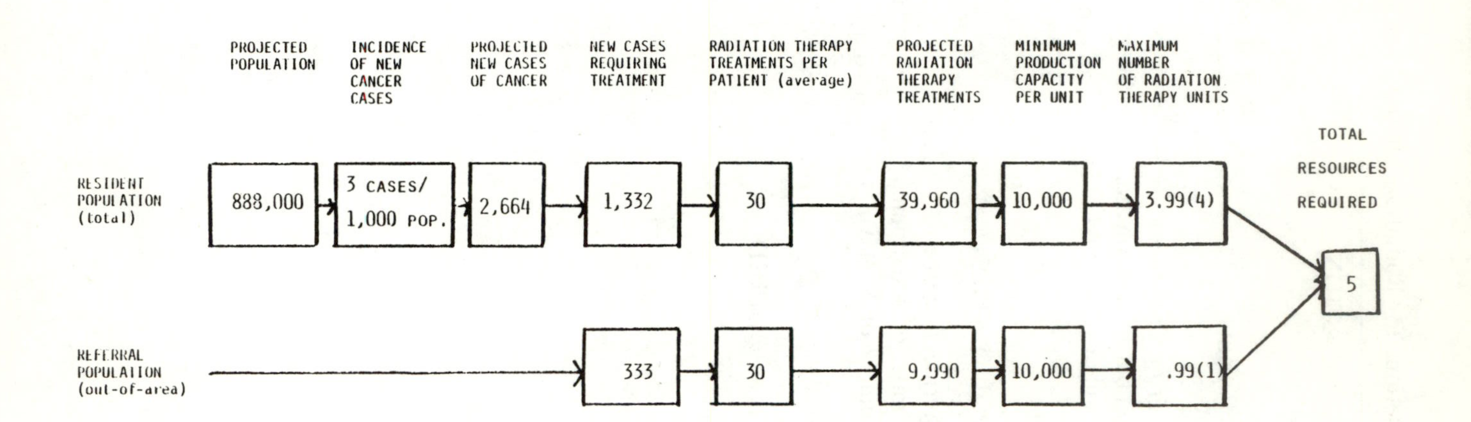

Table 8A-8 Calculations for CT Scanning Resource Requirements, 1983

A. RESIDENT POPULATION

Projected Population	= 888,000
CT Scanner/Population Ratio	= 1/200,000
CT Scanners Required	$= \dfrac{888{,}000 \times 1}{200{,}000} = 4.44$

B. OUT-OF-AREA POPULATION

Projected Population	= 4,300
CT Scanner/Population Ratio	= 1/3,000
CT Scanners Required	$= \dfrac{4{,}300 \times 1}{300{,}000} = 1.43$

C. TOTAL CT SCANNERS REQUIRED

4.44 + 1.43 = 5.87 or 6 CT Scanners

Figure 8A-8 CT Scanning Resource Requirements for 1983, Health Service Area 1

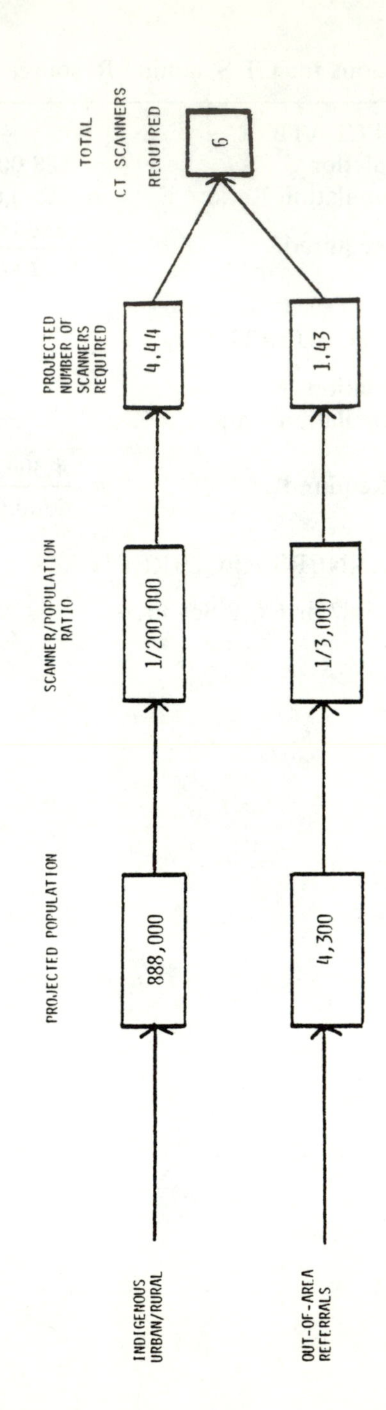

NOTES

1. The bulk of the material for this section is abstracted from Government Studies and Systems, *State-of-the-Art Report, Methods to Determine Geographic/Population Boundaries for Specific Health Services,* DHEW Contract No. HRA-231-77-0055 (Philadelphia: April 1978), pp. 5–6. The author was a consultant in the production of this volume.

2. G. J. Meneley et al., *Methodologies for Delimiting Health Service Areas* (Iowa City, Iowa: Health Services Research Center, the University of Iowa, Jan. 1977), p. 53.

3. Ibid.

4. Ibid.

5. Ibid.

6. D. L. Drosness and J. W. Lubin, "Planning Can Be Based on Patient Travel," *Modern Hospital* 106 (April 1966), pp. 92–94.

7. G. W. Shannon and G. E. A. Dever, *Health Care Delivery—Spatial Perspectives* (New York: McGraw-Hill Book Co., 1974), p. 139.

8. Ibid.

9. Rhode Island Dept. of Health, "Proposed Health Services Planning Subareas for Rhode Island, Health Planning and Resources Development, Tech. Report No. 7," Mimeographed (March 1977), p. 69.

10. Ibid., pp. 45–46.

11. Eleanor Poland and P. A. Lembcke, *Delineation of Hospital Service Districts,* U.S. Public Health Service, No. W-14 (1967), p. 895.

12. This section is modified from a letter from Dr. Frank Houser, District Health Officer, Georgia Dept. of Human Resources, Dalton, Georgia, 1978.

13. Meneley et al., *Methodologies,* p. 53.

14. J. N. Meade, "A Mathematical Model for Deriving Hospital Service Areas," *International Journal of Health Services* 4, no. 2 (Spring 1974): 353–364; and Meade, "Validity of Reporting Patient Origin Studies for Rural Hospitals," *Public Health Reports* 91, no. 1 (Jan./Feb. 1976): 62–66.

15. Government Studies and Systems, *State-of-the-Art Report,* pp. 23–25.

16. I would like to express appreciation to Gerry Rushton and Joe Meneley for their contributions in completing an accessibility analysis for Oklahoma that provided the nucleus for this section.

17. D. Eaton, R. Church, and C. ReVelle, "Location Analysis: A New Tool for Health Planners," Agency for International Development (A.I.D.), Washington, D.C., no. 53 (May 1977), p. 42.

18. G. Rushton et al., *A Statewide Plan for Regional Primary Medical and Dental Care Centers in Iowa,* Institute for Urban and Regional Research and Health Services Research Center (University of Iowa, Aug. 6, 1976), p. 82.

19. W. McClure, *Reducing Excess Hospital Capacity,* Bureau of Health Planning and Resource Development, DHEW (Oct. 15, 1976), p. 71.

20. See *National Guidelines for Health Planning,* DHEW (HRA) 78-643, March 28, 1978, for criteria reflecting population-based standards. Also, see Table 8-8 for standard-specific adjustments which may be applied to population-based planning.

21. McClure, *Reducing Excess Hospital Capacity,* p. 75.

22. Ibid., p. 76.

23. Ibid., p. 79.

24. This section on Oklahoma Hospital Planning could not have been accomplished without the services of Ann Ashmore and Karen VanWagner of the Oklahoma Health System Agency and Gerry Rushton and Joseph Meneley of the University of Iowa, Iowa City, Iowa.

25. Midwest Center for Health Planning, 702 North Blackhawk Avenue, Madison, Wisconsin 53705, "Application of the National Guidelines for Health Planning" and "Application and Adjustment Procedures Manual," Sept. 1978, 59, pp. 24–28. The Midwest Center is to be commended for producing such a fine document.

26. Ibid., pp. 26–28.

27. William E. DeBardlaben, "Basic Methods for Determining Community Resource Requirements," *Selected Methodological Approaches to Address the National Guidelines for Health Planning in Local and State Health Plan Development, A Workbook for Planners,* Health Planning and Development Center, Inc., Region IV, Atlanta, Georgia, January 1979, pp. 41–63, 186. I would like to thank the HPDC for permission to reprint selected parts of this document.

28. Ibid., pp. 45, 46.

29. Ibid., p. 46.

30. Ibid., p. 50.

31. Ibid., p. 51.

32. Ibid., p. 54.

33. Ibid.

34. Ibid., p. 60.

35. Government Studies and Systems, *State-of-the-Art Report,* pp. 29–61.

36. This appendix is abridged from William E. DeBardlaben, "Essential Analytic Steps by Specialty Areas," *Methodological Approaches to Address the National Guidelines for Health Planning in Local and State Health Plan Development, A Workbook for Planners,* Health Planning and Development Center, Inc., published by HPDC, Atlanta, Georgia, January 1979, pp. 91–134. I would like to thank the HPDC for permission to reprint selected parts of the document.

APPENDIX 8B
REFERENCES LOCATION/ALLOCATION PROBLEMS

1. Abernathy, William J., and Hershey, John C. "A Spatial-Allocation Model for Regional Health-Services Planning." *Operations Research* 20 (1972): 629–642.

2. Chapelle, R. A. "Location of Central Facilities, Heuristic Algorithms for Large Systems," Ph.D. Dissertation, Norman, Okla.: University of Oklahoma, 1970.

3. Church, Richard, and ReVelle, Charles. "The Maximal Covering Location Problem." *Papers of the Regional Science Association* 32 (Fall 1974): 101–118.

4. Dee, Norbert, and Liebman, Jon C. "Optimal Location of Public Facilities." *Naval Research Logistics Quarterly* 19 (1972): 753–759.

5. Ellwein, Leon B., and Kalberen, John T., Jr. "Optimal Location of Cancer Centers on the Basis of Population Access." *Federation Proceedings* 34 (1975): 1411–1416.

6. El-Shaieb, A. M. "A New Algorithm for Locating Sources Among Destinations." *Management Science* 20 (Oct. 1973): 221–231.

7. Francis, R. L., and Goldstein, J. N. "Location Theory: A Selective Bibliography." *Operations Research* 22 (1974): 400–410.

8. Garfinkel, R. S.; Neebe, A. W.; and Rao, M. R. "An Algorithm for the M-Medium Plant Location Problem." *Transportation* Science 8 (1974): 217–236.

9. Health Planning Research Services. *Introduction and Sample Methodology* and *A Report on the State of the Art. A Manual for Evaluating the Location of a Health Service,* vols. 1 and 2. Washington, Pa., 1976. Mimeographed.

10. Lea, A. C. "Location-Allocation Systems: An Annotated Bibliography." Discussion Paper No. 13. Dept. of Geography. Toronto: University of Toronto, May 1973.

11. ReVelle, Charles; Marks, Davis; and Liebman, Jon C. "An Analysis of Private and Public Sector Location Models." *Management Science* 16 (1970): 492–707.

12. Revelle, Charles; Toregas, Constantine; and Falkson, Louis. "Applications of the Location Set-Covering Problem." *Geographical Analysis* 8 (1976): 65–76.

13. Scott, Allen J. "Dynamic Location-Allocation Systems: Some Basic Planning Strategies." *Environment and Planning* 3 (1971): 73–82.

14. Scott, Allen J. "Location-Allocation Systems: A Review." *Geographical Analysis* 2 (April 1970): 95–119.

15. Shannon, Gary W., and Dever, G. E. Alan. *Health Care Delivery: Spatial Perspectives.* New York: McGraw-Hill Book Co., 1974.

16. Shannon, Gary W.; Spurlock, Carl W.; Gladin, Steven T.; and Skinner, James L. "A Method for Evaluating the Geographic Accessibility of Health Service." *The Professional Geographer* 27 (February 1975): 30–36.

17. Shuman, Larry J.; Hardwick, C. Patrick; and Huber, George A. "Location of Ambulatory Care Centers in a Metropolitan Area." *Health Services Research* 8 (Summer 1973): 121–138.

18. Tapiero, Charles S. "Transportation-Location-Allocation Problems Over Time." *Journal of Regional Science* 11 (December 1971): 377–384.

19. Toregas, Constantine, and Revelle, Charles. "Optimal Location under Time or Distance Constraints." *Papers of the Regional Science Assn.* 28 (Fall 1972): 133–143.

20. Toregas, Constantine; Swain, Ralph; Revelle, Charles; and Bergman, Lawrence. "The Location of Emergency Service Facilities." *Operations Research* 19 (1971): 1363–1373.

21. Wesolowsky, George O. "Dynamic Facility Location." *Management Science* 19 (1973): 1241–1248.

22. Wesolowsky, George O., and Truscott, William G. "The Multiperiod Location-Allocation Problem with Relocation of Facilities." *Management Science* 22 (September 1975): 57–65.

23. Zimmerman, James P. "Service Areas and Their Needs Must be Reassessed." *Hospitals* 49 (Sept. 1975): 46–48.

Chapter 9

Computer Graphics in Health Planning

BACKGROUND

Many trends are impacting on the changing scene of health care in this country: the shift from medical to social epidemiology, the shift from infectious to chronic disease patterns, the emergence of community health with emphasis on population groups in communities rather than individuals in clinics, and the use of computer graphics as a tool for community administrative decision making. The present chapter is concerned with the latter trend.

Medical care in this country has traditionally focused on the patient or the individual. This tradition has evolved from an infectious disease pattern in which cause-and-effect relationships were single and simple. Disease patterns are no longer infectious, however. Now they are chronic and noninfectious, and the causes and effects are not single and simple, but multiple and complex. Consequently, the dimension of the community had to be added to medical care.

In the 1980s, the focus on the community—the new health recipient—will be crucial to the holistic and wellness policies outlined previously. This new direction, however, suggests the need for new approaches to present community health information. One such approach, computer graphs, is not new, per se, but its application to community health usually has been limited and not well represented.

The practical use of computer graphics has been pioneered predominantly through avant-garde engineering technology by persons associated with the aerospace industry.[1] In the past, the medium of graphics has created the representation of geographic phenomena primarily for visualization. More recently, however, some administrative and planning applications of computer graphics output have surfaced in the health and health-related literature.[2 3 4] Researchers, planners, and administrators in the community health field are just beginning, however, to employ health-oriented, computer-generated graphics for planning, evaluation, and decision making. For the most part, such applications have not been well documented in the professional literature; yet they are well represented in local and state government publications and in many health systems agency plans.[5] The latter plans have integrated health planning with health statistics by utilizing computer graphics as a communication format. They have thus been able to present basic patterns and trends which aid in evaluation, decisionmaking, and policy formulation. These plans have also emphasized the importance of having the data on health variables translated into visual information to achieve effective applications.

Thus, though traditional graphics is still very much with us, computer graphics is able to translate health planning and health statistics into an effective format that various levels of management can use to determine appropriate needs of the future.

TRADITIONAL GRAPHICS

The graphic depiction of health data has usually taken the traditional forms of tables, hand-drawn charts, graphs, and maps. However, the laborious accumulation, reduction, and formulation of health data into such finished products frequently consumed many person-hours. Reproduction of the results was often tailored to publication requirements rather than to adequate graphic presentation of the data. The end products were sometimes "soft" (inaccurate), nonuniform, "not quite right" for the accompanying text, or lacking in audience appeal. Moreover, the text and the accompanying graphics were often research oriented and consequently not immediately applicable to current health program planning or to community health problems.

Graphics produced by traditional methods is still useful for some purposes. But they have become essentially obsolete for the production of the display and data communications necessary to major planning, policy, and evaluation decisions. For instance, policy decisions affecting health programming are often based on highly specialized, up-to-date maps of ephemeral subject matter that may be used only a few times. The slow procedures and tremendous costs of producing many traditional graphics definitely do not satisfy such health administration and planning needs. Indeed, the graphics may not even be available when decisions are being made. Of course, 5, 10, or even 15 timely computer maps will not guarantee improvement over one well-conceived, traditionally produced map. Nevertheless, by automating the graphics process and by improving the material, equipment, and techniques, it has been possible to produce more maps in less time and at lower cost.

COMPUTER GRAPHICS

The proliferation of health data has produced a need to comprehend information, especially "fragile" information, produced from such data in a rapid, accurate, and discerning fashion. Administrators in problem-oriented, crisis-producing, health-associated industries, such as health planning, hospitals, health systems agencies (HSAs), and community epidemiological programs must depend upon the absorption and the digestion of precise, opportune information. Computer-generated graphics, presented in quick, accurate, versatile, and interactive formats, is a viable response to this requirement. Computer-generated graphics is not, of course, a panacea for absorption information, but it does provide a method to produce uniform and timely presentation of information. In any event, before undertaking the expenditure of funds and manpower for integrating computer graphics hardware and software into the program mainstream, one should be aware of the advantages and disadvantages of the procedures involved.

Advantages of Computer Graphics

As health problems and the information needed to understand and deal with them multiply in scale, variety, intensity, and complexity, better means are needed to analyze, display, and communicate health information.[6] Computer graphics has distinct advantages because it allows a user to deal with the problems of scale, variety, intensity, and complexity through better visual communication. Following are some advantages to the user:

1. The method is fast, efficient, simple, and economical.
2. Computer-generated maps may provide a clearer view of information than most tables or charts.
3. Data changing with time may be followed with a series of maps.
4. Several variables that are spatially identical and contiguous may be analyzed simultaneously.
5. It is relatively easy to select and display various sample data sets.
6. The scale of the map and the data range levels of the computer graphics may be selected according to the user's need.
7. Computer graphics can be interactive in that a trial product may be viewed before it is final, thus avoiding costly production errors.

8. By mapping, the user is able to visualize rapidly large volumes of data.

These advantages indicate that computer graphics has considerable merit compared to traditional graphics. The major advantage of computer graphics is its capability to integrate health statistics with health services for effective administration, planning, and policy decisionmaking.

Disadvantages of Computer Graphics

As with most methods or techniques, there are disadvantages to the use of computer graphics:

1. The majority of time is spent coding the data to be mapped. The "base map" also must be digitized. If done by hand, this is time-consuming. Automatic digitizers are available, however, to complete this part of the task.
2. Considerable initial time may be spent reducing the data to fit available equipment and software programs.
3. It is difficult to avoid the pitfall of attempting to map everything.
4. Unless a user has basic knowledge of the techniques of mapmaking and graphic illustration, many problems will arise relative to the scale of the map, choice of symbols, type of map, selection of the legend, and level of measurement to use (that is, nominal, ordinal, interval, or ratio).
5. The user may not know the usefulness of the output or, for that matter, may not even be aware of the quality of the input.
6. It is difficult to select the most appropriate map or graphic for the presentation of data. (Chapter 5 provides a guide to the selection of various methods of illustration.)
7. Interpretation of data is critical, and caution is warranted at this stage.
8. The hardware and software must be tailored to the user's needs.

In light of these disadvantages, it must be stressed that computer-generated maps and graphics are no better than the quality of the data put into them. Most of these limitations are not crucial if the appropriate personnel are recruited to produce the graphics. There will be a major emerging need to recognize this type of professional as part of an agency's organizational structure for community health in the 1980s. Because the advantages far outweigh the disadvantages, the above limitations should not represent insurmountable barriers to implementing computer graphics.

The Problem of Noise

Another aspect of computer graphics that could be considered a disadvantage is noise. This problem is not limited to the visualization and communication process which graphics promotes. Noise may, in fact, take three forms: (1) visual noise, (2) statistical noise, and (3) semantic noise. Visual and statistical noises are related to the effective presentation of information. For instance, removing various types of statistical noise from the data prior to mapping can often improve substantially the final map product. The removal can be done by smoothing, massaging, or filtering the data in premap operations to reduce or eliminate excessive statistical presentation stemming from data error. In a strict statistical sense, noise results when complex and complicated formulas are used to convey a point when, in fact, a simple, uncomplicated procedure can provide the same results.

After resolving the problem of statistical noise, one may also face the problem of visual noise. This is the excessive accumulation of symbols, patterns, and legends, leading to graphic information overload. In this case, so much information is presented on a map that the result is a poor, cluttered, and unstructured graphic with low communication value. The map is essentially useless, and the reader is left confused as to its actual purpose. Because a basic reason for using graphics is to present information visually for effective communication, graphics should at all costs avoid the problem of visual noise. A picture is indeed worth a thousand words.

Semantic noise results from the writer's verbosity and a language structure that is difficult to comprehend. Here, terse and uncomplicated word structures are needed to effect the desired results. The growth of computer graphics may, in fact, be attributed partially to the need to overcome semantic noise. Certainly, one approach toward overcoming this problem is to produce a clear and concise computer graphic. Nevertheless, the concept of semantic noise, as well as visual and statistical noise, is inherent in the presentation of effective and efficient computer-generated graphics.

TYPES OF COMPUTER GRAPHICS

Three basic, generally available computer techniques may be used to produce graphics: (1) character-printed, (2) line-drawn or plotted, and (3) output on cathode ray tubes.[7]

Character-Printed Maps

Character-printed maps are represented by typewriter characters and produced on standard computer paper (Figure 9-1). When a map to be produced is larger than the width of the printout, the printing is done in sections and joined to form the complete map. Boundaries of such maps are only approximated and, therefore, are inadequately delineated. In most cases, this is not a serious hindrance in the presentation of health information, however, since much of the material is not dependent upon exact locations. Shading to present areal data is accomplished by overprinting characters. To represent areas, however, it may be more practical to show the actual data on the map as points rather than do shading. The major benefit of producing character-printed maps is that a plotting device is not needed. Most computer systems have the software capability to produce some form of character-printed map or graphic.

Line-Drawn Graphics

Line-drawn graphics and maps may be produced as plots from drum or flatbed plotters (Figure 9-2). Unlike the character-printed map, the line-drawn map exercises boundary accuracy, and specific lines may be drawn to represent various spatial arrangements. Thus, a line-drawn map may provide health information details by points, lines, or areas. A three-dimensional diagram will show magnitude, while the character-printed map is generally useful only for denoting points or areas. The distinction between character-printed and line-drawn maps reflects differences in hardware capability and versatility in presenting health information for community analysis. If the user has a choice, the line-drawn map is recommended.

Interactive Graphics

Interactive graphics, or output on the cathode ray tube (CRT), has been available for several years, but its application in health planning has only recently been developed.[8] Graphics on the CRT are generated with electronic plotters. Because the graphic can be viewed on the CRT screen, it can be manipulated in several ways, for example, by changing the scale, the horizontal angle, or the rotation. This type of graphic displays lines and points very well, but it produces complex areal patterns only with difficulty.[9] For perspective views, a vertical exaggeration of the graphic can be provided. The user controls these various changes with a light pen through the keyboard. Thus, the interactive capability allows the user to

Figure 9-1 Medical Resources: Manpower, General Practitioners, 1970

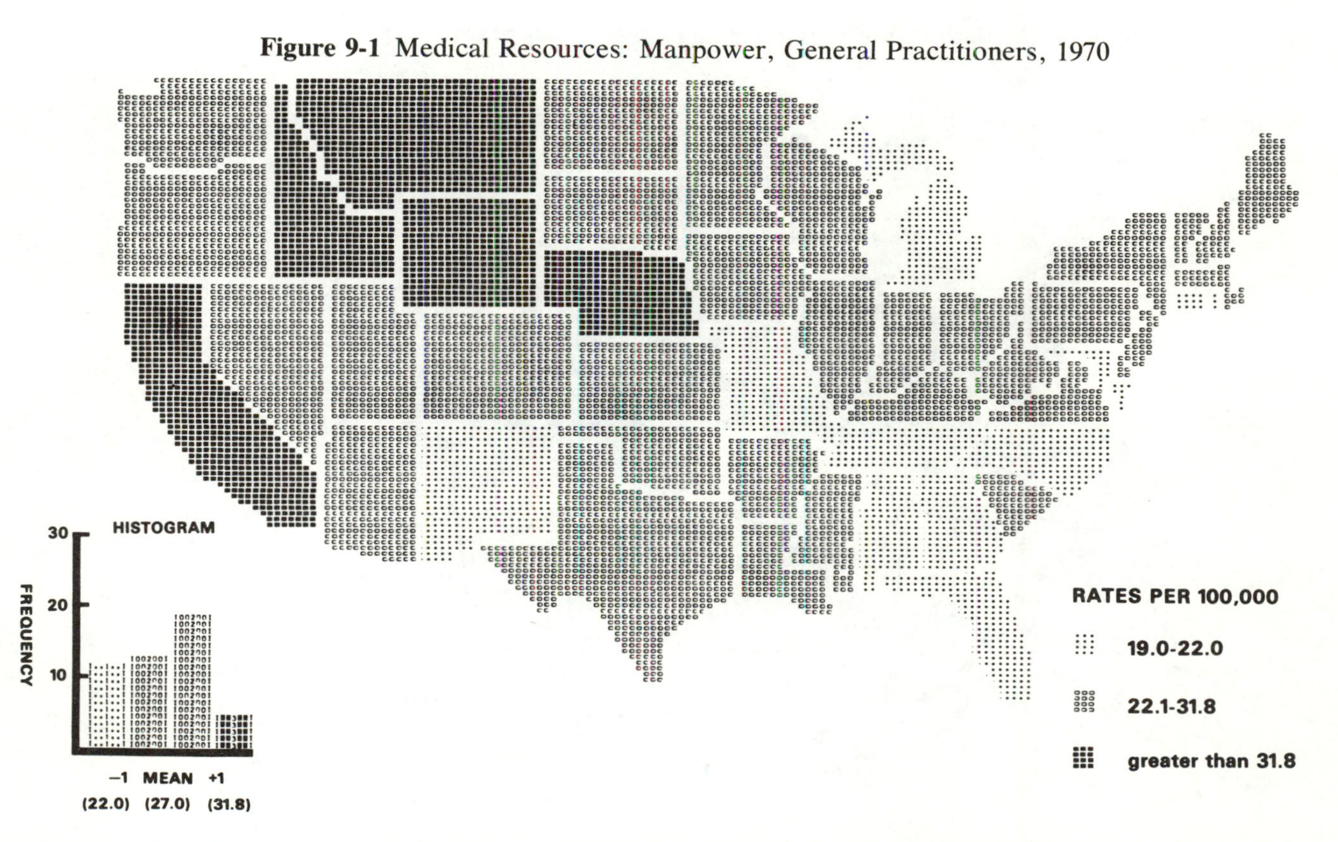

Source: G. E. A. Dever, "Locational Characteristics of Selected Manpower in the United States," *Atlanta Economic Review* 24 (1974), p. 44.

Figure 9-2 Lay Midwives

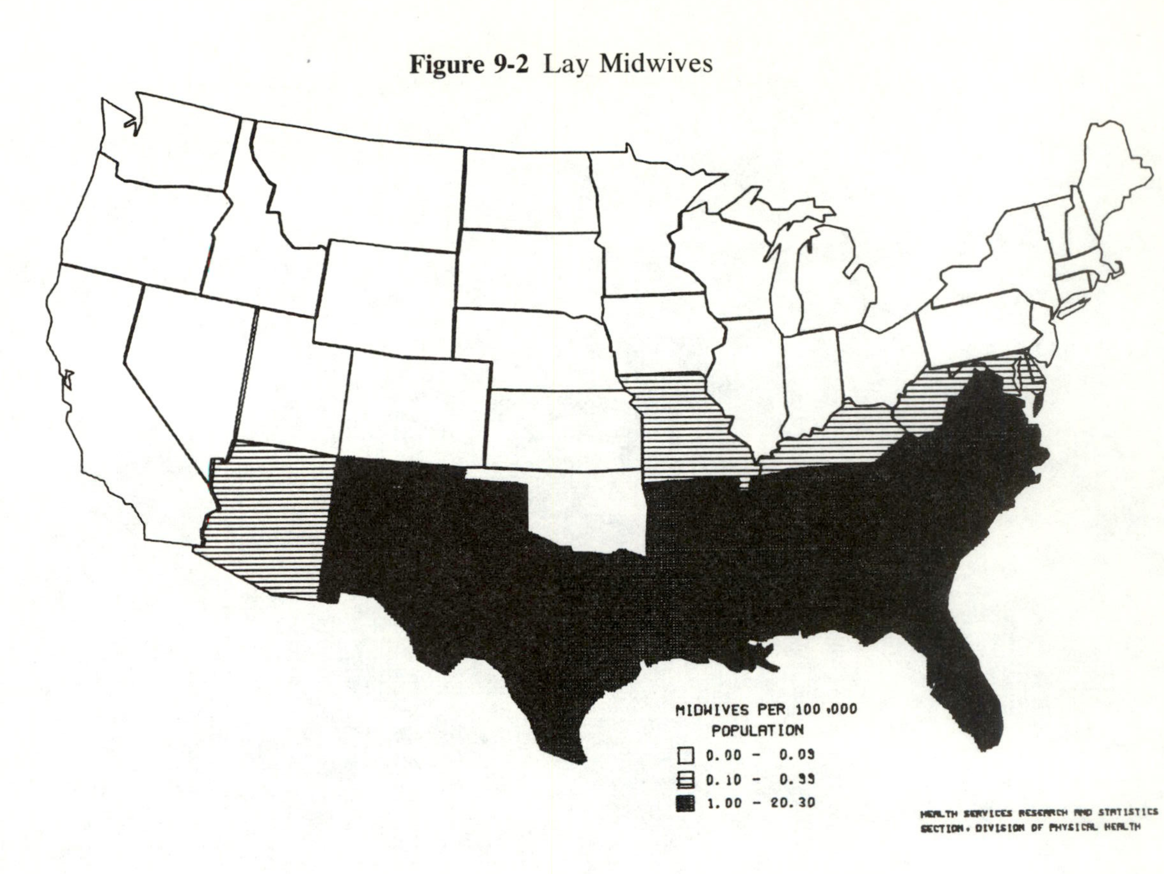

Source: Health Services Research and Statistics Section, Division of Physical Health, Georgia Department of Human Resources (1974).

experiment with the graphic until the right product is achieved. The final product may then be reproduced as a hard copy.

Perhaps the only disadvantage to CRT interactive graphics is the cost. Interactive graphics is, however, generally not as readily available as line printers or plotters. In addition, the size of the CRT screen inhibits the size of the display, requiring the user to decide on either a total display with little detail or a partial display of an area with considerable detail.

COMMUNITY HEALTH ANALYSIS AND COMPUTER GRAPHICS

Though practical involvement with computer-generated graphics in the management of community health programs is not widespread at present, the resurgence of interest in health care in the past decade has opened many fruitful areas for using computer graphics. One such area, as outlined in recent legislation, is in the health systems agencies (HSAs).[10] The HSA offers a clear potential for computer-generated displays because it is required to assemble, analyze, communicate, and display data concerning the following:

1. The health status, including the determinants of health status, of service area residents. (A holistic/wellness model is recommended for this in Chapter 1.)
2. The status of the health care delivery system and the area residents' use of that system.
3. The effects of the health care delivery system on the health of area residents.
4. The number, type, and location of the area's health resources, including services, manpower, and facilities.
5. The pattern of utilization of the area's health resources.
6. The factors of environmental and occupational exposure which effect immediate and long-term health conditions.

If the HSA is to provide answers in these areas, it must exploit its potential for using computer-generated graphics. Not all HSAs, of course, will need or want to establish ongoing mechanisms for developing computer graphics. Many resources associated with universities and consultants are available for completing computer graphics. Indeed, it is frequently more advantageous—and advisable—to employ outside resources with experience in the health field. In addition to the six areas noted above, there are other areas related to community health (hospitals, health departments, health maintenance organizations, insurance companies) in which more sophisticated analyses may be provided. For example:

1. The basic functional aspects of hospital accessibility—time, cost, and distance—can be mapped to show areas of high or low accessibility. This approach is valid for determining patient accessibility to emergency rooms, neighborhood health clinics, county public health departments, patient-physician visits, and nursing homes.
2. Medical trade areas or hospital service areas may be delineated through patient-origin studies. Such studies may identify patients as points or line flows indicating volume or as areas using circles with variable radii or ellipses based on the standard deviation of an areal distribution.
3. Manpower data may be mapped to illustrate underserviced, scarcity, and oversupplied areas. The map would aid in making decisions as to the development and location of satellite clinics and mobile health vans. Moreover, strategies in the recruitment process could be based on locational needs for medical and paramedical personnel. (Location/allocation methods are examined more thoroughly in Chapter 8.)
4. Disease patterns may be mapped in relationship to facility and manpower distribution. If the health-planning organization possesses the appropriate expertise, it may initiate studies dealing with the measurement and assessment of health status related to available resources.

The trend in health planning toward a greater attention to population groups in communities than on individuals in clinics has facilitated the above uses of computer graphics. The shift in disease patterns from infectious to chronic diseases has also stimulated more widespread interest in these areas of use. In the case of morbidity or mortality data, computer graphics has functional uses in addition to those presented above. It can, for example, aid in:

1. Identifying high or low risk areas for specified diseases. There is a critical need to reduce the potential for random variability in the data in such presentations. This can be accomplished either by expanding the time period of the study or by aggregating the areal units being investigated.
2. Rating a community on the health status of the population by providing a community diagnosis. This is similar to the above use, except that periodic community epidemiological studies would be expected.

3. Setting priorities for allocation of resources in health programs by developing policy for state and district programs.
4. Planning health and social programs.
5. Making reports or presentations of information to state legislators, special governors' councils, boards of health, planning agencies, consumer groups, and news media.
6. Periodically updating baseline or benchmark epidemiological data, or other health data to indicate changes in evaluation measures from one time frame to another.

In spite of the multiple uses of computer-generated maps and graphics, the technique is by no means the panacea for solving the health problems facing this country. It is basically merely an efficient and effective way of communicating and displaying pertinent information.

APPLICATION OF COMPUTER GRAPHICS IN COMMUNITY HEALTH

The major uses of computer graphics can be best demonstrated by showing practical applications in community health at three scales of analysis, national, state, and city, considering in each case its uses in health planning and health policy.

The National Scale

At the national scale, the data are usually aggregated by counties, by state economic areas, or by states to illustrate geographical patterns of health information. The selected administrative units show the relative differences in pattern perception and information content. Computer-generated graphs can further illustrate the data by providing different methods of information display.

Manpower Distributions

The two maps in Figures 9-1 and 9-2 illustrate manpower distribution by state. Figure 9-1 is produced by the SYMAP procedure (character printed), while Figure 9-2 is plotted (line drawn) from a Calforms package.[11] The two maps illustrate patterns of need for specific types of manpower at the national scale. Figure 9-1 includes a histogram providing the frequency distribution of the data. Federal and regional offices may use the spatial portrayal of the rates for manpower planning and for formalizing health policy in decision strategies for manpower needs.

Mortality Distributions

Maps for this purpose were produced by an automated cartography system developed at the National Institutes of Health. The system interfaces with an integrated graphics software package with output to COM (computer output on microfilm). Images are produced on a cathode ray tube (CRT) and photographed. Color separation negatives are used in the preparation of the printing plots. The illustrations in the *Atlas of Cancer Mortality for U.S. Counties*[12] and the *Atlas of Cancer Mortality Among U.S. Nonwhites*[13] show age-adjusted death rates of various types of cancers for the white and nonwhite population, aggregated by state economic areas (SEA), from 1959 to 1969. The maps in these publications are strikingly unique in the method of reproduction and the visual impact conveyed by color. While demonstrating present descriptive epidemiology, they also provide stimulus to future analytical investigations. For example, the Center for Disease Control has begun regional and local investigations of cancer of the lung, mouth, and throat. The maps could also be used for interregional mortality comparisons to set national standards for establishing realistic goals and objectives for health status measurement. The legends on the maps show relative measures of significance in the U.S. rates.

Figures 9-3 through 9-5 are examples of graphics from *Patterns in Cancer Mortality in the United States.*[14] Figure 9-3 shows four line-printer maps (SYMAP) of lung cancer mortality for white and nonwhite males and females in 1950–67. A plotted graph in Figure 9-4 shows age-specific death rates of lung cancer by five-year age groups for white and nonwhite males and females. Figure 9-5 shows age-adjusted death rates for lung cancer for white and nonwhite males and females in 1950–67. When combined, the three figures illustrate risk factors for lung cancer mortality relative to age, sex, race, geography, and time, and also provide a description of the epidemiology of lung cancer. These graphic illustrations of lung cancer mortality are unique in that they have been plotted or printed by computer to provide a detailed level of information.

The State Scale

The state scale illustrates data which delineate more precise patterns and relationships. Interpretation at this scale of investigation (county administrative units) is most beneficial to community epidemiologists, state and local health program managers, HSA planners, and health policy formulators.

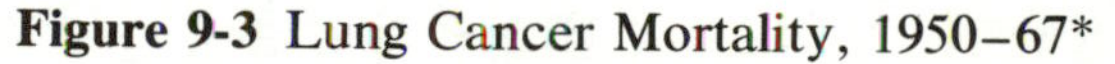

Figure 9-3 Lung Cancer Mortality, 1950–67*

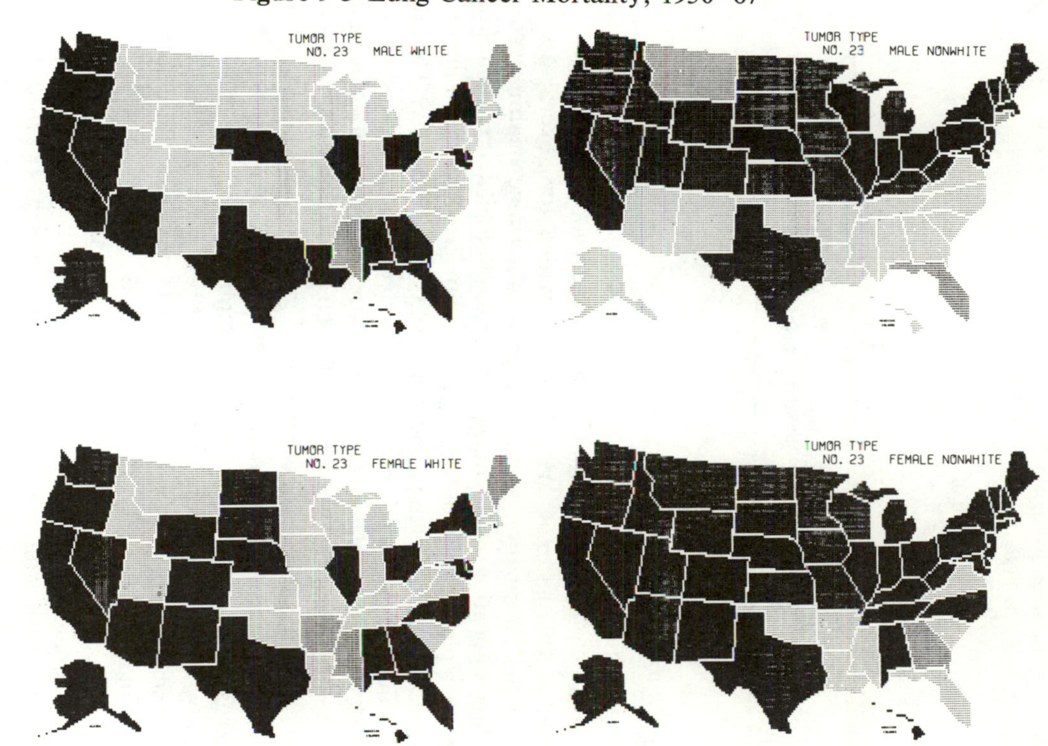

*See page 320 for shading key.

Source: Fred Burbank, *Patterns in Cancer Mortality in the U.S.: 1950–67* (Washington: U.S. Government Printing Office, 1971), p. 207.

Figure 9-3 continued

Static geographic distribution significance codes

Code No.	Meaning
1	Lower at $P < 0.002$
2	Lower at $P < 0.02$
3	No difference at $P > 0.02$
4	Higher at $P < 0.02$
5	Higher at $P < 0.002$

	1	2	3	4	5
SHADING SYMBOLS					

Mortality Analysis

Figures 9-6 through 9-8 provide the user with a varied information display, demonstrating risk factors for lung cancer mortality by age, sex, race, time, and geographic area. When provided for several disease categories, this information may be used to determine health program policies, fund allocations, and community epidemiological investigations.

Figure 9-6, a plotter map, depicts age-sex adjusted death rates, illustrating the spatial pattern of lung cancer mortality for 1970–74.[15] The map also shows the rates as being above average, average, and below average relative to the state's average. Figure 9-7 is a plotter graph, illustrating male and female crude death rates per 100,000 population for lung cancer for 1950–74.[16] Figure 9-8 is another plotted graphic, a disease pyramid, showing lung cancer deaths as percentages, by age, race, and sex.[17]

An interesting application of computer graphics at the national scale is illustrated by Schnell and Monmonier (Figure 9-9).[18] Geographic associations are exhibited between the birth and death rates, and a third category shows the mortality-fertility ratio. The maps also present four time periods, suggesting change over time and variation in space. These three-dimensional block diagrams show quite vividly the regional pattern of birth and death rates. The line-plotter maps were produced by SYMVU, a computer program which generates three-dimensional statistical surfaces. To allow for comparison among the time periods and between the two rates, the same vertical scale was used for all maps in the first two columns. A constant vertical scale was used for the remaining maps in the third column. The results clearly indicate a decline in the birth rate (note the decrease in height of the graphics), while the death rate

Figure 9-4 Death Rates for Lung Cancer, by Age Group, 1950–67

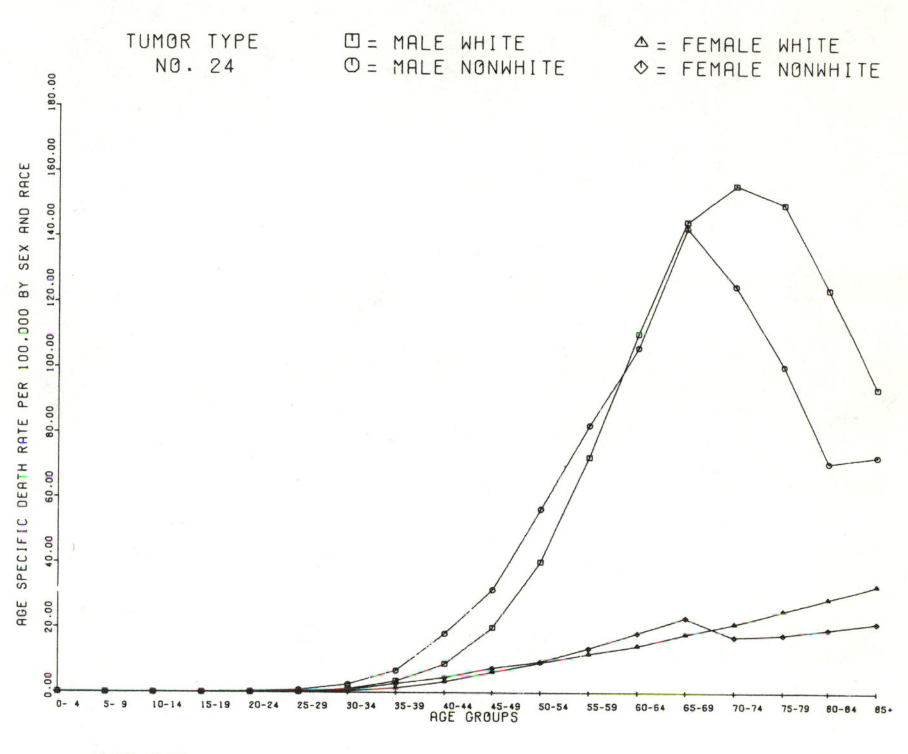

TUMOR TYPE NO. 24	MALE		FEMALE	
	WHITE	NONWHITE	WHITE	NONWHITE
0- 4	0.0251*	0.0521	0.0162	0.0316
5- 9	0.0114	0.0227	0.0099	0.0113
10-14	0.0143	0.0389	0.0128	0.0648
15-19	0.0296	0.0639	0.0424	0.0
20-24	0.1155	0.2124	0.0545	0.1642
25-29	0.2628	0.6787	0.1419	0.3299
30-34	1.1541	2.4542	0.5234	0.6897
35-39	3.5769	6.7087	1.4749	2.6866
40-44	8.8587	18.0784	3.4166	4.5519
45-49	20.0387	31.5792	6.3793	7.5197
50-54	40.1848	56.4175	9.2650	9.4150
55-59	72.4367	82.2068	12.0157	13.6203
60-64	110.3197	106.0460	14.4815	18.3200
65-69	144.5569	142.6089	18.1084	23.0590
70-74	155.6987	124.8469	21.2886	17.1338
75-79	149.8107	100.3662	25.2924	17.7921
80-84	123.8201	70.6254	28.9840	19.5135
85+	93.5631	72.6301	33.0680	21.4256

* AGE SPECIFIC DEATH RATE PER 100,000

Source: Fred Burbank, *Patterns in Cancer Mortality in the U.S.:* 1950–67 (Washington: U.S. Government Printing Office, 1971), p. 208.

Figure 9-5 Age-Adjusted Death Rates for Lung Cancer, 1950–67

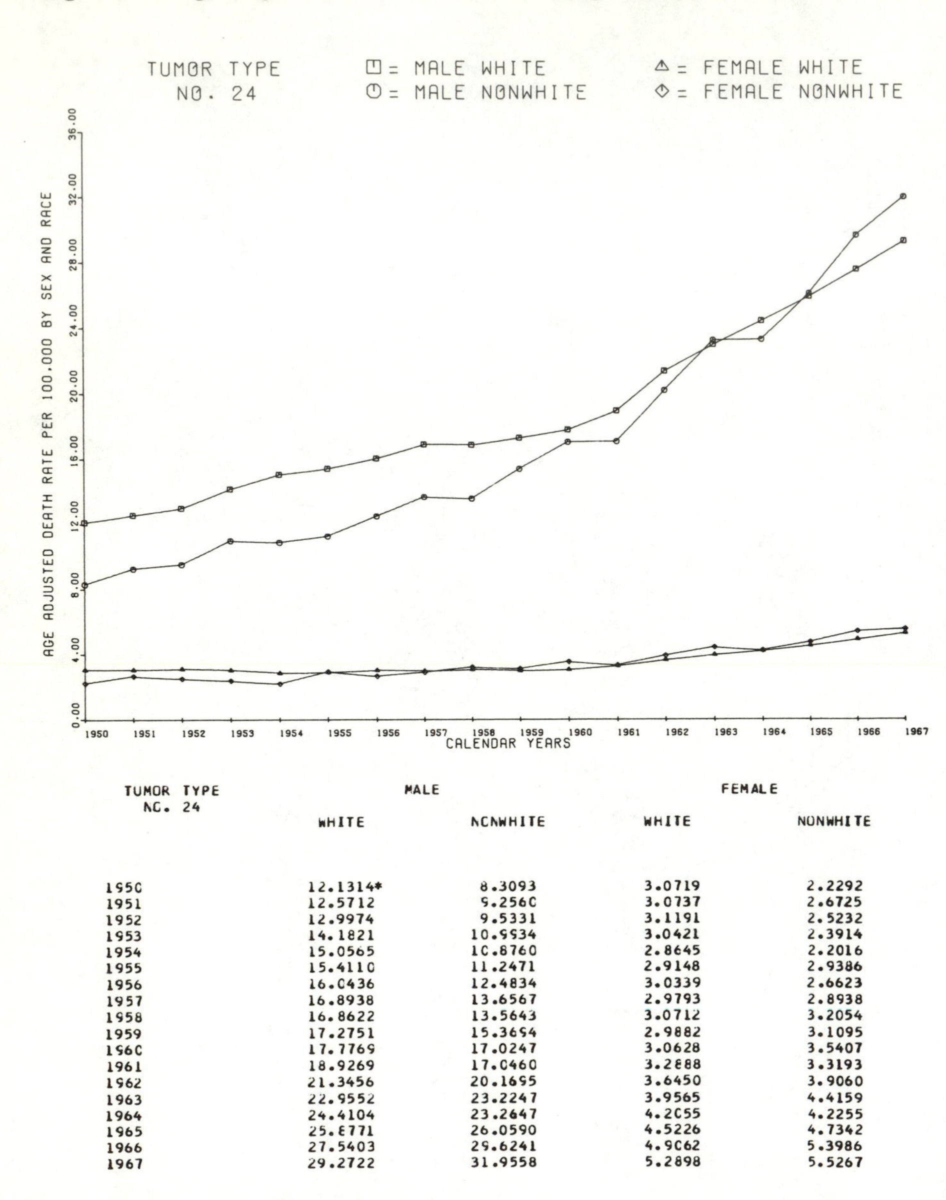

TUMOR TYPE NO. 24	MALE		FEMALE	
	WHITE	NONWHITE	WHITE	NONWHITE
1950	12.1314*	8.3093	3.0719	2.2292
1951	12.5712	9.2560	3.0737	2.6725
1952	12.9974	9.5331	3.1191	2.5232
1953	14.1821	10.9934	3.0421	2.3914
1954	15.0565	10.8760	2.8645	2.2016
1955	15.4110	11.2471	2.9148	2.9386
1956	16.0436	12.4834	3.0339	2.6623
1957	16.8938	13.6567	2.9793	2.8938
1958	16.8622	13.5643	3.0712	3.2054
1959	17.2751	15.3694	2.9882	3.1095
1960	17.7769	17.0247	3.0628	3.5407
1961	18.9269	17.0460	3.2888	3.3193
1962	21.3456	20.1695	3.6450	3.9060
1963	22.9552	23.2247	3.9565	4.4159
1964	24.4104	23.2647	4.2055	4.2255
1965	25.8771	26.0590	4.5226	4.7342
1966	27.5403	29.6241	4.9062	5.3986
1967	29.2722	31.9558	5.2898	5.5267

* AGE ADJUSTED DEATH RATE PER 100,000

Source: Fred Burbank, *Patterns in Cancer Mortality in the U.S.: 1950–67* (Washington: U.S. Government Printing Office, 1971), p. 209.

Figure 9-6 Cancer of the Trachea, Bronchus, and Lung, 1970–1974

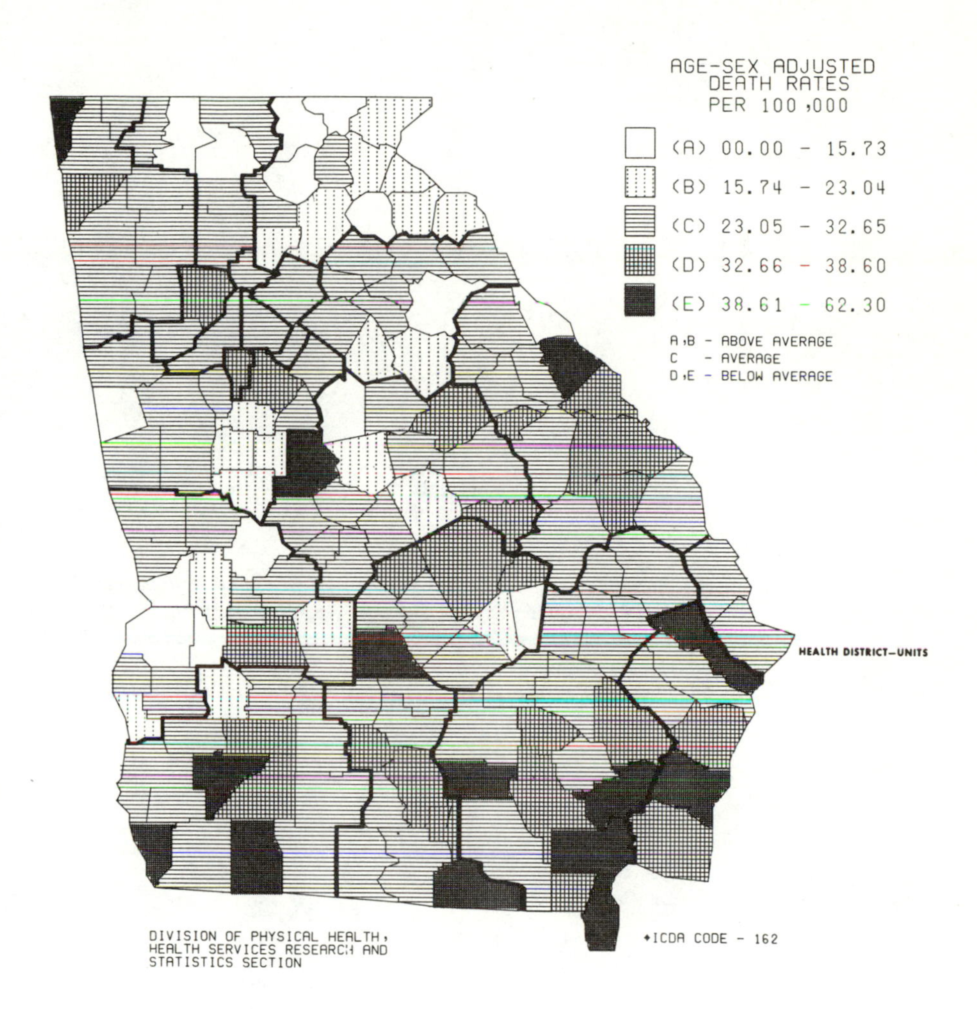

Source: Office of Health Services Research and Statistics, *Disease Patterns of the 70s* (Atlanta: Ga. Dept. of Human Resources, Div. of Physical Health, Aug. 1976), p. 89.

Figure 9-7 Cancer of the Trachea, Bronchus, and Lung, 1950–1974

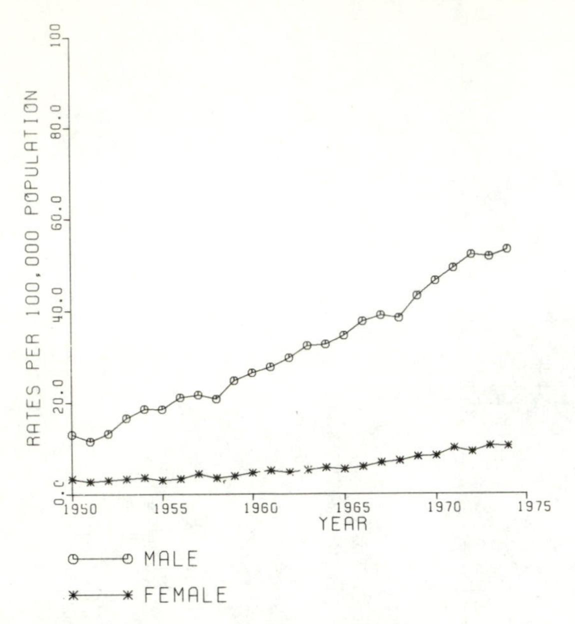

Source: Office of Health Services Research and Statistics, *Disease Patterns of the 70s* (Atlanta: Ga. Dept. of Human Resources, Div. of Physical Health, Aug. 1976), p. 90.

Figure 9-8 Cancer of the Trachea, Bronchus, and Lung, 1970–1974

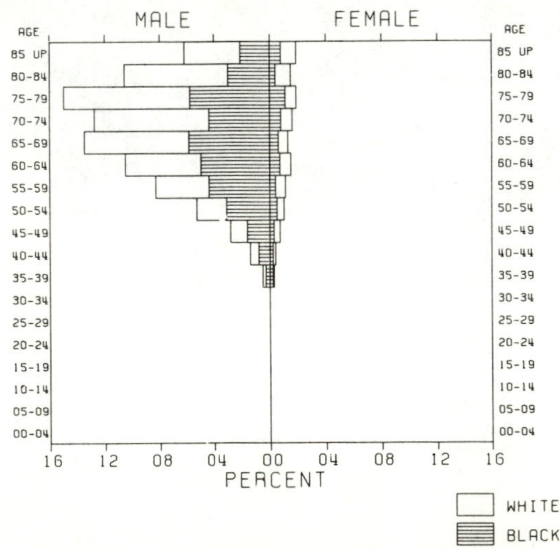

Source: Office of Health Services Research and Statistics, *Disease Patterns of the 70s* (Atlanta: Ga. Dept. of Human Resources, Div. of Physical Health, Aug. 1976), p. 90.

Figure 9-9 The Changing Topography of U.S. Vital Rates

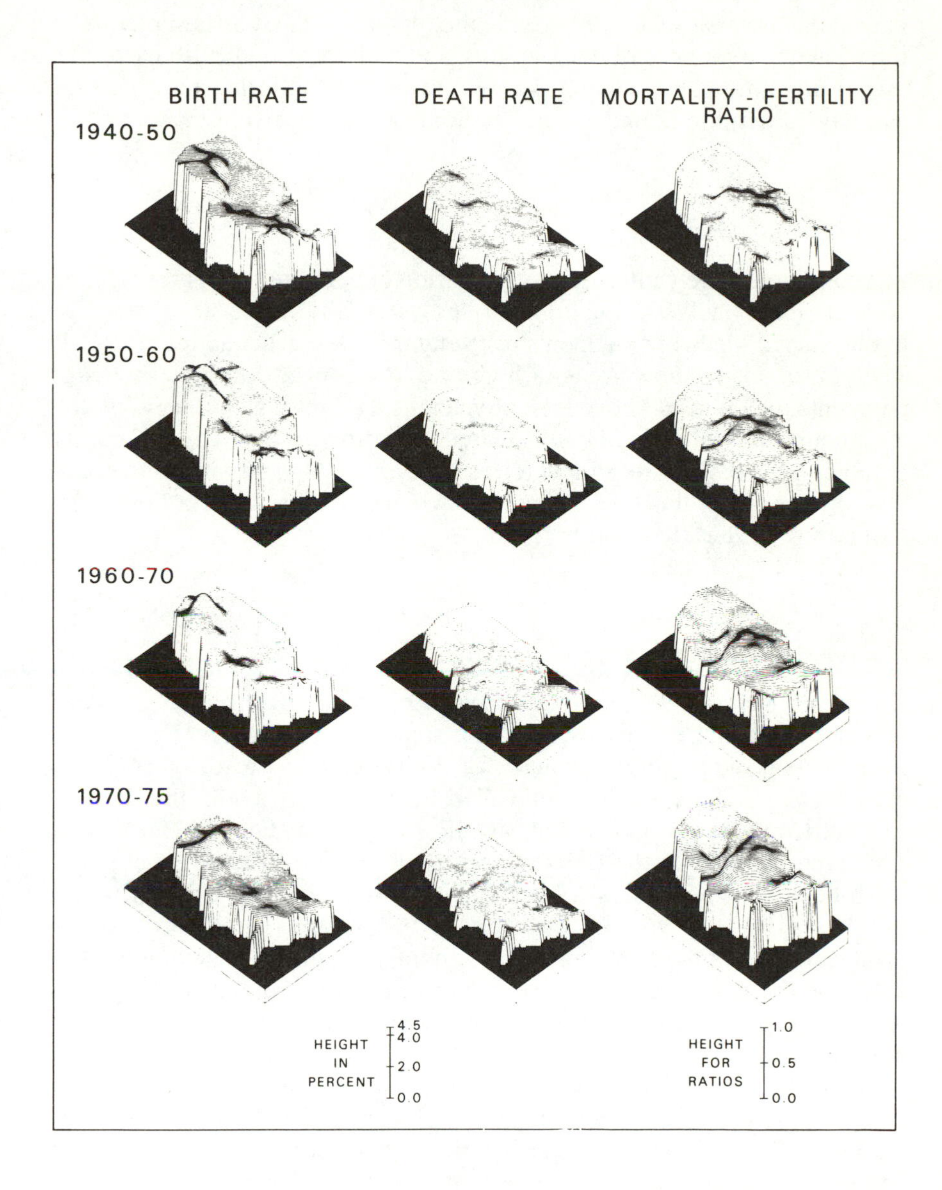

Source: George A. Schnell and Mark S. Monmonier, *Intercom* 6, No. 8 (Aug. 1978) p. 9; from "The Mortality-Fertility Ratio: A Useful Measure for Describing Demographic Change in the U.S., 1940–1975," *Geographical Survey,* in press.

remains relatively constant. The ratio between the two increased greatly over the time periods. The application of this kind of three-dimensional map at the national scale can provide the planner with an instant picture of the changing dynamics of demography and its impact on health care. The use of multiple maps showing various rates over differing time periods can have a definite impact on policy analysis and decision making.

Fiscal Health Analysis

Another extremely interesting application of computer graphics is in the area of fiscal analysis. Figure 9-10 shows a fiscal analysis of average Medicaid and Medicare payments per vendor in Georgia counties in 1972.[19] The plotted maps show areas of high and low concentrations of average payments to vendors—hospitals, physicians, and nursing homes—in dollar amounts. By showing health-related cash flow in this way, computer graphics can present areas in which to investigate high payments to counties. As a result of this type of analysis, Georgia did, in fact, initiate strict monitoring of the Medicaid program.

Manpower Analysis

Figures 9-11 and 9-12 show two types of graphics, three-dimensional and graduated circles, representing the same set of data. The Figure 9-11 three-dimensional map on primary care physicians in Iowa in 1972 was generated by a mapping program called SYMVU, written by the Laboratory for Computer Graphics and Spatial Analysis of Harvard University. This program utilizes the Calcomp drum plotter for output.

Three-dimensional maps are useful in showing the relative magnitude of the data. Also, "views" of the data can be "rotated" or "elevated" to produce different aspects from various compass points or elevations. Because of the complexity of interpretation, however, application of this type of graphic representation to decisionmaking in the health field is quite limited.

Figure 9-12 shows the same data, represented by graduated circles. This map was produced by a mapping program called POWRMAP, written by Phillip Frankland.[20] Given specified input, the program locates the corresponding place on the map and plots the appropriate size of circle. This graphic is very easily understood by the user and is of considerable use in location/allocation problems involving manpower, facilities, and other health resources.

Figure 9-10 Medicaid and Medicare Payments Per Vendor, By County, Georgia, 1972

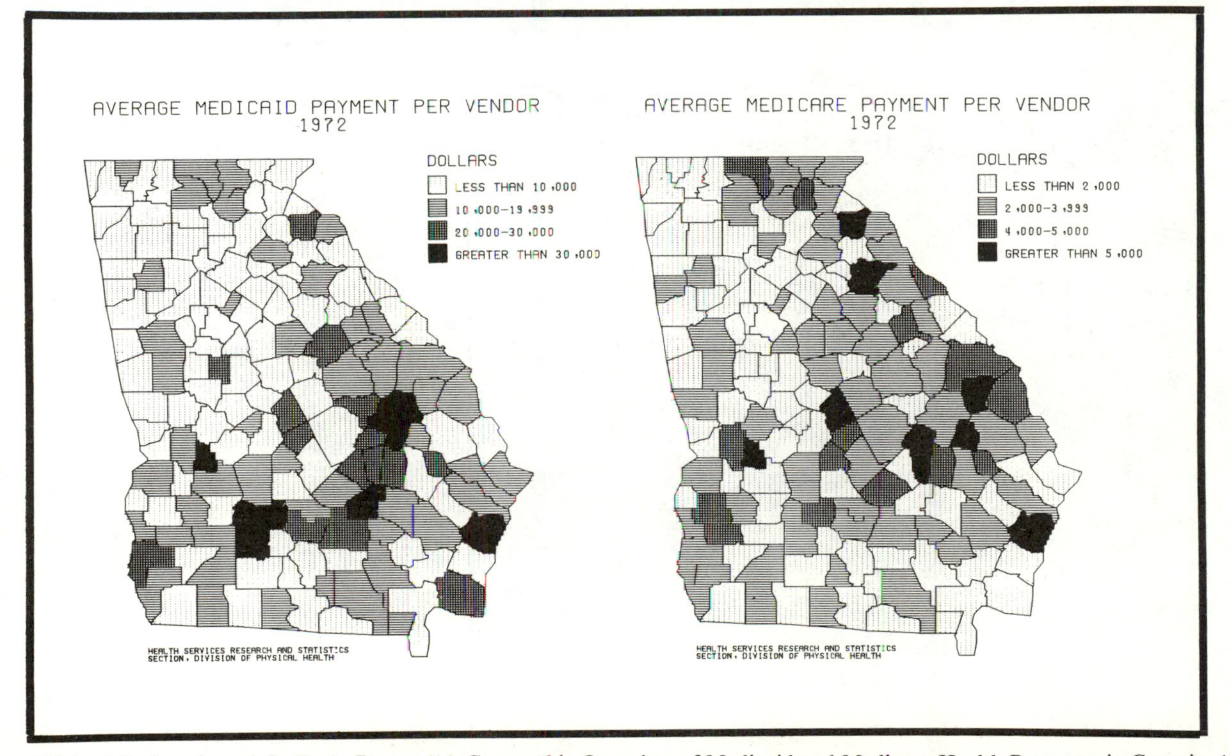

Source: Michael R. Lavoie and G. E. A. Dever, "A Geographic Overview of Medicaid and Medicare Health Programs in Georgia, 1972," *Atlanta Economic Review* 25 (1975): 25.

Figure 9-11 Primary Care Physicians, Iowa, 1972

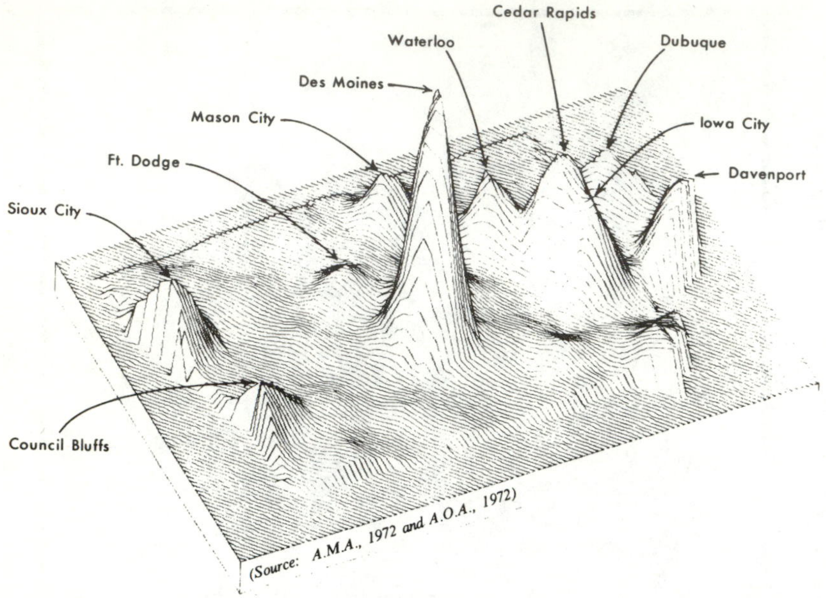

Source: Phillip Frankland, *Atlas of Primary Medical and Dental Manpower in Iowa,* Technical Report No. 50 (Iowa City Center for Locational Analysis, Institute of Urban and Regional Research, University of Iowa, April 1976), p. 4.

The Urban or Metropolitan Scale

This scale of analysis deals with graphic presentations aggregated at the urban, metropolitan, or city scale. Illustrations at this scale are useful for intraurban epidemiological investigations to identify city health problems, target areas, resource placement, and for program planning. At this scale it is essential to analyze the data by census tract, block, or even by individual street addresses (that is, housing units). The following examples demonstrate approaches to graphic presentation at this scale.

Morbidity and Mortality Analysis

Figures 9-13 and 9-14 show data portrayed by census tracts. Figure 9-13 depicts age-specific morbidity rates for measles in Akron, Ohio, 1971.[21] Figure 9-14 shows the percentage of population five years of age and

Figure 9-12 Primary Care Physicians, Iowa, 1972

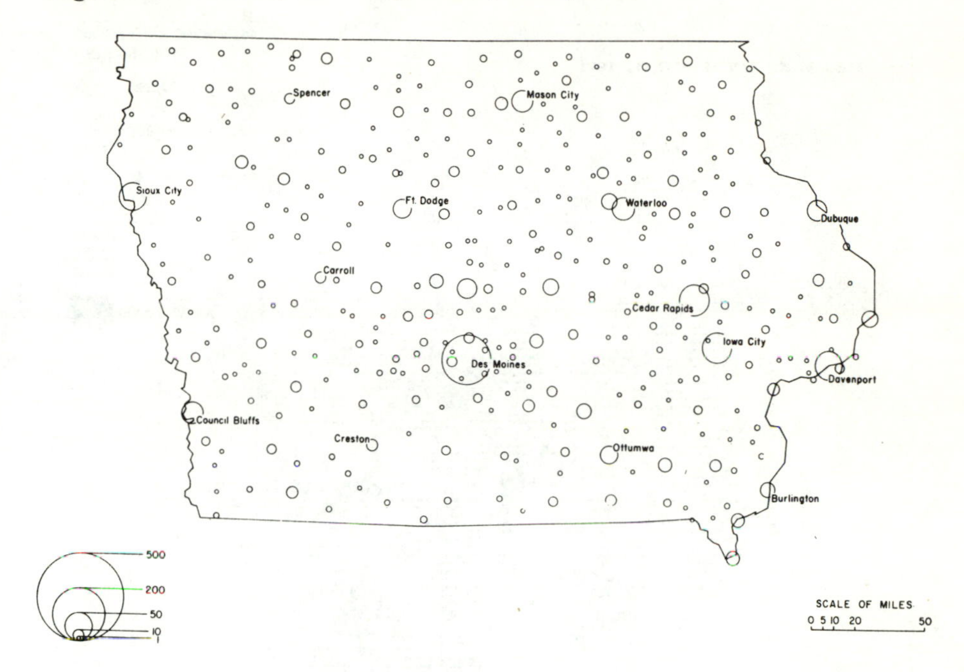

Primary care physicians, 1972.

town size class	no. of towns	no. of towns with PCPs	% of towns in class	no. of PCPs	% of total PCPs
under 500	853	41	5	46	3
501- 1000	213	89	42	105	7
1001- 2000	112	92	82	146	10
2001- 4000	62	55	89	176	12
4001- 8000	37	36	97	209	14
8001- 16000	18	18	100	155	10
16001- 32000	9	9	100	132	9
32001- 64000	6	6	100	171	11
64001-128000	4	4	100	196	13
128001 & over	1	1	100	158	11
total	1315	351		1494	100

Source: Phillip Frankland, *Atlas of Primary Medical and Dental Manpower in Iowa,* Technical Report No. 50 (Iowa City Center for Locational Analysis, Institute of Urban and Regional Research, University of Iowa, April 1976), pp. 4–5.

Figure 9-13 Morbidity Rates, Measles Epidemic, Akron, Ohio, 1971

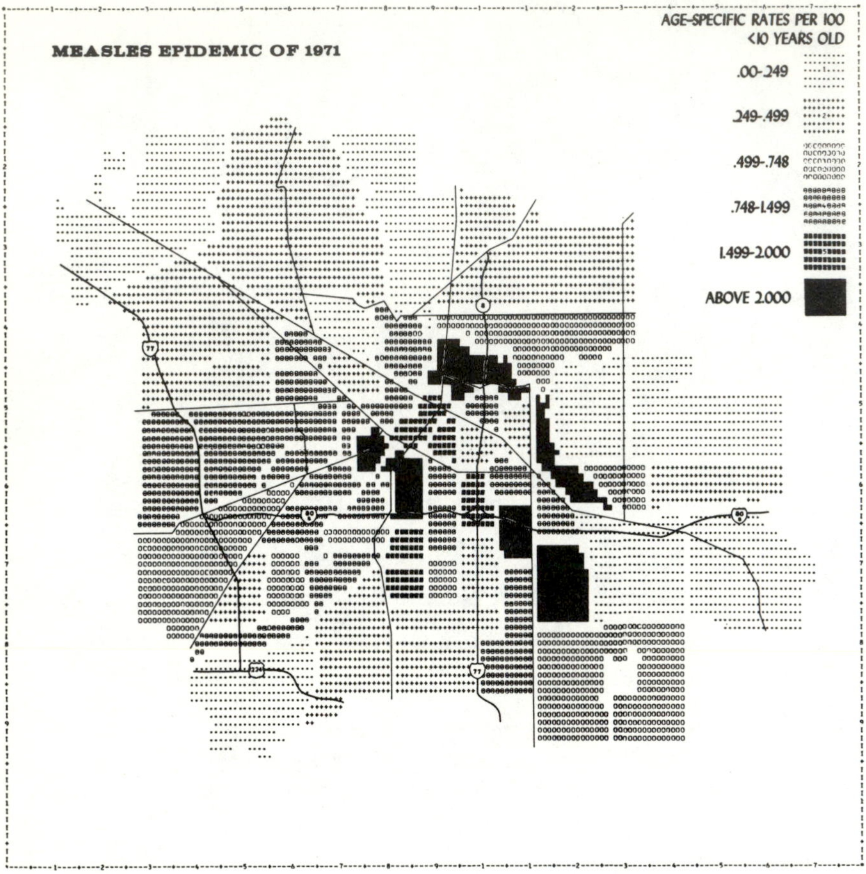

Source: Gerald F. Pyle, *Measles as an Urban Health Problem: The Akron Example* (paper presented to the 11th Commission in Medical Geography, Guelph, Ontario, Canada, 1972), p. 19.

---

below in Fresno, California.[22] Both figures are SYMAPS with additional material in the titles and legends. The map on measles can define high and low risk areas. The population map of Fresno could be particularly useful in defining target areas of high risk for screening programs for lead poisoning and immunizations and for early and periodic screening, diagnosis, and treatment (EPSDT).

Figure 9-15 is a plotted map of hospital discharge data portrayed by census tract.[23] The map shows the average length of stay by location of

Figure 9-14 Population, 5 years and below, Fresno Metropolitan Area, 1970

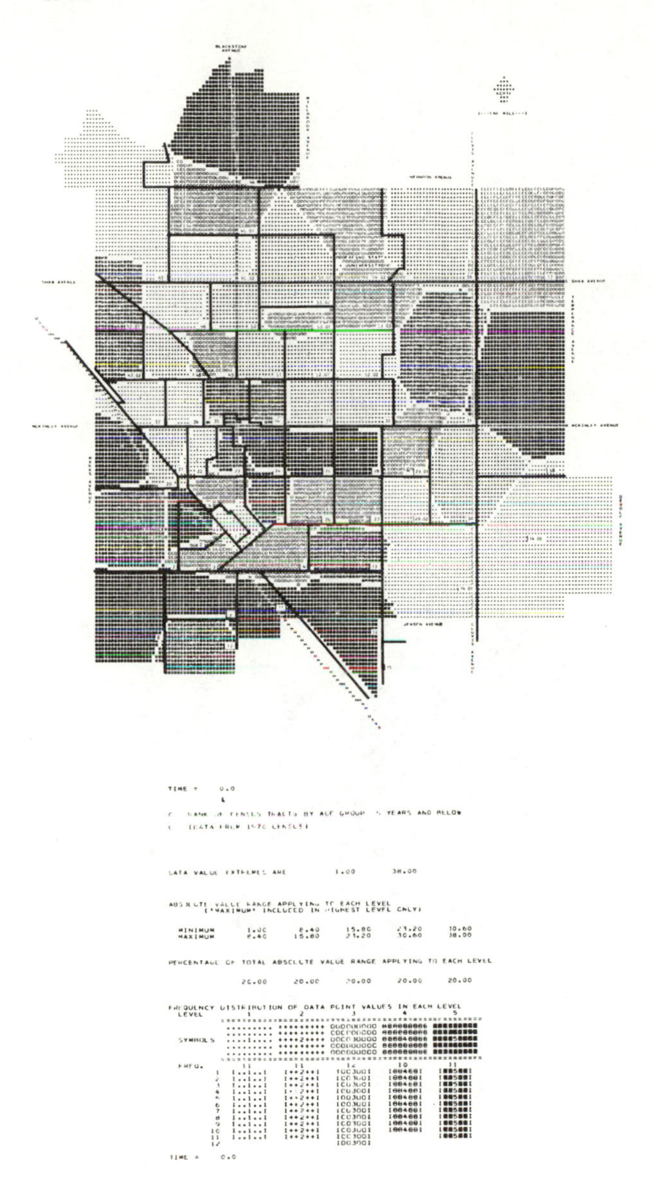

Source: Management Systems Offices, *Community Profile, 1973* (Fresno: City of Fresno Administration Management, 1973), p. 9.

Figure 9-15 Hospsital Discharges, by Tucson Census Tracts, 1973

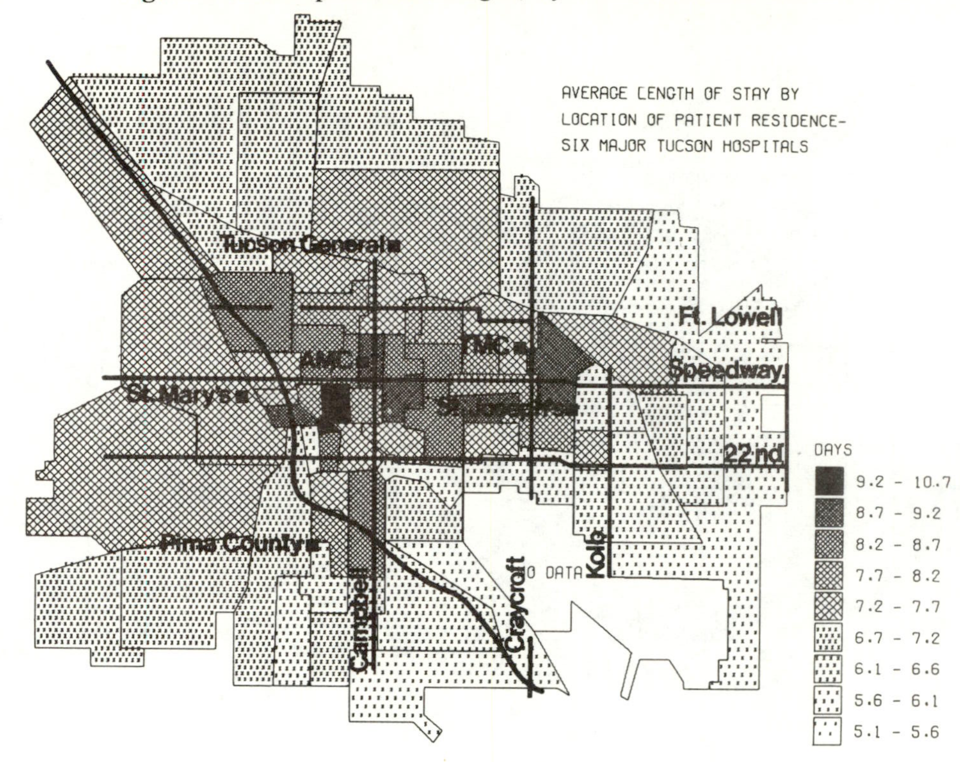

Source: Alan B. Humphrey, *The Cooperative Health Statistics Project,* Hospital Discharge Data System, Pima County Community Profile (University of Arizona, 1973), p. 33.

the patient's residence in Tucson, Arizona. This map could be employed for patient-origin studies, hospital catchment area investigations, morbidity analyses, and health policy analyses. The map could also aid in determining potential problems connected with hospital availability and accessibility.

A minor difficulty in using the Figure 9-15 data, however, is that the number of symbols (nine) are too many and, therefore, difficult to interpret (high visual noise). A user must always maintain a balance between the number of symbols and the number of units (for example, census tracts) to be analyzed.

Population-at-Risk Analysis

Figures 9-16 and 9-17 are plotted maps which show problems encountered in computer mapping.[24] Neither map indicates the population-at-risk with reference to the category being mapped, that is, incidence rates are not calculated. This is a serious omission; if the information is to be meaningful for evaluation and decision making, the population-at-risk must be related to the frequency of the event. These examples suggest that cartographic expertise is needed to determine the proper relationship of symbols, map type, and scale of analysis.

Figure 9-16 shows the location of females with urinary infection in Pima County, Arizona, in 1973. Apparently each point represents a case of urinary infection, but no reference is made to the population-at-risk. In intraurban epidemiological investigations, the display of cases as points can be a valid way to determine if such cases cluster in time or space, thereby suggesting an infectious disease process. In this instance, however, there are too few cases for this purpose; investigations of this type require more data to be viewed over a longer period of time.

Figure 9-17 represents the same basic problem. In this case, a question immediately arises: What were the total number of deliveries in relationship to those who had normal deliveries? The map does, however, use dot symbolization well. Other possible means of displaying point data are with the use of graduated circles, a shorter sample time period, different dot sizes, different symbols for each hospital, a change of scale, or individual maps for each hospital's data. In this instance, high visual noise obscures the data from each of the seven hospitals, tending to destroy the purpose of the map.

Neither of the maps in Figures 9-16 and 9-17 contains a legend to explain symbol values. It is therefore difficult to determine the primary objective of each map procedure. The two maps do, however, represent the first use of individual street addresses to show exact locations, a process done by geocoding with ADMATCH.[25]

Figure 9-16 Location of Females with Urinary Infections, Pima County, Arizona, 1973

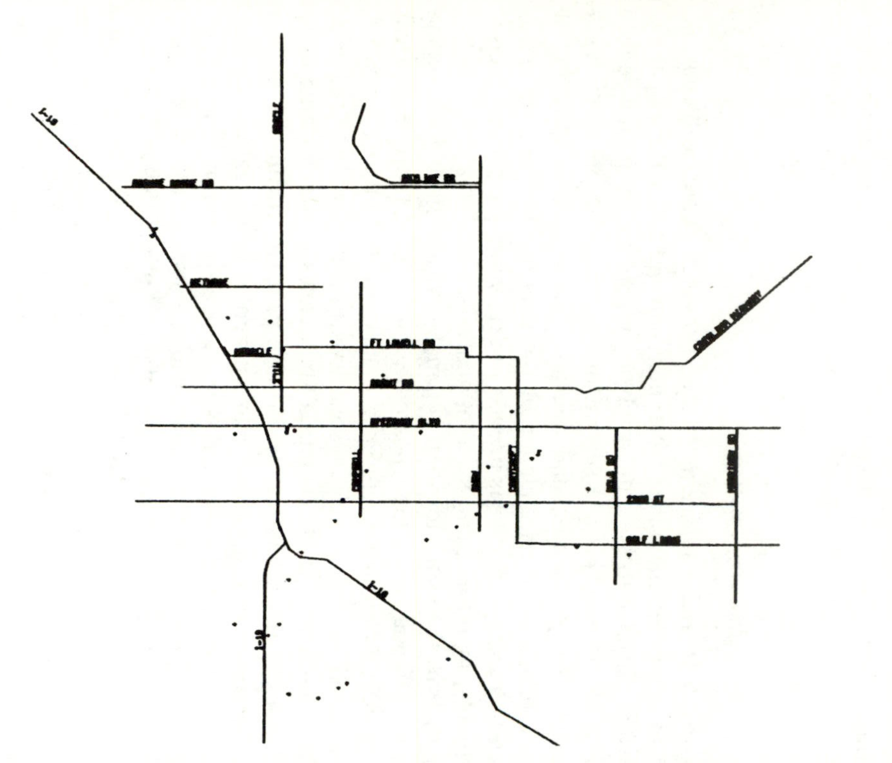

Source: Alan B. Humphrey, *The Cooperative Health Statistics Project,* Hospital Discharge Data System, Pima County Community Profile (University of Arizona, 1973), p. 35.

Figure 9-17 Location of Females with Normal Deliveries, Pima County, Arizona, 1973

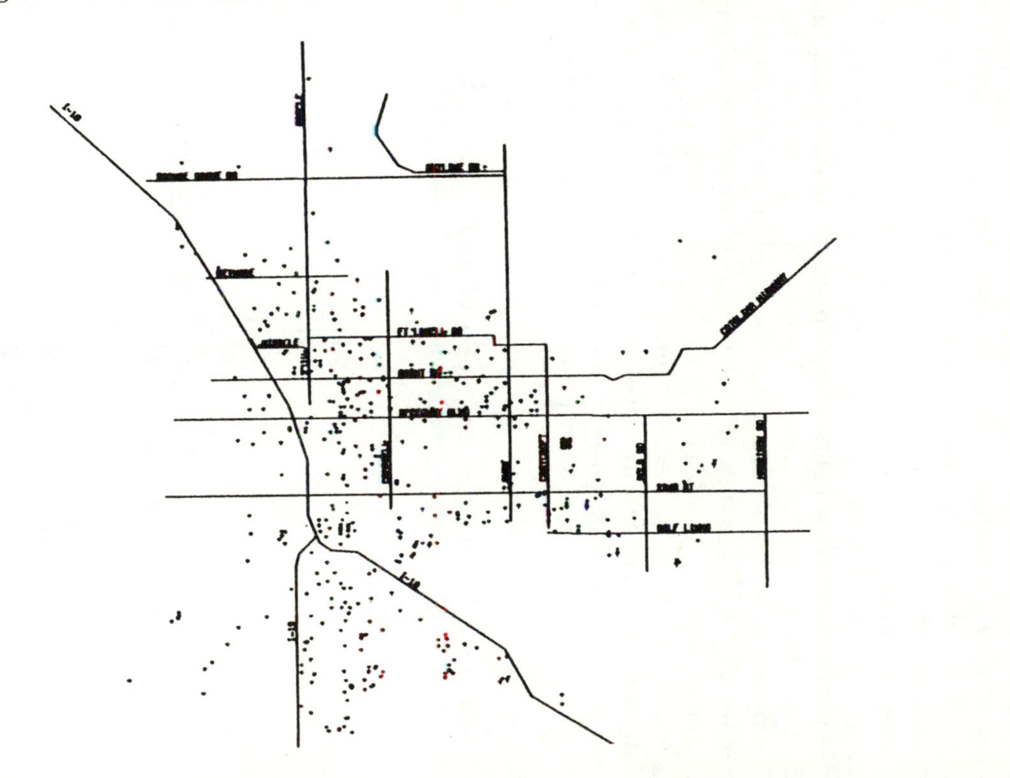

Source: Alan B. Humphrey, *The Cooperative Health Statistics Project in Arizona*, Hospital Discharge Data System, 1973 (paper presented at the American Public Health Association, October 1974).

Advanced Data Analysis

Though emphasis should be on a simple and straightforward presentation of health data, there are more advanced data analysis techniques with which one should at least become familiar. Such techniques, although more difficult to produce, provide quite practical means for planning facilities, predicting health-poor areas, showing time/space trends, illustrating potential disease distribution areas, and depicting measures of health care effectiveness.

The map in Figure 9-18, produced by CRT graphic techniques, shows information through three-dimensional grid cells. This graphic clearly indicates the magnitude of the hours worked by nurses of the visiting nurse association.[26] Because it shows areas of utilization, it could be of value in health program resource planning. It would not be of use in fiscal allocations, however, because of the lack of data to define established administrative units.

Figure 9-19 shows another series of three-dimensional plotted maps.[27] The three graphics show the diffusion of a health care plan, but they could just as easily show the diffusion and magnitude of a disease (for example, influenza) or predict areas of further diffusion of the selected disease in time and space.

Figure 9-18 Hours Worked by Nurses of a Visiting Nurses Association, New Haven, Connecticut

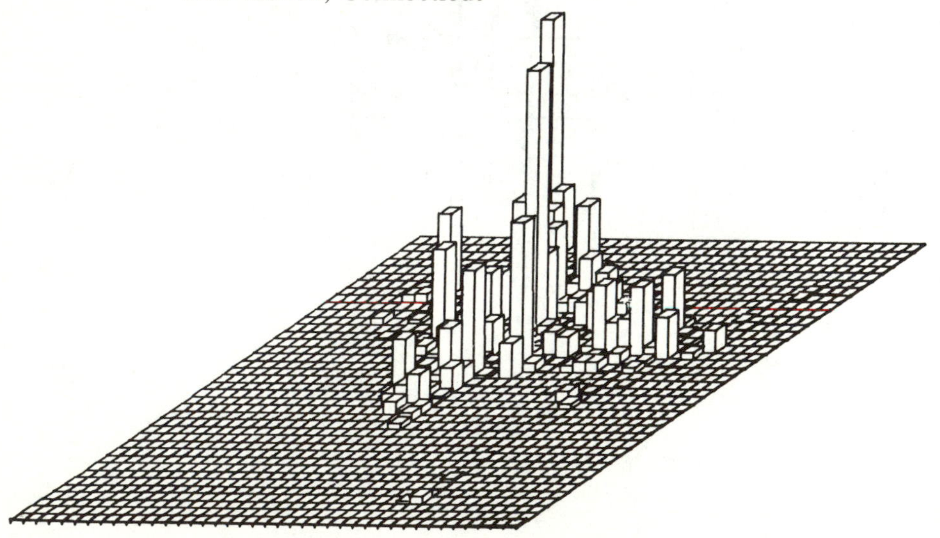

Source: U.S. Bureau of the Census, *Census Use Study: Computer Mapping*, Report No. 2 (Washington: Dept. of Commerce, 1969), pp. 39, 49.

Figure 9-19 Cumulative Spatial Diffusion of a Health Care Plan

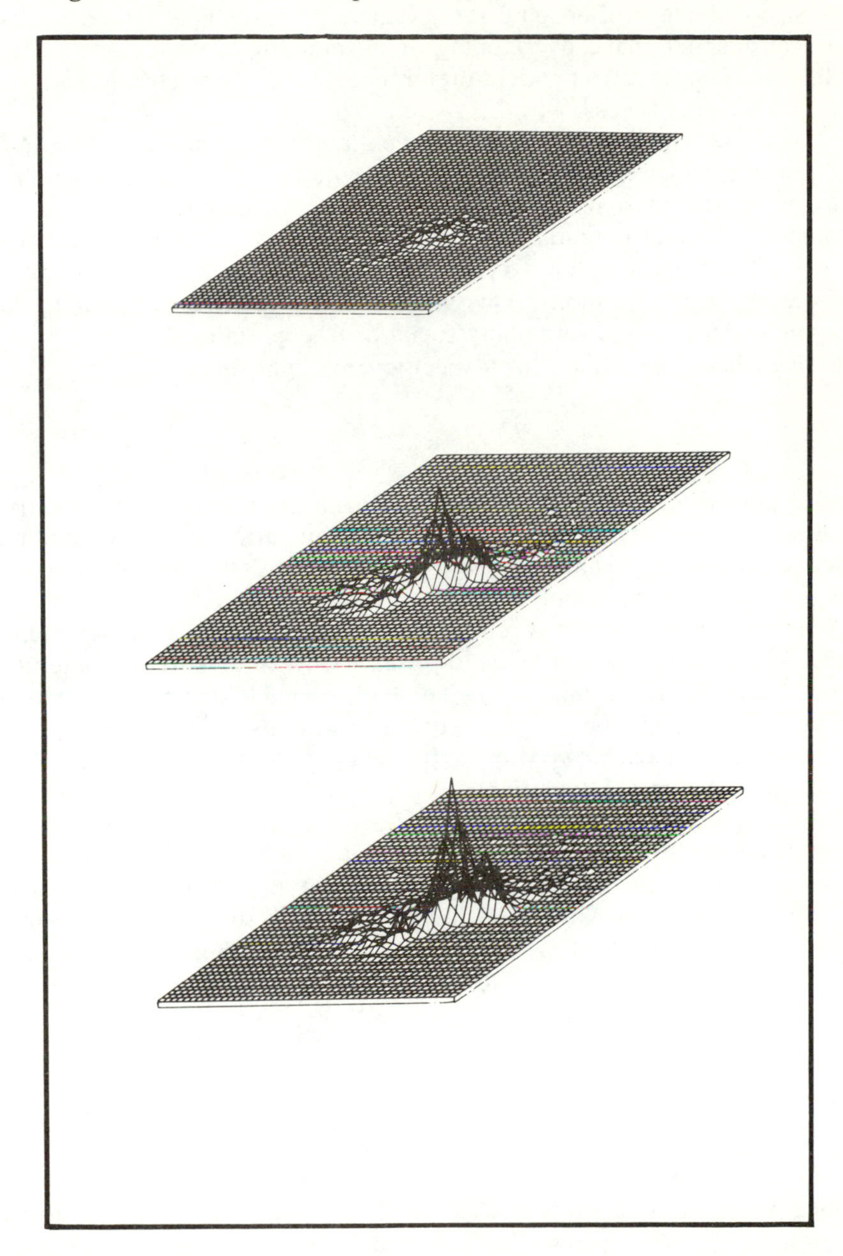

Source: G. W. Shannon and G. E. Alan Dever, *Health Care Delivery, Spatial Perspectives* (New York: McGraw-Hill, 1974), p. 133.

The map in Figure 9-20 employs standard deviational ellipses to define the size and shape of hospital service areas.[28] The ellipses indicate that several hospitals have overlapping or asymmetrical service areas. The ellipsoidal shapes reflect patient preference, facility competition, and barriers to hospital access.

Figure 9-21 shows the distribution of patients around alternate locations of a neighborhood health clinic.[29] The map plots two series of concentric circles around alternate locations of the clinics. The circles enclose the home locations of potential clinic patients at three specified percentage ranges. The map thus shows a considerable difference in the accessibility of the two clinic locations. This graphic could be used in planning the location of facilities, overcoming social or transportation barriers, or assessing clinic accessibility for a specific geographic area.

Patient-Origin Data Analysis

Patient-origin studies have generally suffered from unimaginative methods to portray results needed for administrative decisionmaking. Schneider and others have explored alternatives to origin-destination data in the context of transportation planning.[30] The application of this approach to health planning is remarkably simple. The two graphics in Figures 9-22 and 9-23 were produced primarily by a computer graphic program CENVUE used initially by Tobler.[31] Noguchi and Schneider later developed several innovative approaches to the use of CENVUE.[32]

Figure 9-22 displays two ways to present patient-origin data. The upper map illustrates travel by patients to a hospital in Zone 10, using vectors and histograms. In this instance, the height of the histogram shows the volume of the flow. The lower map illustrates the identical data, but here the vectors express the volume of flow. Both types of graphics are obviously extremely expensive. Individuals reacting to these displays seemed to prefer the upper display because of clarity and comprehensibility. The viewpoint at which the graphic is set to be produced is critical to the presentation of these data.

Analysis with Contour Displays

One method by which travel time and accessibility surfaces can be graphically displayed is with contour maps showing travel times plotted along minimum time paths from a single origin. A contour line-drawn map has been developed by C. Gehner using the minimum path-gridding and contouring procedure.[33] This type of graphic could, for example, show accessibility limits of 30 minutes from a primary health care center.

Figure 9-20 Hospital Service Areas, by Emergency Room Visits, Herkimer County, New York, 1970

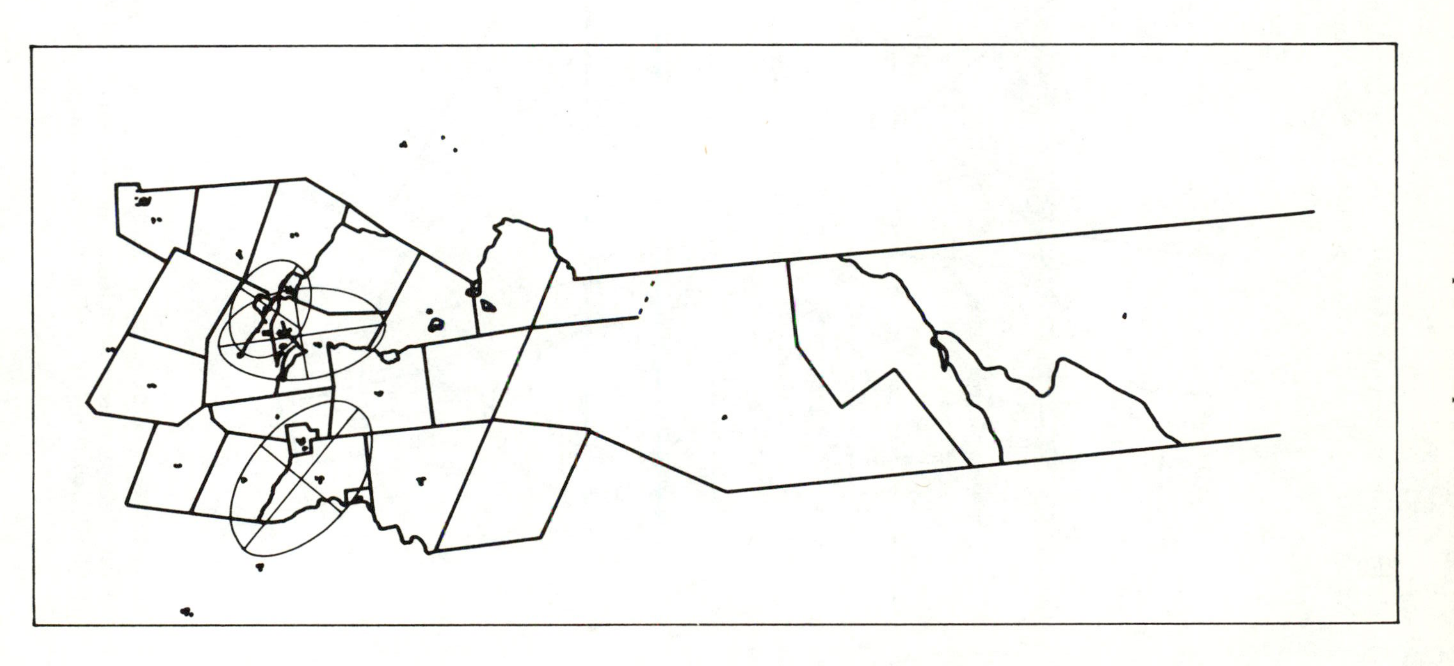

Source: H. A. Sultz, DHEW Community Health Services, Community Profile Data Center, Community Health Profiles, Technical Report Series #2 (Buffalo, New York, 1973), p. 37.

Figure 9-21 Distribution of Patients Around Alternate Locations for a Neighborhood Health Center in Buffalo, New York

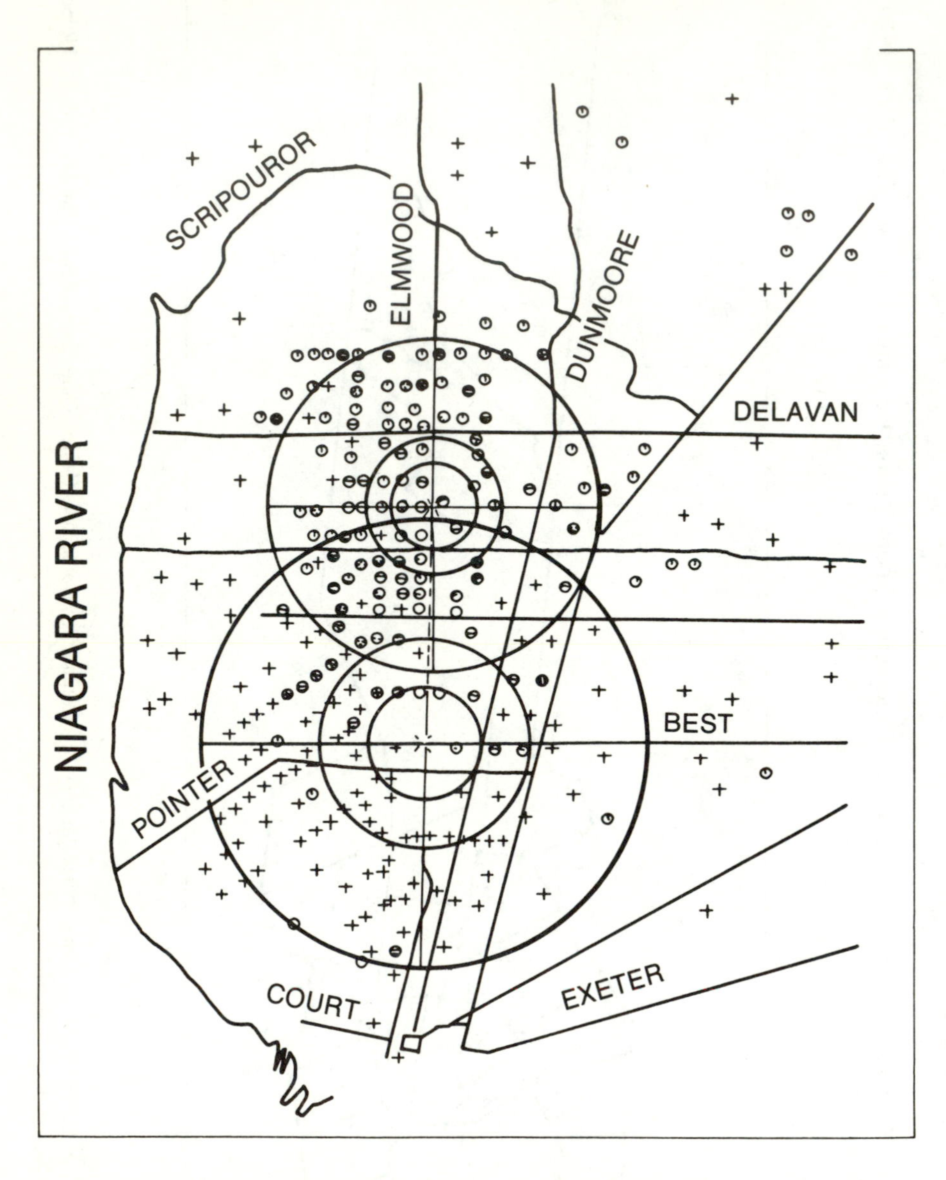

Source: A CHIP System Based on Computer Graphics. Presented at the 99th Annual Meeting, American Public Health Association, Minneapolis, Minnesota, October 12, 1971. From H. A. Sultz, DHEW Community Profile Data Center, Community Health Profiles, Technical Report Series #2 (Buffalo, New York, 1973), p. 36.

Figure 9-22 Potentially Alternate Ways of Displaying Travel by Patients to a Hospital in Denver

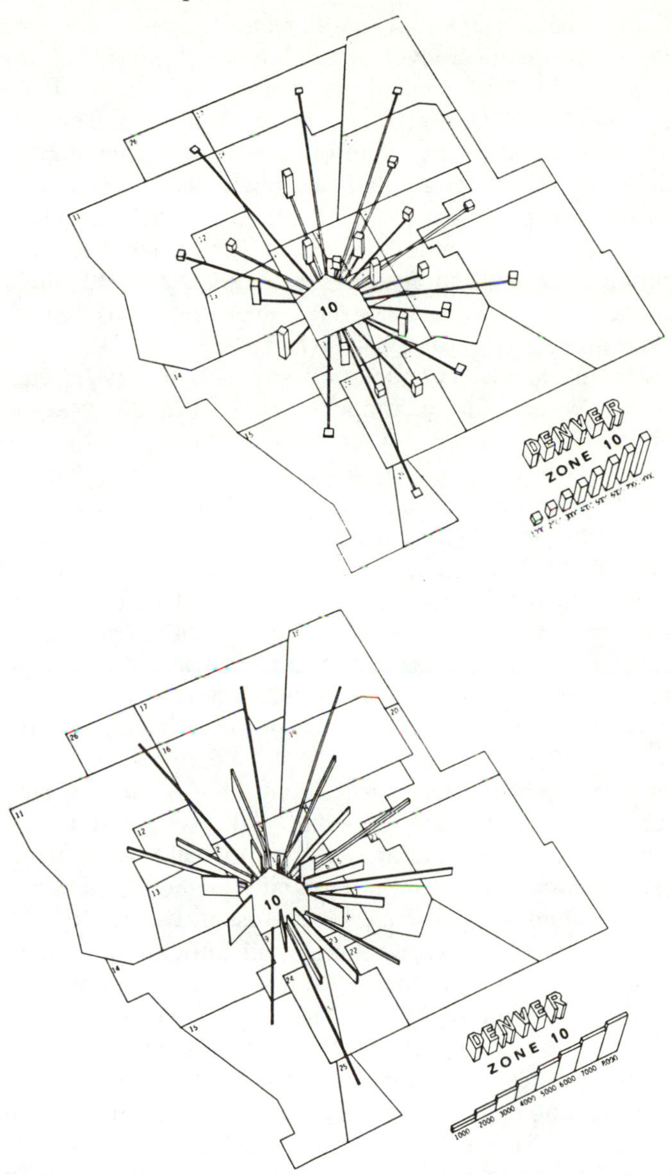

Source: Reprinted by permission from J. B. Schneider et al., *Data Display Techniques for Transportation Planners: Experiments and Applications*, rev. ed. (Seattle, Washington: University of Washington, Department of Civil Engineering, Urban Planning and Architecture, July 1978), pp. 36–39.

SUMMARY

The uses of computer graphics in health planning apply on a continuum from the national to the local level. At each level, different solutions are necessary to solve the various health problems facing decisionmakers. In this context, computer-generated maps, charts, and graphs have the potential to present community health information with visual impact, clarity, and timeliness. Computer graphics are relatively inexpensive to produce, once front-end hardware and software are installed, and they are repetitively accurate and versatile and can produce production-ready copies in minutes. Table 9-1 summarizes the major types and applications of computer graphics. Each graphic is rated on a scale from one to three to give the reader an indication of its quality.

The needs of the highly technocratic society of the 1960s and 1970s produced rapid advances in the computer graphics field. These achievements, however, have been slow to reach the health care field. Nevertheless, technological advances will continue. Ink jet plotters, line graphics, and high increment speeds with high resolution and compactness, will be developed.[34] In the 1980s, health managers will utilize computer technology to display health information for community planning, monitoring, and evaluation, and for conducting epidemiological investigations. The judicious and practical application of computer-generated graphics will thus, hopefully, ease a health agency's planning and policy problems as the technology enters the mainstream of decisionmaking.

However, the job of advancing computer graphics in community health does not lie with the manufacturers or developers of hardware and software but with the health field profession—that is, in "peopleware." The contribution computer graphics can make to community health programs—planning and evaluation, epidemiological investigations, policy decisions, and morbidity monitoring—must be determined by health program managers and decisionmakers. At present, the increased flow of patient information can be overwhelming and difficult to comprehend. Adequate computer graphics hardware, software, and "peopleware" can help to alleviate this condition. Beyond that, the wise health manager can make widespread use of computer-generated graphics to aid in assessing health problems and devising solutions.

Thus, as the technology of resource persons and computer hardware and software become widespread and more available in the coming years, the practical application of computer graphics will become common practice at levels of health management.

Table 9-1 A Summary of Computer Graphics and Their Use and Application in Community Health Analysis

Fig.	Type of Graphic	Type of Program	Application	Use	Scale	Admin. Units	Quality of Graphics
9-1	Character printed (map)	SYMAP	General Practitioners	Identify areas of scarcity and oversupply of medical manpower Manpower policy	National	State	2
9-2	Line drawn (map)	CALCOMP	Lay Midwives	Identify areas of concentration for lay midwives	National	State	3
9-3	Character printed (map)	SYMAP	Lung cancer, male/female, white/nonwhite	High/low risk areas Epidemiological analysis	National	State	3
9-4	Line drawn (graph)	CALCOMP (line graph)	Lung cancer, age-specific death rates, male/female	Population at risk, by age, sex, and race	N/A	N/A	1
9-5	Line drawn (graph)	CALCOMP	Age-adjusted death rates, male/female, white/nonwhite	Population at risk, sex, race Trend analysis Health planning	National	N/A	1
9-6	Line drawn (map)	CALCOMP	Lung cancer, age-sex adjusted rates	Epidemiological analysis High/low risk areas Health planning	State	County health district	1

Table 9-1 continued

Fig.	Type of Graphic	Type of Program	Application	Use	Scale	Admin. Units	Quality of Graphics
9-7	Line drawn (graph)	CALCOMP	Crude death rates, lung cancer, male/female	Trend analysis Health planning	N/A	N/A	2
9-8	Line drawn (disease pyramid)	CALCOMP	Lung cancer, age, race, sex, by percentages	Risk factor analysis	N/A	N/A	1
9-9	Line drawn (map)	SYMVU	Birth and death rates, mortality-fertility ratio (4 time periods)	Geographic associations Regional variation Temporal trends Health planning	National	State	1
9-10	Line drawn (map)	CALCOMP	Medicaid, medical payments to vendors in dollars	Cash flow analysis High/low concentrations of payments	State	County	2
9-11	Line drawn (3-dimensional map)	SYMVU	Primary care physicians	Magnitude of data Scarcity and over-supply areas	State	City	2
9-12	Line drawn (graduated-circle map)	POWRMAP	Primary care physicians	Scarcity and over-supply areas Policy analysis	State	City	1

9-13	Character printed (map)	SYMAP	Measles morbidity	High/low risk areas Immunization programs	City	Census tract	3
9-14	Character printed (map)	SYMAP	Population under 5 years	Target areas for childhood disease screening programs Health planning	City	Census tract	3
9-15	Line drawn (map)	CALCOMP	Hospital discharge data, average length of stay	Patient-origin studies Hospital service area analysis Hospital availability/ accessibility	City	Census tract	2
9-16	Line drawn (point map)	CALCOMP ADMATCH	Urinary infection	Epidemiological investigations	City	Street address	3
9-17	Line drawn (point map)	CALCOMP ADMATCH	Normal deliveries	Health planning	City	Street address	3
9-18	Line drawn (3-dimensional grid cells)	Advanced CRT	Hours spent by Visiting Nurse Association	Magnitude of data Health resource planning Resource utilization	City	Grid cells	3
9-19	Line drawn (3-dimensional grid cells)	SYMVU	Diffusion of a health care plan	Diffusion of health innovation	City	Grid cells	3
9-20	Line drawn (map with standard ellipses)	CALCOMP	Hospital service areas	Hospital accessibility	City	Standard deviation ellipses	1

Table 9-1 continued

Fig.	Type of Graphic	Type of Program	Application	Use	Scale	Admin. Units	Quality of Graphics
9-21	Line drawn (map with concentric zones)	CALCOMP	Hospital service areas	Facility planning In-depth social/ transportation barriers Assessing clinic accessibility	City	Concen-tric zones	2
9-22	Line drawn (3-dimen-sional maps)	CENVUE	Origin/destination data	Patient-origin studies Hospital discharge studies Mortality/morbidity/ disability	City	Census tract	1

1 = Excellent
2 = Good
3 = Adequate

NOTES

1. R. Eliot Green and R. D. Parslow, *Computer Graphics in Management* (Princeton: Auerbach Publications, 1970), pp. 97, 140.

2. Robert A. Greenes and Victor W. Sidel, "The Use of Computer Mapping in Health Research," *Health Services Research* (1967):.243–258.

3. Robert Lewis and Lawrence Chadzynski, "Evolutionary Changes in the Environment, Population, and Health Affairs in Detroit, 1968–71," *Environmental Changes* 64 (1974): 557–567.

4. Howard Fisher, "The Use of Computer Graphics in Planning" (Paper presented at the National Planning Conference of the American Society of Planning Officials, Harvard University, Cambridge, Mass., April 1970), p. 7.

5. In a recent Applied Statistics Training Institute series of maps of health data, 13 states were found to be using computer graphics (geocoding health data) at the county level or below. See Applied Statistics Training Institute Series (St. Louis, Mo.: September 28–29, 1977), p. 12. For more detailed information about this and subsequent series, contact Alan B. Humphrey, University of Rhode Island, Kingston, R.I.

6. R. E. Mytinger and A. White, "Communicating Complexity: A Health Policy Analysis Framework," (Paper presented at the Data Use Conference, Phoenix, Arizona, November 1978) pp. II-19–II-41.

7. U.S. Bureau of the Census, "Census Use Study: Computer Mapping," *Report No. 2,* Washington, D.C. 1969, p. 44.

8. D. D. Achabal et al., "Designing and Evaluating a Health Care Delivery System Through the Use of Interactive Computer Graphics," *Social Science and Medicine* 12 (1978): 1–6.

9. M. A. Murray and F. Drago, "A Decade of Computer Mapping," *Atlanta Economic Review* Vol. 26, No. 6 (1976): 31–38.

10. The National Health and Resources Development Act of 1974 (P.L. 93–641) was established to create at least one Health Systems Agency in each state. The basic function of the HSA is to assure health care that is affordable, accessible, available, qualitative, continuous, and acceptable.

11. G. E. A. Dever, "Locational Characteristics of Selected Manpower in the United States," *Atlanta Economic Review* 24 (1974): 41–47. The Calforms package was produced by the Office of Health Services Research and Statistics, Division of Physical Health, Georgia Department of Human Resources, 1974.

12. Thomas J. Mason et al., *Atlas of Cancer Mortality for U.S. Counties: 1950–69,* DHEW Pub. No. (NIH) 75-780 (Washington, D.C.: U.S. Government Printing Office, 1975), pp. 14, 24, 37.

13. Mason et al., *Atlas of Cancer Mortality Among U.S. Nonwhites, 1950–69,* DHEW Pub. No. 76-1204 (Washington, D.C.: U.S. Superintendent of Documents, 1976), p. 142.

14. Fred Burbank, *Patterns in Cancer Mortality in the U.S.: 1950–67* (Washington, D.C.: U.S. Government Printing Office, 1971), pp. 199–206.

15. Office of Health Services Research and Statistics, *Disease Patterns of the '70s* (Atlanta: Georgia Dept. of Human Resources, Div. of Physical Health, Aug. 1976), p. 167.

16. Ibid.

17. Ibid.

18. George A. Schnell and Mark S. Monmonier, *Intercom* 6, no. 8 (Aug. 1978); pp. 8–10; from Schnell and Monmonier, "The Mortality-Fertility Ratio: A Useful Measure for Describing Demographic Change in the U.S., 1940–1974," *Geographical Survey,* in press.

19. Michael R. Lavoie and G. E. A. Dever, "A Geographic Overview of Medicaid and Medicare Health Programs in Georgia, 1972," *Atlanta Economic Review* 25 (1975): 25.

20. Phillip Frankland, *Atlas of Primary Medical and Dental Manpower in Iowa,* Technical Report No. 58 (Iowa City: Center for Locational Analysis, Institute of Urban and Regional Research, Univ. of Iowa, April 1976), p. 103.

21. Gerald F. Pyle, "Measles as an Urban Health Problem: The Akron Example" (Paper presented to the IGU Commission on Medical Geography, Guelph, Ontario, Canada, 1972), p. 19.

22. Management Systems Office, *Community Profile, 1973* (Fresno: City of Fresno, Administration Management, 1973), p. 9.

23. Alan B. Humphrey, The Cooperative Health Statistics Project, *Hospital Discharge Data System: Pima County Community Profile, 1973* (Arizona Medical Center, Tucson, Arizona, Univ. of Arizona, 1973), pp. 33, 35.

24. Alan B. Humphrey, "The Cooperative Health Statistics Project in Arizona: Hospital Discharge Data System, 1973" (Paper presented at the New Orleans, Louisiana American Public Health Association, Oct. 1974), p. 7.

25. ADMATCH is an address-matching system capable of geocoding computer-readable records containing street addresses. Local records are matched to a geographic base file (GBF) via a coding file which is an address coding guide (ACG). ACG files contain block side records for all streets within a particular Standard Metropolitan Statistical Area (SMSA). Problems with the ACG led to the development of the Dual Independent Map Encoding (DIME) file. A basic difference between the ACG and the DIME is that ACG records contain codes for one side of a street, whereas DIME records contain codes for both sides of a street. For more detailed information on geocoding of health information, see the following: U.S. Bureau of the Census, Census Use Study, *DIME: A Geographic Base File Package,* Report No. 4 (Washington, D.C., 1970), p. 161; U.S. Bureau of the Census, Census Use Study, *Geocoding with ADMATCH,* Report No. 14 (Washington, D.C., 1971), p. 23; U.S. Bureau of the Census, *Use of Address Coding Guides in Geographic Coding, Case Studies, Conference Proceedings, Wichita, Kansas, Nov. 19–20, 1970* (Washington, D.C., Jan. 1971), p. 70; Richard M. Levy, *"Use of a Geographic Base File in a Health Information System," U.S. Base of the American Geographic Base File System—Uses, Maintenance, Problem Solving* (Report GE No. 3, Nov. 16–17, 1971, Arlington, Texas (Washington, D.C., 1972), p. 123; Anthony Oreglia, *The Uses of Census Data for Health Services Planning and Management,* Health Services Research and Training Program (Indiana: Dept. of Sociology, Purdue Univ., 1973) pp. 121–149; and Kenneth J. Ducker et al., *A Geocoded Statewide Information System for Primary Medical and Dental Planning,* Institute of Urban and Regional Research and Health Services Research Center, Tech. Report No. 2: Univ. of Iowa, May 1976), p. 46. The most recent information available on the geocoding of health information is in Proceedings of an Applied Statistics Training Institute Seminar, mimeographed (St. Louis, Mo., Sept. 28–29, 1977), p. 12.

26. U.S. Bureau of the Census, *Census Use Study: Computer Mapping,* Report No. 2 (Washington, D.C.: Dept. of Commerce, 1969), pp. 39, 49.

27. Gary W. Shannon and G. E. A. Dever, *Health Care Delivery: Spatial Perspectives* (New York: McGraw-Hill Book Co., 1974), p. 133.

28. Harry A. Sultz, *Community Profile Data Center,* Tech. Paper Series #2 (Buffalo: Suny, 1973), p. 26.

29. Ibid., p. 25.

30. J. B. Schneider et al., *Data Display Techniques for Transportation Planners: Experiments and Applications,* rev. ed. (Seattle, Wash.: Univ. of Washington, Dept. of Civil Engineering, Urban Planning and Architecture, July 1978), pp. 36–39.

31. W. Tobler, "Select Computer Programs," mimeographed, Dept. of Geography, Univ. of Michigan, Ann Arbor, 1970.

32. T. Noguchi and J. Schneider, "Data Display Techniques for Transportation Analysis and Planning: An Investigation of Three Computer Produced Graphics," *Research Report 762,* Univ. of Washington, Seattle, June 1976, p. 59.

33. C. Gehner, "Utilizing Geographic Benefiles for Transportation Analysis: A Network Benefile System," Research Report 77-3, Urban Transportation Program, Department of Civil Engineering and Urban Planning, University of Washington, Seattle. (Paper presented at Transportation Research Board, Washington, D.C., 1978). *Transportation Research Record* forthcoming.

34. C. H. Hertz and T. Orhuag, "The Ink Jet Plotter: A Computer Peripheral for Producing Hard Copy Color Imagery," *Computer Graphics and Image Processing: An International Journal* 5 (1976): 1.

BIBLIOGRAPHY

Halpern, J. W. "Computer Graphics." *Research News* 21, (1970): p. 26.

Keates, J. S. *Cartographic Design and Production.* New York: John Wiley & Sons, 1973, p. 240.

Laboratory for Computer Graphics and Spatial Analysis. *SYMAP, Reference Manual for Synographic Computer Mapping V.* Cambridge, Mass.: Harvard University Graduate School of Design, p. 55.

Muehrcke, P. "Thematic Cartography," Resource Paper No. 19 (Washington, D.C.: Association of American Geographers, 1972), p. 66.

Peucker, T. K. "Computer Cartography," Resource Paper No. 17. (Washington, D.C.: Association of American Geographers, 1972) p. 70.

Proceedings, Conference on Geographic Information Systems and Automated Mapping," July 31–Aug. 1, 1974. Arizona State University, p. 32.

Chapter 10

Holistic Health—Process and Risk-Factor Analyses

This chapter builds on the holistic and wellness models presented in Chapters 1 and 2. The holistic-health process model and risk-factor analysis models presented below can be used at any level of organization. The models could involve a health department, an HSA, or an individual. The basic epidemiological models, proposed by Lalonde and amplified by the author, incorporate life style, environment, biology, and the medical care system as the elements of a comprehensive risk-factor analysis. The process model for analyzing risk factors grew out of the author's association with the Community Health Task Force in the Georgia Department of Human Resources from 1972 to 1977. The application of the process, or the holistic-health, risk-factor analysis model, resulted from his consultation with the Oklahoma Health Systems Agency in 1978.

THE PROCESS MODEL

The process model, which has worked effectively in the Georgia Public Health Agency and in the Oklahoma Health Systems Agency, may be divided into two phases. Phase One assesses the current health issues and asks, Why a new health outlook embodying a holistic approach? To answer this question, it is necessary to address three factors, each with inherent problem areas: system, people, and community. Each factor must be subdivided to demonstrate specifically where the problems exist.

NOTE

1. Material in this section is drawn from a paper prepared by the Oklahoma HSA, based in part on the author's consultative work with the agency. The author wishes to thank Karen Van Wagner and Larry DePriest of the Oklahoma HSA for their permission to reproduce an abridged edition of the plan.

Thus, system problem areas or variables are cost, availability, accessibility, continuity, accountability, and quality. People variables are stress, tension, lack of exercise, smoking, alcohol and drug abuse, obesity, and malnutrition. Community variables are illnesses causing morbidity, disability, and mortality. The objective of Phase One, then, is to utilize the three factors and to justify a new holistic health outlook or a change in our belief systems about health. In this phase, it is recommended that the agency organize a slide presentation to point out the problems within each of the set components of system, people, and community. (This type of presentation has already been organized on a national scale by the author.) The final product of Phase One is a justification for the agency to adopt a new direction in community health care planning.

If the agency is convinced of the need for a new approach, Phase Two provides the process for planning and implementing it. In this phase, the success of the model will depend upon the level of local community organization and participation. The community must have a definite sense of ownership in the process. If it does not, the adoption of the new holistic health outlook may be accepted but implementation will not occur. Phase Two of the holistic process model, the community health task force analysis, can be developed by following the following steps:

1. Formulate the community health task force.
   a. Identify a broad range of participants (by age, sex, race, occupation): consumers, professionals (nurses, physicians), public health officials, hospital officials, subarea councils, HSA boards, education officials, private industry representatives, and insurance industry representatives.
   b. Select a chairperson.
2. Establish objectives. At a minimum, this should require the following:
   a. Establishment of priorities for disease analysis.
   b. Identification of causes and risk factors.
   c. Analysis of risk factors in terms of life style, environment, biology, and health care system.
   d. Determination of the potential for reducing problems by eliminating risk factors.
   e. Development of recommendations for plans.
3. Determine what diseases are to be investigated. The analysis should be limited to the diseases which are crippling and killing the population. For this, data are needed to support decisions for disease selection; for example, leading causes of mortality death rates, morbidity rates, and disability rates.

4. Establish subcommittees. The number will depend on the total number of participants, the number of diseases selected for investigation, and the interests of the task force at large. Chairpersons should be selected for subcommittee task forces.
5. Ensure provision of information by the agency staff to the subcommittees. This will require data to support decisions relative to the disease being investigated, that is, information on disease rates by age, sex, race, time, and geographical area (descriptive epidemiology). It will also require pertinent literature relating to causes and risks for the diseases and the identification of a resource person from staff to provide additional information as requested.
6. Develop a matrix (Analysis 1) to permit orderly analysis of risk factors contributing to the disease (Figure 10-1). The matrix should reflect four elements: life style, environment, biology, and the health care system. The various causes and risks for each selected disease should then be identified and listed. Finally, the potential for reduction of the disease which can be allocated to each of the four elements should be determined, using percentages (this is basically a subjective analysis).
7. Develop an additional matrix (Analysis 2) for each disease investigated in Step 6. This matrix will reflect the risk factors identified and listed in Step 6. The other part of the matrix will reflect the four elements of life style, environment, biology, and health care system.
8. Determine the potential for programs aimed at reducing the risk factors in terms of the four elements (Table 10-1). This involves the following substeps (caution should be exercised here, since mistakes will occur):
   a. Develop a method for allocating the risk factor to each of the four elements. Possible approaches include the use of high, medium, low (H, M, L) values, number values, or ranks.
   b. Determine if each risk factor is detectable, if it is alterable, and if intervention is accepted or feasible (Table 10-2).
   c. Complete the matrix.
9. Share the results of the completed matrix for all diseases at a statewide conference or workshop.
   a. The chairperson should present results to the participants.
   b. Feedback should occur for creative exchange and updating of the matrix.
   c. New members may be added to the task force.
   d. Workshop sessions should focus on matrix changes and begin to formulate program recommendations (Table 10-3).

Figure 10-1 An Example of a Matrix for Evaluating the Reasons for Mortality

DISEASE	REASONS FOR MORTALITY (List the various reasons under each reportable type)	HEALTH FIELD CATEGORIES (Use Percentages)			
		Life Style	Environ-ment	Biology	Health Care System
Heart disease					
Cancer					
Hypertension and stroke					
Accidents, motor vehicle					
Accidents, other					

Source: Georgia's New Health Outlook, Community Health Task Force, Division of Physical Health, Georgia Department of Human Resources, June 1976, p. 238.

10. Develop program recommendations into a written document, which will be given to the agency for incorporation into the health plan. With this, the task force will have completed its work.
11. Publish an agency plan containing the following for each disease:
    a. Introduction (overview).
    b. Background (statistical analysis).
    c. Causes and risk factors (Matrix Analysis 1).
    d. Relationship of contributing factors to the four elements (Matrix Analysis 2).
    e. Recommended programs.
    f. Summary (risk factors and programs cited in more than one report).
12. Organize a statewide health meeting to unveil the new holistic health outlook.
    a. Invite all task force members and recognize their input.
    b. Invite four speakers, each to talk about one of the individual elements: life style, environment, biology, and health care system.

c. Alert the news media to the significance of the program.
d. Present copies of the new document to all participants.
e. Congratulate yourselves on a task well done.

13. Prepare for the next cycle. In implementation, the process should be duplicated at the district or subarea level. The issues to be addressed should include:
    - Legislation
    - Education
    - Marketing health (Madison Avenue)
    - Why and how people change (belief systems, imitation, force (policy, peer pressure)
    - Themes in Prevention (TIPs)
    - Health Hazard Appraisal (HHA)
    - Improving life style or decreasing risks

Table 10-1 Analysis of Risk Factors of Immature Infants by Health Field Concept Components

Risk Factors	Potential for Programs Aimed at Risk Factors				Potential for Reducing Problems by Eliminating Risk Factors
	Biological	Environ-mental	Life Style	System of Health Care	
Maternal Age	Moderate	Moderate	High	Low	High
Previous Pregnancy	Moderate	High	High	Moderate	High
Poverty	None	Moderate	High	High	Moderate
Educational Level	None	Low	Moderate	Moderate	Moderate
Availability of Care	None	Moderate	Low	Moderate	High
Quality of Care	None	Moderate	Moderate	High	High
Cigarette Smoking	Moderate	Moderate	High	Low	Moderate
Diet	Moderate	Moderate	High	Moderate	High
Family Mores	None	Low	High	Low	High

Source: Adapted from *Georgia's New Health Outlook,* Community Health Task Force, Division of Physical Health, Georgia Department of Human Resources, June 1976, p. 88.

Table 10-2 Lung Cancer Risk Factors by Health Field Elements and Program Potential

Risk Factors	Presence Detectable	Factor Alterable	Intervention Accepted/ Feasible	Impact of Intervention on Lung Cancer
Life Style				
Cigarette Smoking	Y	Y	Y	[H]
Alcohol Abuse	Y	Y	Y	L
Environment				
Industrial Chem.	Y	Y	Y	[M]
Air Pollution	Y	Y	Y	[M]
Geographic Location	Y	Y	N	L
Biology				
Age	Y	N	N/A	N/A
Race	Y	N	N/A	N/A
Sex	Y	N	N/A	N/A
Health Care System	N/A	N/A	N/A	N/A

Y = Yes
N = No
N/A = Not Applicable
L = Low
M = Moderate
H = High
□ = Greatest Potential
COPD = Chronic Obstructive

Source: Adapted from *Georgia's New Health Outlook*, Community Health Task Force, Division of Physical Health, Georgia Department of Human Resources, June 1976, p. 135.

THE RISK-FACTOR ANALYSIS MODEL

This section focuses on a grass-roots application of the above process in a holistic-health risk-factor analysis model in Oklahoma. In this model, the four major determinants of health—life style, environment, biology, and the health care system—work together to influence a person's health.[1] Accordingly, if a program is to make an impact on community health status, it must examine the causes related to each disease or wellness level. By investigating each health determinant, a range of either risk or enhancing factors associated with illness or wellness will be discovered.

Table 10-3 Risk Factors and Programs Cited in More Than One Subcommittee Report

Risk Factors and Recommended Programs	Disease Task Forces							
	Cardio-vascular	Cancer (Resp., Breast, Cervix)	COPD	Suicide/ Homocide/ Alcohol-ism	Motor Vehicle Accidents	Sexually Transmit-ted Diseases	Dental	Prema-ture Births
Common Risk Factors								
Cigarettes	X	X	X		X		X	X
Poverty	X					X	X	X
Pollution (Env.)		X	X		X			
Pollution (People)	X			X	X	X		
Exercise	X		X					
Emotional Stress	X			X	X			
Diet	X	X		X			X	X
Drugs				X	X	X	X	X
Predisposing Family History	X	X	X					X
Nonuse of Services	X	X	X	X		X	X	X
Alcohol	X	X	X	X	X	X		X

Table 10-3 continued

Risk Factors and Recommended Programs	Disease Task Forces							
	Cardio-vascular	Cancer (Resp., Breast, Cervix)	COPD	Suicide/ Homocide/ Alcohol-ism	Motor Vehicle Accidents	Sexually Transmit-ted Diseases	Dental	Prema-ture Births
Common Recommended Programs								
Methods of Payment							X	X
Data Collection	X	X	X	X	X	X		X
Increased Detection/ Prevention	X	X	X	X	X	X	X	X
Nutrition	X		X	X			X	X
Coordination of Agencies	X	X		X	X		X	X
Consumer Education	X	X	X	X	X	X	X	X
Provider Education	X	X	X		X	X	X	X
Increased Exercise/ Physical Fitness	X		X					
Specialized Clinics	X	X	X			X	X	X
Rehab. Services	X		X	X	X			
Public Recreation Facilities	X		X	X		X		

Source: Modified from *Georgia's New Health Outlook,* Community Health Task Force, Division of Physical Health, Georgia Department of Human Resources, June 1976, p. 230.

In April 1978, using these concepts as a foundation, the Oklahoma HSA approved the formation of a Health Status Task Force to deal with priority health status issues. The issues were to be selected by the HSA's Board of Trustees with input from Subarea Councils.

During February and March of 1978, each Subarea Council determined the five health status priority areas in its location. A listing of the priority areas is shown in Table 10-4. Table 10-5 shows the decision-making criteria used for selecting the priority areas. The priority areas were submitted to the Board of Trustees for selection of statewide health-status priority issues. The board selected the following health status issues for initial analysis by the Health Status Task Force: (1) circulatory system diseases (heart, hypertension, stroke), (2) substance abuse, and (3) lung cancer.

Following the selection of the priorities, the board issued the following charge to the task force:

> The charge of this health status task force is to analyze the risk factors associated with the leading killers and cripplers in the state of Oklahoma and decide which of the four determinants of health contribute most directly to that disease or disability being a problem. In addition, the task force is charged with developing a plan of action based on their findings which will reduce death and disability from each killing or crippling disease.

The Health Status Task Force served as an advisory committee to the Oklahoma HSA's Board of Trustees. The task force was mandated to meet over a period of two years. In the first year, the task force was to conduct risk-factor analyses of the three health-status issues cited above. In this task, the task force was to use the health field concept as its guiding framework. This framework, as noted, assumes that the four basic areas affect a person's health. Finally, in performing its role, the task force was to incorporate the concept of wellness, or positive health in its procedures. Thus, the product of the task force was to reflect not only the identification of risk factors but also to deal with the identification of enhancement factors, or with the question, What can be done to increase a person's health beyond the mere absence of disease or disorder?

At the end of its first year, the task force was required to produce a report covering the following points:

1. Identification and compilation of the risk factors associated with each disease or disability under consideration.

Table 10-4 Health Status Priorities by Subarea Councils, Oklahoma, 1978

SAC I
1. Cancer
2. Alcoholism
3. Heart, Stroke
4. Wellness, Accidents (tied)
5. Diabetes, Arthritis (tied)

SAC II
1. Heart
2. Stroke
3. Cancer
4. Mental Illness
5. Wellness

SAC III
1. Hypertension, Heart Disease, Stroke
2. Cancer of the:
   a. Cervix
   b. Lung
   c. Uterus
   d. Prostate
3. Alcohol and Drug Abuse
4. Infant Health:
   a. Perinatal
   b. Neonatal
5. Wellness

SAC IV
1. Alcoholism (Mental Health)
2. Circulatory System
3. Cancer of the:
   a. Lung
   b. Prostate
   c. Large Intestine
   d. Breast
4. Infant Care
5. Accidents, Respiratory Diseases (tied)

SAC V
1. Circulatory System Diseases
2. Cancer
3. Substance Abuse
4. Accidents
5. Mental Health

SAC VI
1. Cardiovascular Disease
2. Cancer
3. Degenerative Disease (Geriatrics)
4. Substance Abuse
5. Maternal Health Status

Source: By permission from the Oklahoma Health Systems Agency. Health Status Task Force Report, October 1978, pp. 4–6.

2. Identification and compilation of the enhancement factors which increase a person's chances of premature death or disability from disease.
3. The relative impact of each risk factor on each status issue.
4. A determination of which health field (life style, environment, biology, or health care delivery system) affords the best opportunity for intervention and reduction of death and disability as well as for the promotion of wellness.

Table 10-5 Health Status Criteria for Priority Setting

1. Do we have the knowledge to impact on this issue?
   Yes - 5 No - 1

2. In the next ten years, this problem is expected to get better (1), stay the same (3), get worse (5).
   Get better - 1 Stay the same - 3 Get worse - 5

3. If this issue is selected, will we be successful in coming up with something concrete for the people of Oklahoma?
   Yes - 5 No - 1

4. Public awareness of this problem is low (1), medium (3), high (5).
   Low - 1 Medium - 3 High - 5

5. Are attitudes of state and local political bodies towards solving this issue favorable?
   Yes - 1 No - 1

6. Is this a mortality or morbidity problem?
   Yes - 2 No - 3

7. Data from killers and cripplers (this was available from a data supplement).

Source: By permission of the Oklahoma Health Systems Agency. Modified from the Oklahoma Health Systems Agency, Health Status Task Force Report, October 1978, pp. 4–6.

5. Health-status objectives for each status issue, specifying required quantitative changes if death and disability resulting from the issue are to be reduced.

The end product of the second year was to be a development of specific plans of action for these status issues. The plans were to concentrate on identifying those objectives and intervention strategies for the selected health field which had the most impact upon the particular diseases and disabilities. The plans of action developed during the second year were to be included in the Health Systems Plan and the Annual Implementation Plan.

The holistic-health risk-factor model may be established using the following step-by-step procedure:

1. A listing of risk factors for the disease being studied. Risk factors and causes should be listed in sufficient detail to allow for group consensus concerning what is actually meant. For example, the problem of barriers to health care needs further elaboration on the type of barrier. Some examples might be:
   a. Patient acceptability/compliance to treatment protocols
   b. Third party payment policy
   c. Provider bias and territoriality
   d. Accessibility to quality care, that is, prehospital/prevention, disease management, or rehabilitation
2. An estimation of the amount of influence each health field element has on each risk factor, that is, where does most of the problem lie? In this step, an "X" should be recorded under each health field element (life style, environment, biology, health care delivery system) that contributes to the existence of the risk factor. Then, the following questions apply:
   a. Does the risk factor exist because of heredity, maturation, or growth? If so, then biology plays a role in the risk factor.
   b. Does the risk factor occur because of some personal action over which the individual has direct control? If so, then the risk factor has a basis in the life style element.
   c. Does the risk factor exist in the physical or social environment (external to the individual), and is it beyond the individual's control? If so, then the environment is a basis for the risk factor.
   d. Does the risk factor come from the quantity, quality, arrangement, nature, and relationship of people and resources providing health care? If so, the health care delivery system would be a basis for the risk factor.

   After deciding which health field element plays a role in creating the risk factor, the amount of influence the health field elements have on that risk factor should be identified, using the code indicated in Table 10-6, to determine how much of the problem lies in what areas.
3. Grouping risk factors by health status impact potential. Here one should determine by how much the levels of death and disability would be reduced if the risk factor is reduced or eliminated. Place an H (high), M (moderate), or L (low) in the appropriate box to signify the potential for disease reduction if the risk factor is eliminated or reduced. Use N/A if the risk factor cannot be reduced. An example is given in Table 10-7.

4. Program development potential by health field components. Three questions must be answered to determine the potential of the program in light of health field components:
   a. Is the risk factor's presence detectable?
   b. If detectable, is the risk factor alterable?
   c. If detectable and alterable, is intervention acceptable or feasible?
   Indicate in the space provided the answers to the above questions, using the codes on Table 10-8, and then indicate what the potential of the program development will be. A format for this is given in Table 10-8.

Table 10-6 The Effect of Health Field Elements on Risk Factors

Code	Percentage	Risk Factor	Health Field Elements			
			Bio.	L.S.	Env.	HCDS
0.	0%	Smoking	0	x3	x1	0
1.	1%– 25%					
2.	26%– 50%	Race	x4	0	0	0
3.	51%– 75%					
4.	76%–100%	Barriers	0	x1	x1	x2

Note: The rows do not necessarily add to 100% because of the use of ranges.
Source: By permission from the Oklahoma Health Systems Agency. Health Status Task Force Report, October 1978, pp. 3–7.

Table 10-7 Effect of a Change on Disease if Risk Factors Are Reduced.

Risk Factor	Potential Impact on Disease if Risk Factor is Reduced
Smoking	H
Race	N/A
Obesity	M
Birth Control Pills	L

Source: By permission from the Oklahoma Health Systems Agency. Health Status Task Force Report, October 1978, pp. 3–7.

Table 10-8 Program Development Potential by Health Field Element

Risk Factors by Health Field Element	Presence Detectable	Factor Alterable	Intervention Accepted/ Feasible	Program Development Potential
Biology				
Race	H	N	N/A	N/A
Sex	H	N	N/A	N/A
Life Style				
Smoking	H	M	H	H
B.C. Pills	H	L	L	M
Environment				
Smoking	H	M	H	M
HCDS				
B.C. Pills	H	M	L	M

L = low H = high
M = moderate N = none

Source: By permission from the Oklahoma Health Systems Agency. Health Status Task Force Report, October 1978, pp. 3–7.

A Risk-Factor Analysis of Lung Cancer and Chronic Obstructive Pulmonary Disease

Utilizing the four basic steps outlined by the Oklahoma Health Systems Agency, the Health Status Task Force, directed by the Oklahoma HSA Board of Trustees, was asked to examine cancer as their third health status problem. They decided to study the biggest killer in the cancer group: cancer of the lung. Because of major similarities in risk factors, chronic obstructive pulmonary disease (COPD) was also addressed in the study. The problem was dealt with in the following steps.

Nature of the Problem

Cancer of the lung and COPD accounted for 7.9% of the 26,766 total deaths occurring during 1977 in Oklahoma.

Cancer of the Lung. Of all cancers in Oklahoma, lung cancer had the highest death rate. For the years 1970–1976, the average age-sex adjusted death rate was 45.68 per 100,000 population. As shown in Figure 10-2, Subarea I, with a rate of 50.65, had the highest risk, followed closely by Subarea II with a rate of 49.12. The area of lowest risk was the northwest corner of the state. County rates ranged from 11.68 in Ellis County to 66.48 in Ottawa County.

Figure 10-2 Cancer of the Lung, 1970–1976

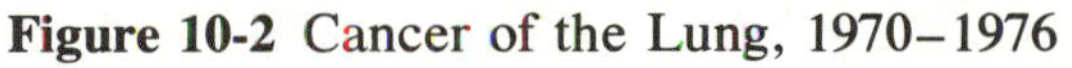

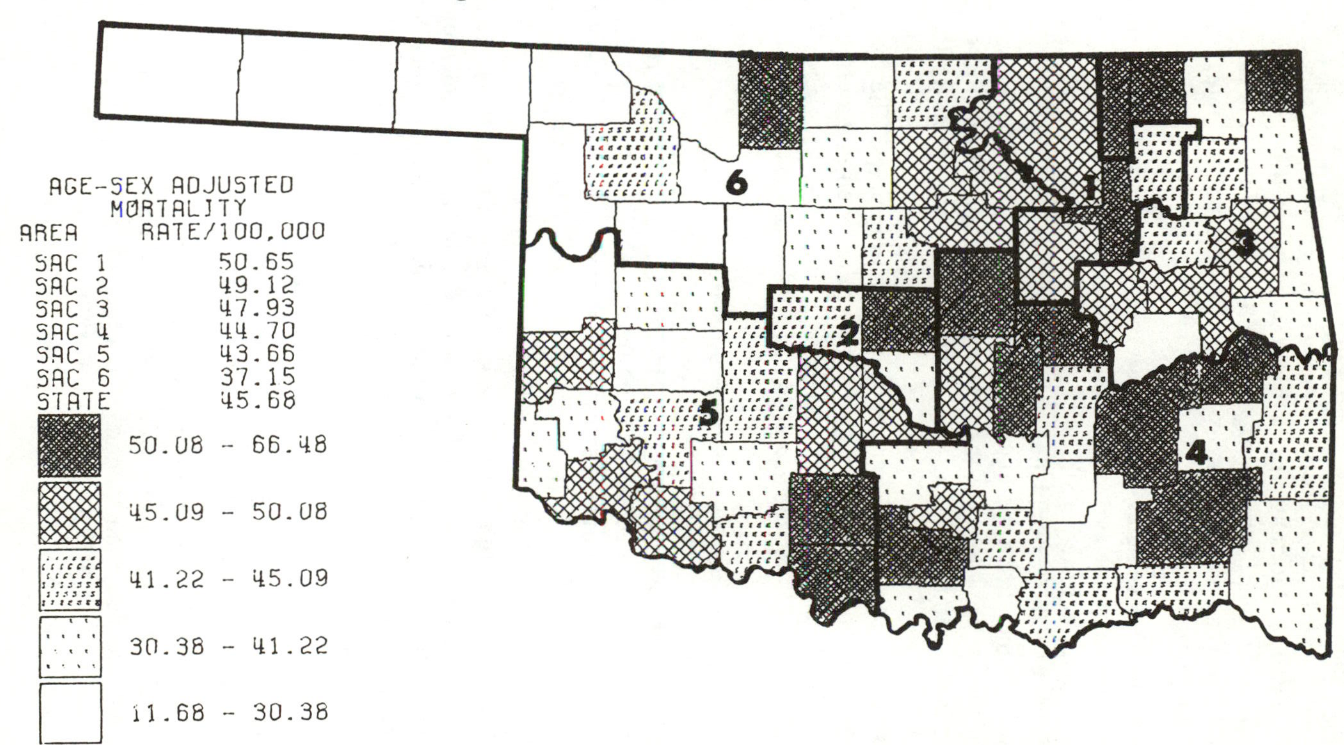

Source: A Plan for Health in Oklahoma, Oklahoma Health Systems Agency, Health Status Data Supplement, Killers and Cripplers, 1970–76, January 1979, p. 25.

Death rates for lung cancer increased for both sexes. Males had higher death rates than females. The death rates for females increased by 69 percent over the last seven years, however, compared to an increase of 40 percent for males. Mortality for both sexes began in the mid-1930s and increased to the highest risk at ages 65–69. Early detection was vital, since the five-year survival rate was only 8 percent for males and 12 percent for women.

Chronic Obstructive Pulmonary Disease. COPD is a composite term for the diseases of chronic bronchitis, emphysema, and asthma. In Figure 10-3, the age-sex adjusted death rate for COPD for Oklahoma was shown to be 25.02 per 100,000 population. As with lung cancer, the urban areas of Subareas I and II had the highest rates (26.01 and 26.26). Subarea VI (25.72) also had a higher rate than the state average. The highest rates occurred in the panhandle. The highest county rate was 74.72 for Beaver County.

Males consistently had higher death rates than females. The rates for both sexes were shown to have increased over the seven-year period from 1970 to 1976. Deaths for males and females began at ages 25–29 and increased to ages 75–79, the age group at highest risk.

Causes of and Risk Factors in Lung Cancer and COPD

Identification of Risk Factors. The Health Status Task Force received information on lung cancer and COPD from speakers with expertise on the subjects and from journal articles on these topics. With this overview, members of the task force listed the risk factors related to lung cancer and COPD in a format illustrated in Table 10-9.

Risk Factors by Health Field Elements. After the individual risk factors and causes were listed, the task force members determined which of the four health field elements influenced the risk factors. Risk factors could have come from one or a combination of the four health field elements. A percentage range was assigned to signify where and how much each health field element influenced the risk factor. Using the example cited above, the risk factor of heredity was estimated as 100 percent biologically based. The results of the task force analysis of risk factors by health field elements are contained in Tables 10-10 through 10-15.

Potential for Reduction of Disease Incidence. Once the risk factors and the health field elements from which they originated were identified, the task force proceeded to an examination of the potential impact of the risk factor on the disease or disorder. This was done using a coding system of high (H), moderate (M), and low (L) values. If the risk factor affected the

Figure 10-3 Chronic Obstructive Pulmonary Disease, 1970–1976

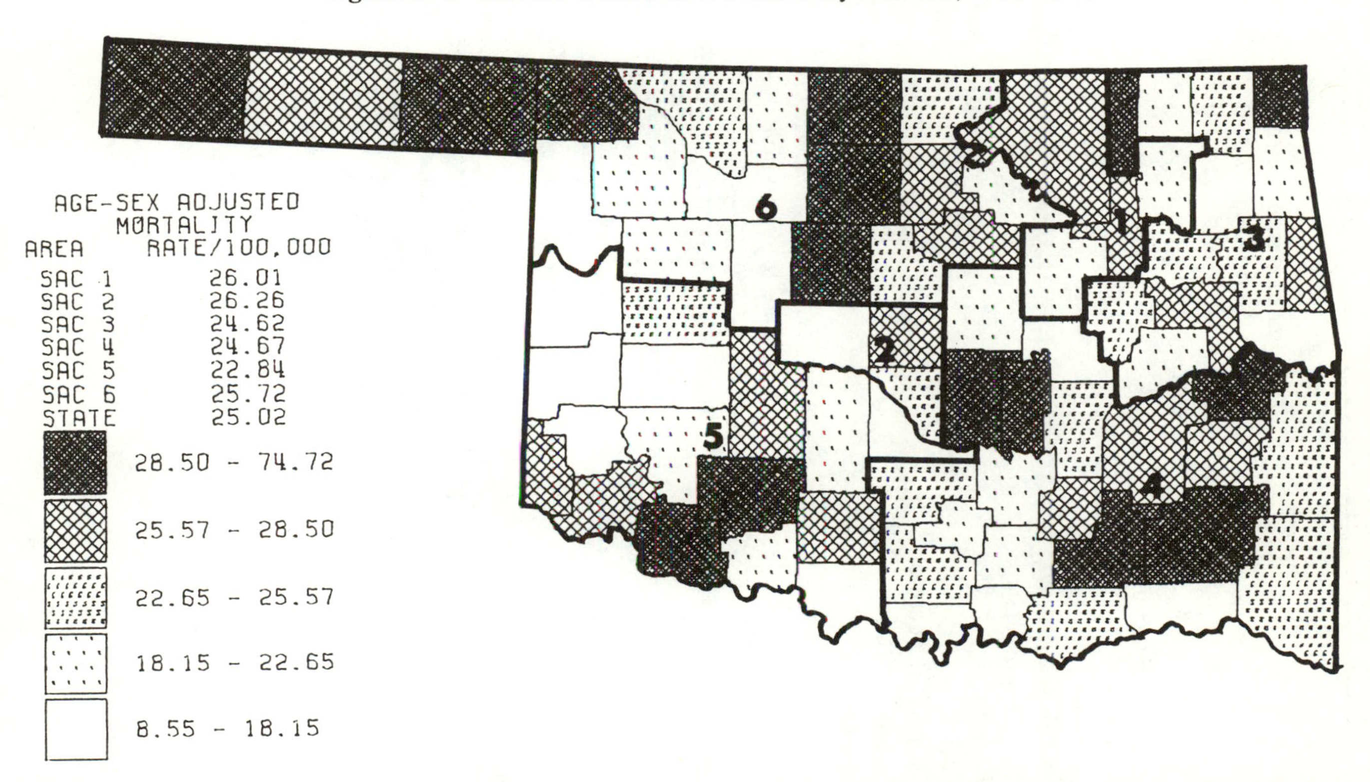

Source: A Plan for Health in Oklahoma, Oklahoma Health Systems Agency, Health Status Data Supplement, Killers and Cripplers, 1970–76, January 1979, p. 75.

Table 10-9 Risk Factors of Lung Cancer and COPD

Smoking	
Heredity	*The inheritance of certain traits which may induce carcinogens and also a family history of lung cancer.*
Occupational Exposure 1. Asbestos 2. Chromium 3. Nickel 4. Radiation (ionizing) 5. Silicates 6. Coal 7. Farming, dust/cotton 8. Potters, craftsmen	
Air Pollution	
Personality	*Suppression of emotions, use of denial and repression, impaired self-awareness, etc.*
Geographic—Urban/Rural	*Where a person lives.*
Sex	
Age	
Race	
Marital Status	
Socioeconomic Status	
Stress	*An expenditure of energy used in adapting to a situation which, if too prolonged/large, may be detrimental.*
Accessibility to Health Care Services:	
1. Screening	*Screening of persons for COPD.*
2. Modeling	*Role models as provided by health care professionals.*
3. Educational (Professional)	*Lung cancer education that is accessible to health care professionals.*

Table 10-9 continued

4. Treatment Services	
Media:	
1. Advertising	
2. Influential Role Models	*Smoking by esteemed individuals of society.*
Alcohol Abuse	
Infection	
Allergic Reaction	
Attitudes (Social)	*Ambivalent attitudes about smoking and health.*
Attitudes (Political)	*E.g., funding tobacco industry subsidy while acknowledging the health hazards of smoking.*
Economics	*The taxes that are received from cigarettes along with jobs and income from the tobacco industry.*
Energy Crisis	*The use of fuels that promote air pollution.*
Smoking:	
1. Lack of Knowledge	*Concerning the physical hazards of smoking.*
2. Lack of Motivation	*That leads to nonsmoking behavior.*

Source: By permission from the Oklahoma Health Systems Agency. Health Status Task Force Report, October 1978, pp. 60–61.

incidence of disease in a major way, the reduction or elimination of that risk factor would be scored as having a high (H) impact on disease incidence. If no change in the risk factor were possible, N/A was scored. The scoring process was done for each risk factor. The results appear in Table 10-16.

Risk factors having high impact upon the status problems of lung cancer and COPD were identified as smoking; occupational exposure to asbestos; air pollution; media advertising and support of other detrimental risk

Table 10-10 Risk Factors Influenced by Life Style and Environment

Risk Factor	L.S.	Env.	Bio.	HCDS
Geographic, Urban/Rural	2	3		
Marital Status	4	1		
Socioeconomic Status	2	3		
Attitudes (Social)	3	2		
Energy Crisis	3	2		

0 0%
1 1%– 25%
2 26%– 50%
3 51%– 75%
4 76%–100%

Source: By permission from the Oklahoma Health System Agency. Health Status Task Force Report, October 1978, pp. 62–64.

Table 10-11 Risk Factors Influenced by Biology, Life Style, and Environment

Risk Factor	Bio.	L.S.	Env.	HCDS
Air Pollution	1	2	3	
Personality	1	3	2	
Alcohol Abuse	1	3	2	
Allergic Reaction	2	2	2	

0 0%
1 1%– 25%
2 26%– 50%
3 51%– 75%
4 76%–100%

Source: By permission from the Oklahoma Health Systems Agency. Health Status Task Force Report, October 1978, pp. 62–64.

factors; social attitudes allowing for the existence of cigarettes and other harmful occupational risk factors; political attitudes involving the economics in the smoking issue; and lack of motivation by individuals. Accessibility to health care services, such as screening and the role of providers as models to discourage smoking, were felt to have a medium

Table 10-12 Risk Factors Influenced by Life Style, Environment, and the Health Care Delivery System

Risk Factor	Bio.	L.S.	Env.	HCDS
Smoking		3	2	1
Occupational Exposure		2	3	1
Accessibility to Health Care Services				
a. screening		1	2	3
b. education (professional)		1	1	3
c. treatment		1	1	3
Media				
a. advertising		1	4	1
b. influential role models		2	3	1
Political Attitudes		1	3	1
Economics		1	3	1
Smoking				
a. lack of knowledge		1	3	2
b. lack of motivation		3	2	1

0 0%
1 1%– 25%
2 26%– 50%
3 51%– 75%
4 76%–100%

Source: By permission from the Oklahoma Health Systems Agency. Health Status Task Force Report, October 1978, pp. 62–64.

potential impact on the health status problem. Stress, occupational exposure to coal, and a lack of knowledge about the effects of smoking and occupational dangers were felt to be of moderate or medium importance in reducing the risk of lung cancer and COPD. Accessibility to existing health care services designed to provide treatment was considered to have only a low potential for reducing the incidence of deaths and disabilities due to lung cancer and COPD.

A second method of examining the risk factors' status impact potential along with the health field element influence on that risk factor is shown in Table 10-17. This summarizes the last two steps of the analysis done by the Health Status Task Force.

Table 10-13 Risk Factors Influenced by All Four Health Field Elements

Risk Factor	Bio.	L.S.	Env.	HCDS
Stress	1	2	2	1
Infection	1	2	2	1

0 0%
1 1%– 25%
2 26%– 50%
3 51%– 75%
4 76%–100%

Source: By permission from the Oklahoma Health Systems Agency. Health Status Task Force Report, October 1978, pp. 62–64.

Program Development Potential. After determining the potential for reduction of disease incidence, the Health Status Task Force turned its attention to the determination of the potential for program development. In this stage, each risk factor and the health field element that influenced it were considered in relation to five basic questions:

1. What is the probability that the presence of a health field's influence on the risk factor could be detected and measured?
2. To what degree could the risk factor, through intervention from this health field, be changed by existing state-of-the-art know-how?
3. To what degree would intervention aimed at the risk factor be acceptable or feasible (that is, acceptable to the population in general, except where noted as concerned only with the at-risk population, and feasible to the degree technology and money were available to impact on the risk factor)?
4. Could, in fact, the program be developed?
5. If a program were developed, what would be its potential for success?

Each question had four possible answers, with the exception of question number four, which was answered either yes or no. The four answers were: to a high degree—H, to a moderate degree—M, to a low degree—L, no or none—N. If, in order of presentation, any question were answered no or none, the process was stopped for that risk factor.

Status-Impact/Program-Potential Relationship. The task force also studied the relationships between the health-status impact of a risk factor and its potential for program development. These relationships are sum-

Table 10-14 Risk Factors Influenced by the Health Care Delivery System

Risk Factor	Bio.	L.S.	Env.	HCDS
Accessibility to Health Care Services: Modeling				4

0 0%
1 1%– 25%
2 26%– 50%
3 51%– 75%
4 76%–100%

Source: By permission from the Oklahoma Health Systems Agency. Health Status Task Force Report, October 1978, pp. 62–64.

Table 10-15 Risk Factors Influenced by Biology

Risk Factor	Bio.	L.S.	Env.	HCDS
Heredity	4			
Sex	4			
Age	4			
Race	4			

Source: By permission from the Oklahoma Health Systems Agency. Health Status Task Force Report, October 1978, pp. 62–64.
0 0%
1 1%– 25%
2 26%– 50%
3 51%– 75%
4 76%–100%

marized in Table 10-18. The table shows that the following factors were considered by the task force to have high-status impact and high program potential in regard to lung cancer and COPD: occupational exposure to asbestos, smoking, air pollution, media (advertising), and social and political attitudes. Additional risk factors with a high program-development potential of moderate status impact were stress, smoking (lack of knowledge), screening, media, influential role models, and occupational exposure to coal, chromium, nickel, radiation, silicates, cotton, dust, and the workplace environments of potters and craftsmen. Only one low status impact risk factor, radiation, was shown to have a high potential for program development.

Table 10-16 Lung Cancer and COPD, Potential for Reduction of Disease Incidence

HIGH	MODERATE	LOW
SMOKING OCCUPATIONAL EXPOSURE a. ASBESTOS AIR POLLUTION MEDIA: a. ADVERTISING SOCIAL ATTITUDES POLITICAL ATTITUDES ECONOMICS b. LACK OF MOTIVATION	OCCUPATIONAL EXPOSURE f. COAL STRESS ACCESSIBILITY TO HEALTH CARE SERVICES: a. SCREENING b. MODELING MEDIA b. INFLUENTIAL ROLE MODELS SMOKING a. LACK OF KNOWLEDGE	HEREDITY OCCUPATIONAL EXPOSURE b. CHROMIUM c. NICKEL d. RADIATION e. SILICATES g. FARMING (COTTON/DUST) h. POTTERS/CRAFTSMEN PERSONALITY GEOGRAPHIC (URBAN/RURAL) MARITAL STATUS SOCIOECONOMIC STATUS ACCESSIBILITY TO HEALTH SERVICES c. EDUCATION (PROFESSIONAL) d. TREATMENT ALCOHOL ABUSE INFECTION ALLERGIC REACTION ENERGY CRISIS
		NONAPPLICABLE
		SEX AGE RACE

Source: By permission from the Oklahoma Health Systems Agency. Health Status Task Force Report, October 1978, pp. 65–68.

Recommendations and Conclusions

The final tasks called for in the Health Status Task Force's risk-factor analysis were selection of areas for future programmatic planning (next year); compilation of recommendations for selected diseases, health field elements, and risk factors; and the listing of factors to enhance an individual's health. A selection of areas for future programmatic planning was

Table 10-17 Lung Cancer and COPD Risk Factors by Health Field Element Influence and Potential for Reduction of Disease Incidence

Risk Factors	Amount of Influence of Health Field Element				Potential for Reduction of Disease Incidence
	Bio.	L.S.	Env.	HCDS	
Smoking	0	3	2	1	H
Occupational Exposure:	0	2	3	1	
a. asbestos					H
Air Pollution	1	2	3	0	H
Media:					
a. advertising	0	1	4	1	H
Attitudes (Social)	0	3	2	0	H
Political Attitudes	0	1	3	1	H
Economics	0	1	3	1	H
Smoking:					
a. lack of motivation	0	3	2	1	H
Occupational Exposure:	0	2	3	1	
f. coal					M
Stress	1	2	2	1	M
Accessibility to Health Care Services:					
a. screening	0	1	2	3	M*
b. modeling	0	0	0	4	M
Media:					
b. influencial role models	0	2	3	1	M
Smoking:					
a. lack of knowledge	0	1	3	2	M
Heredity	4				L
Occupational Exposure:	0	2	3	1	
b. chromium					L
c. nickel					L
d. radiation					L
e. silicates					L
g. farming-cotton/dust					L
h. potters/craftsmen					L
Personality	1	3	2	0	L
Geographic-urban/rural	0	2	3	0	L

Table 10-17 continued

Risk Factors	Amount of Influence of Health Field Element				Potential for Reduction of Disease Incidence
	Bio.	L.S.	Env.	HCDS	
Marital Status	0	4	1	0	L
Socioeconomic Status	0	2	3	0	L
Accessibility to Health Care Services:					
c. education (PRO)	0	1	1	3	L
d. treatment	0	1	1	3	L
Alcohol Abuse	1	3	2	0	L
Infection	1	2	2	1	L
Allergic Reaction	2	2	2	0	L
Energy Crisis	0	3	2	0	L
Sex	4				N/A
Age	4				N/A
Race	4				N/A

*High Risk COPD

Code for Amount of Influence:

1. 1% to 25% — Bio. = Biology
2. 26% to 50% — L.S. = Life Style
3. 51% to 75% — Env. = Environment
4. 76% to 100% — HCDS = Health Care Delivery System

Numbers do not add up to 100% due to the use of ranges.

Source: By permission from the Oklahoma Health Systems Agency. Health Status Task Force Report, October 1978, p. 69.

necessary because of the large number and variety of risk factors associated with each disease. The task force had neither the resources nor the time to do further in-depth analysis and planning for all risk factors listed.

In analyzing risk factors, the task force members became aware of the many areas affecting health. The task force wanted to impress upon various groups and individuals the importance their actions might have on the reduction of disease and disability. The members thus compiled a set of

Table 10-18 Health Status Impact and Program Development Potential for Lung Cancer and COPD

	HIGH STATUS IMPACT	MODERATE STATUS IMPACT	LOW STATUS IMPACT
High Program Potential	*Life Style:* Smoking *Environment:* Smoking (2) Occupational Exposure: asbestos (3) Air Pollution (3) Media: advertising (4) Social Attitudes (2) Political Attitudes (3) *HCDS:* Smoking (1)	*Life Style:* Occupational Exposure (2) Stress (2) Smoking: lack of knowledge (3) *Environment:* Occupational Exposure: coal (3) Screening (2) Media: influential role models (3) Smoking: lack of knowledge (3) *HCDS:* Education of the public with regard to occupational hazards of exposure to coal, chromium, nickel, radiation, silicates, cotton, dust, potters/craftsmen, stress, and smoking	*Life Style:* Radiation (2)

Table 10-18 continued

	HIGH STATUS IMPACT	MODERATE STATUS IMPACT	LOW STATUS IMPACT
Moderate Program Potential	*Life Style:* Occupational Exposure: asbestos (2) Air Pollution (2) Media: advertising (1) Smoking: lack of motivation	*Life Style:* Screening: (COPD) (1) Media: influential role models (2)	*Life Style:* Occupational Exposure: chromium (2) nickel (2) silicates (2) farming (cotton/dust) (2) potters/craftsmen (2) Infection (2) Alcohol Abuse (3) Energy Crisis (3) Treatment (1) Allergic Reactions (2)
	Environment: Economics (3)	*Environment:* Stress	*Environment:* chromium (3) nickel (3) radiation (3) silicates (3) farming (3) potters/craftsmen (3) Personality (2) Education (professional) (1) Treatment (1)
		HCDS: Accessibility to Health Care Services: COPD screening (3) COPD education (3) Modeling (1)	

Low Program Potential	*Life Style:* Social Attitudes (3) Political Attitudes (1) Economics (1)	*Life Style:* Screening: Lung Cancer (1)	*Biology:* Personality (1) *Life Style:* Personality (3) Geographic-urban/rural Socioeconomic Status (2) *Environment:* Socioeconomic Status (3) Alcohol Abuse (2) Infection (2) Allergic Reaction (2) Energy Crisis (2) *HCDS:* Treatment (3)

Source: By permission from the Oklahoma Health Systems Agency. Health Systems Task Force Report, October 1978, pp. 70–71.

recommendations pointed at certain sectors of Oklahoma society in an attempt to focus attention on what those sectors could do to enhance health and reduce disease. Beyond that, a listing of health enhancement factors was needed to reinforce the idea that the values and behaviors a person chooses will increase the chances of avoiding disease. Such factors, when actively pursued by the individual, would, it was felt, not only result in less disease but would also enhance health beyond the mere absence of disease.

Selected Areas for Programmatic Planning. In making a selection of areas for further analysis and programmatic planning, the task force examined the health field elements and the risk-factor analyses for lung cancer, COPD, circulatory disease, and substance abuse. In each case, the primary risk factors were identified in terms of program development potential, status impact potential, and the health field elements generating them.

Summary of Findings: Lung Cancer and COPD. In lung cancer and COPD, it was shown that the best opportunity for intervention is through the health field elements of environment and life style. For lung cancer and COPD, 67 percent of all risk factors were found to be generated through life style (31 percent) and environment (36 percent). This compared with 16 percent of the risk factors influenced by biology and 17 percent by the health care delivery system. When considering only those risk factors that the task force indicated as having high or moderate potential for reduction of disease incidence, life style and environment were found to generate 74 percent of the total influence for lung cancer and COPD. This information was presented for all three priority categories selected for analysis (Table 10-19).

The task force members selected the following as the most significant factors associated with lung cancer and COPD: (1) smoking; (2) media, the advertising of unhealthful products; (3) stress; and (4) occupational exposure to coal and asbestos. Smoking was selected as a primary risk factor because of the tremendous impact it has on lung cancer and COPD. The risk of developing lung cancer is ten times greater for cigarette smokers than for nonsmokers. Cigarette smoking is also the most important cause of COPD, usually encompassing both chronic bronchitis and emphysema. When cigarette smokers are also occupationally exposed to asbestos, they have 8 times the risk of developing lung cancer compared to smokers of the same age who do not work with asbestos and 92 times the risk of men who neither work with asbestos nor smoke cigarettes.

The media was cited as a primary risk factor for lung cancer and COPD because of the presence of smoking role models and the advertisement of cigarettes.

Table 10-19 Percentage of Influence on Diseases Considered by Specific Health Field Element

HEALTH FIELD ELEMENT	CIRCULATORY DISEASE		LUNG CANCER & COPD		SUBSTANCE ABUSE		TOTAL OF 3 DISEASES	
	High/Mod/Low Status	High & Mod Status	High/Mod/Low Status	High & Mod Status	High/Mod/Low Status	High & Mod Status	High/Mod/Low Status	High & Mod Status
LIFE STYLE	33	47	31	30	28	31	30	35
ENVIRONMENT	24	29	36	44	46	49	38	43
BIOLOGY	20	8	16	3	7	2	13	3
HCDS	23	16	17	23	19	18	19	19
TOTAL	100%	100%	100%	100%	100%	100%	100%	100%

Note: Column 1 under each disease includes all risk factors generated through that health field element.
Column 2 indicates the percent of risk factors that are of high or moderate status.

Source: By permission from the Oklahoma Health Systems Agency. Health Status Task Force Report, October 1978, pp. 78–79.

Stress is a risk factor that allows other detrimental behavior patterns to develop and to impact on lung cancer and COPD. An estimated 50 to 80 percent of all illness is psychosomatic or stress-related. In Table 10-9 stress is defined as an expenditure of energy used in adapting to a situation which, if too prolonged or large, may be detrimental to the individual. At present, few data are available on the number of individuals suffering from stress-induced cancer of the lung and COPD. It is likely, however, that stress acts with other risk factors in the creation of lung cancer and COPD problems rather than as a single causal or associated factor.

Risk Factors Across Disease Categories. A summary of the information on lung cancer, COPD, and circulatory disease indicates that certain risk factors are common to more than one disease entity. When comparing results across disease categories, the following becomes evident:

1. Five high impact risk factors are associated with more than one disease. These are smoking, stress, media or the advertising of harmful products and role models, economic incentives to produce harmful products, and attitudes in society supporting unhealthful behavior. An impact on any of these risk factors would significantly reduce death and disability from circulatory disease, substance abuse, lung cancer, or COPD.
2. The data in Table 10-19 indicate that, in general, most of the risk factors with high impact potential are generated through environment and life style. Of all the risk factors listed for the three diseases, 68 percent were generated through environment and life style. In addition, 78 percent of the risk factors rated as having a high or moderate impact on disease incidence were found to originate from these two health field elements. The risk factors generated by biology and the health care delivery system have a lower impact on the killers and cripplers under study than the other two health field elements.
3. The overall findings show that successful intervention through several of the primary risk factors would involve a large amount of individual responsibility. Regardless of the amount of effort by various agencies, program development for these risk factors without the cooperation of the individual would not improve the health status of the population. Programmatic planning that successfully altered the responsibility taken by individuals for their own health would undoubtedly impact on many significant risk factors.

Task Force Planning Areas. After consideration of all information, the task force selected three risk factors for the following year's programmatic planning activities. The three risk factors were: (1) personal responsibility, (2) smoking, and (3) media/advertising. The Health Status Task Force recommended that

> The Health Status Task Force develop programmatic plans of action which would increase an individual's likelihood of assuming responsibility for his/her own health. This plan would emphasize, as starting points, the areas of smoking and media advertising as they affect health attitudes and behaviors.

Because of the impact that implementation of a successful plan would have upon other risk factors for the three diseases, personal responsibility was assigned for future programmatic planning activities. If individuals were persuaded to take responsibility for their own health, much of their unhealthy behavior would be eliminated. Smoking, for example, is a significant factor in substance abuse; its elimination would, in turn, reduce significantly the incidence of lung cancer, COPD, and circulatory disease. Media advertising was selected for programmatic planning because of the encouragement role models and the advertising of abusive substances give to unhealthy behavior.

Task Force Recommendations. After selection of risk factors for further internal planning and program development, the task force turned its attention to formulating recommendations in other areas deemed appropriate by the group. Recommendations could be made for almost anyone whom the task force believed was involved or associated with the risk factors. In this way, efforts to decrease the impact of the disease would extend beyond the activities of the Health Status Task Force and become better coordinated with a greater chance of successful implementation. The recommendations of the task force are detailed in Table 10-20.

Health Enhancement Factors. Many of the risk factors on which the task force made recommendations are associated with behavior that is contrary to wellness and our belief systems about being well. The task force's purpose in dealing with these factors was to decrease the impact a particular factor has on disease or to eliminate the risk factor altogether to improve the health status of the citizens of Oklahoma.

On the positive side, the task force was charged by the OHSA Board to identify those factors which would enhance an individual's health. The enhancement factors selected by the task force were those that either would provide a basis for wise decision making or would represent positive health practices. These aspects could be considered as involving preventive techniques to maintain good health after it has been achieved.

Promotion of the following enhancement factors, selected by the task force, is as important as planning for the reduction of negative risk factors.

Exercise. Individuals who exercise regularly experience a higher level of cardiovascular fitness than those with a sedentary life style. Regular exercise helps to prevent heart attacks and other circulatory disorders and is also a major contributor in maintaining total body fitness, which promotes wellness.

Nutrition. Proper nutrition is imperative for good health. A balanced diet provides the nutrients that are needed for the body to function at its most efficient level. Deprivation of necessary nutrients allows the body to become susceptible to illness.

Individual responsibility. No outside intervention could have as much impact as that of individuals who assume personal responsibility for their health.

Personal and social alternatives. Related to personal responsibility are personal and social alternatives. People must be aware of choices that are available to them beyond those accepted by a particular family, community, or society. A person who is aware of several alternatives for dealing with a stressful situation, for example, can select the one that will most enhance their health.

Preventive services. Health can be enhanced significantly through the use of preventive services. Regular checkups provide individuals with an indication of their personal health status. Such checks might lead to identification of an illness or disease in its early stages. Various treatments for maintaining good health, such as dental cleaning, are also available and can prevent more serious medical complications in the future.

Nonsmoking knowledge and motivation. Cigarette smoking had a high impact on all three of the diseases studied. If they were motivated and were aware of the benefits of nonsmoking, individuals could be prompted toward wiser, more health-enhancing behavior concerning the use of tobacco.

Substance abuse knowledge. Finally, individuals need to understand the possible consequences of substance abuse. It is important for potential abusers to understand as fully as possible why they plan to use the substance. With this information they can make more knowledgeable decisions concerning the use of substances.

Conclusions. Reflecting the activities of the Health Status Task Force's first year, the following conclusions were evident:

1. A significant reorientation is needed in the way the major diseases that are killing and crippling Oklahomans are perceived and treated.

Specifically, individuals must reorient themselves to view these killers and cripplers as stemming from life style and environmental behavior over which they have substantial control. To reduce death and disability from the diseases under study (circulatory, substance abuse, lung cancer, and COPD), Oklahomans should change their behavior patterns. The behavior in our life styles which makes us susceptible to these diseases must be eradicated. Alternative behaviors and activities should be pursued on a regular basis to make us more resistant to these major killers and cripplers.

2. The health care delivery system is, and always will be, necessary to reduce death and disability from the diseases under study. The impact of the system on this objective is relatively small, however, when compared with that produced by changes in life style and environment. Further study is needed to define more clearly how the health care delivery system should be changed to maximize its impact. At this point, however, it is already fairly certain that a general shift will be necessary toward greater emphasis on preventive and more holistic types of health care services within the present health care delivery system.
3. A reallocation of resources is clearly needed. Though, again, further study is needed before exact monetary figures are available, it may be both feasible and desirable to retain the majority of our resources within the health care delivery system for use at the secondary or tertiary level of care. Because some people will always need hospital care regardless of how healthful their lives have been, the majority of the health care dollar may have to be allocated continuously to servicing a minority proportion of the problem and the populace. Still, some reallocation of resources is clearly needed to increase the quality as well as the length of life for the vast majority of Oklahomans who do not need hospital treatment in their fight against the major diseases.
4. Major shifts are needed in the community's belief system about health and the health care delivery system. The following facts must be understood if Oklahomans are to change their behavior successfully and to accomplish a reallocation of resources and a restructuring of health care priorities.
   a. The health care delivery system cannot cure the diseases studied by the task force. Once damage from these diseases has progressed to a certain point, the health care delivery system can do very little to "cure" an individual. Rather, the emphasis must be on repairing as much of the damage as possible.
   b. Oklahomans can control their own health, particularly their sus-

ceptibility to the diseases studied by the task force. By practicing certain good health behavior and avoiding behavior that puts them at greater risk, Oklahomans can increase not only the quality of their personal life style but also their length of life.

c. When receiving treatment from the health care delivery system, individuals should expect to receive counseling and education on the behaviors they can adopt to help reduce risk. The traditional doctor/patient relationship has been passive with regard to the patient's role. To move towards a more productive relationship, consumers of health care must be aware of their right to receive counseling and education as well as treatment.

d. The data collection systems now in existence are highly geared toward collection of "illness" data. Very little quantitative information is available on Oklahomans who have adopted healthful behaviors or life styles. The establishment of a data collection system that stresses the importance of measuring healthful as well as illness behaviors is mandatory in implementing the changes suggested in the task force's report.

The Health Status Task Force found itself at the crossroads of numerous possibilities for future action. The task in developing plans of action for change is monumental. If death and disability can be effectively reduced, however, the effort will prove worthwhile to the people of Oklahoma.

SUMMARY

The process and risk-factor analysis models are excellent tools for developing health plans that focus on wellness and holism. They are designed to encourage consumers, boards, and resource persons to participate in the planning of health at the local level. The general feeling of participation and satisfaction resulting from this approach has aided many individuals to transform and adopt a new belief system that stresses self-responsibility in health.

Health is something we must do for ourselves, not have done for us. The process will be long, but the search for wellness and holistic health will surely become a major movement in this country in years to come.

Table 10-20 Summary of Health Status Task Force Recommendations

No.	Area of Responsibility	Recommendations	Rationale
1	General Policy	Intervention efforts should be aimed at changing individuals' environments and life styles to reduce, most significantly, death and disability from these killers and cripplers.	Based on the risk-factor analysis, the health field elements, life style and environment, generated the largest percentage of risk factors associated with the diseases under study. Life style influenced 30% and environment influenced 38% of all risk factors. These percentages go even higher when only the high or moderate status of disease impact risk factors are examined; 34% of the total high and moderate risk factors come from life style, and 43% come from environment.
1a		There should be a significant increase in resources—monies, manpower, services—allocated to programs designed to reduce death and disability through life style and environment interventions.	
2	Oklahoma HSA	The Oklahoma HSA should give priority consideration to programs utilizing life style and environmental factors in dealing with circulatory disease, lung cancer and COPD, and substance abuse. This policy should be applied to all OHSA functions such as planning, review, development, public education, and public issues.	At present, OHSA is engaged in a wide variety of activities related to health. The Health Status Task Force has determined that the majority of factors influencing health originate from a person's life style and environment. The task force points out that OHSA activities, if directed toward life style and environment intervention, would have a

Table 10-20 continued

No.	Area of Responsibility	Recommendations	Rationale
			greater impact on health status than the pursuit of actions not centered in these two health field elements.
2a		The sections of the HSP dealing with health promotion, health education, and disease detection should receive priority attention for development. In addition, future planning efforts should emphasize the development of plans aimed at increasing possibilities for life style and environmental changes.	
2b		The Facilities and Services Task Force in future years should give priority attention to alternative forms of service delivery both within and outside of the hospital setting. In particular, it is recommended that this task force develop plans of action to stress primary care services and educational/preventive services	

within current facilities, while controlling unnecessary duplication and expansion of the present level of hospital services throughout the state of Oklahoma.

2c The review department should incorporate as a criterion for all reviews the variable of health status impact. Applicants should be required to show, when applying for certificate of need (1122) and participating in appropriateness review, that the services or equipment which they wish to purchase or currently have actually do affect positively the health status problems of their service area. This should be done as quantitatively as possible and should include evidence that alternative forms of treatment have been considered.

2d In implementing objectives, priority attention should be given once again

Table 10-20 continued

No.	Area of Responsibility	Recommendations	Rationale
		to those objectives dealing with life style and environment which are found within the health promotion, disease detection, and health education components of the existing plan.	
2e		OHSA should present to the State Legislature the findings of this task force and educate them as to the importance of life style and environmental change versus usage of the health care delivery system and biological intervention.	
3	Oklahoma Legislature	Give priority for funding to those health programs focusing upon life style and environment in the treatment of circulatory disease, lung cancer and COPD, and substance abuse.	The Oklahoma State Legislature, as shapers of public policy and elected representatives of the people, has the responsibility to be at the forefront in the battle against circulatory disease, lung cancer and COPD, and substance abuse.
3a		Pass state legislation banning smoking in all public buildings and conveyances as well as offices and other	With knowledge now available concerning the causes of these diseases, new direction and emphasis can begin. The

		enclosed work or educational environments.	above recommendations would provide public recognition and clarity as to where the locus of control for impacting these health status problems really falls.
4	Health Care Delivery System	The Oklahoma Health Care Delivery System broaden its focus to include in a more meaningful way investigations of viable preventive techniques for all diseases.	For a long time, the health professionals and the health care system should have had the focus of responsibility for health placed upon them. Whether this was adopted as reality or attached to the health care community by the public, it is now more evident than ever that other systems and elements play an even more important role in the resulting health status of the population. The incorporation of this new awareness by the consumer/client population seeking health care could be bolstered enormously by appropriate techniques from the Health Care Delivery System. The health care providers are in a powerful position to foster personal responsibility
4a		All health professional organizations and associations should determine how to incorporate needed individual life style and environmental change into their clients' lives as part of the normal delivery of primary or secondary levels of care.	
4b		All health professionals and students should be made aware of themselves as role models in smoking, obesity, etc.	

Table 10-20 continued

No.	Area of Responsibility	Recommendations	Rationale
4c		All health professionals should counsel individuals to take the responsibility for their own health.	for health through role model examples and consumer education.
4d		All health professional schools and associations should incorporate, as part of their initial or continuing education, the teaching of wellness techniques.	
5	Insurers	Insurers, particularly third-party reimbursers, should alter their policy structure so as to reward those individuals engaging in healthy behavior, i.e., not smoking, maintaining proper weight, exercising, and require those individuals who choose to engage in unhealthy behavior to bear more of the financial burden.	To further reinforce life style and environmental changes by health care consumers, the insurance industry should realign its reimbursement system from one of rewarding sickness, as is presently the case, to one that rewards persons who remain healthy and participate in healthful behavior. This would also include payment for health education and preventive services which are rarely reimbursed at present.
5a		Cost associated with health education of the consumer/client should be a reimbursable item.	

6	Business	Business and industry should examine the health care benefits provided employees to ensure coverage of health education and preventive services.	Health education, preventive services, exercise, and stress management are all factors contributing to physical and mental wellness. Employers who encourage and provide for such practices are likely to have healthy employees, thus increasing the productivity of their businesses. Breaks for exercise and stress management during the work day allow employees to return to work relaxed and with a clear mind. Health education helps to ensure that individuals know how to maintain a high level of wellness. Health care benefits providing for preventive services also allow employees to obtain the necessary checkups and treatments which also contribute to wellness. All individuals would benefit from these techniques, and business is an excellent way to reach a large percentage of the population.
6a		Business and industry should provide opportunities for exercise and stress management to its employees as called for in the OHSA's Health Systems Plan and Annual Implementation Plan.	
6b		Those businesses required to supply an Environmental Impact Statement should emphasize in that statement an analysis of how their plant will impact on the health of their work force and the surrounding population.	

Table 10-20 continued

No.	Area of Responsibility	Recommendations	Rationale
7	Community and Media	Support should be withdrawn from those sections of the economy fostering health hazards such as tobacco, air pollution, various occupational exposures, either through social or legislative action.	All forms of media advertising or providing role models (television, radio, newspaper, magazines, billboards) have a tremendous impact on the behavior of individuals, particularly smoking behavior. Curtailment of tobacco usage by the media in either of these two forms could possibly decrease the number of individuals using the products. Since the media does impact on behavior, positive health information and programs should replace the negative influences.
7a		Federal tax dollars utilized as subsidies for the tobacco industry should be withdrawn gradually and given to assist development of alternative crops.	
7b		The media should either (1) curtail advertising of all tobacco products or (2) provide equal space or time to ads countering the effects of those tobacco product ads.	Gradual withdrawal of monies from support of health hazards to support of health enhancing products and behaviors would complement the concept that health and its achievement is the responsibility of everyone rather than the sole responsibility of the health care system.
7c		Role models in the media should not be presented using tobacco products.	
7d		The media should present information and programs on positive health behaviors.	

7e		State clean air standards should be enforced.	
8	State Government	The Oklahoma State Departments of Health, Mental Health, Education, and DISRS, should take a more active role in advocating life style and environmental changes with regard to all diseases through their programs and reimbursement mechanisms.	All of these agencies are in daily contact with many Oklahomans and have access to programs and individual contacts which they could use to encourage changes in life style and environment that would enhance health. Life style and environment are shown to have a large influence on the three diseases studied, and these agencies should incorporate that knowledge into their programs so that more Oklahomans can be reached.
9	Individual Oklahomans	People should take responsibility for their own health. This behavior could be greatly encouraged through the media and through opportunities given by employers, the community, and the health care delivery system.	Throughout this entire process, it has been shown that many risk factors exist due to a lack of personal responsibility for health. Positive health practices such as those outlined in Recommendation 9 constitute an excellent program for maintaining wellness. No outside intervention by the health care delivery system can impact upon the health of Oklahomans as
9a		Each individual Oklahoman should develop an individualized program for	

Table 10-20 continued

No.	Area of Responsibility	Recommendations	Rationale
		health to include appropriate nutrition, adequate exercise, sufficient amounts of sleep, appropriate weight, nonsmoking, and the usage of alcoholic beverages only in moderation.	would healthy behavior on the part of each individual. Teaching children positive health behaviors by practicing them in the home helps to ensure that they will continue to practice preventive techniques throughout their lifetime, as opposed to depending on the health care delivery system for intervention.
9b		Parents should take responsibility for instilling in their children a positive attitude toward health and health behaviors by careful supervision of the foods they eat and by setting themselves as healthful examples which their children can follow.	

Source: By permission from the Oklahoma Health Systems Agency. Health Status Task Force Report, October 1978, pp. 86–98.

Index

B

C

T